THE ULTIMATE GUIDE TO BEING NATURALLY GORGEOUS

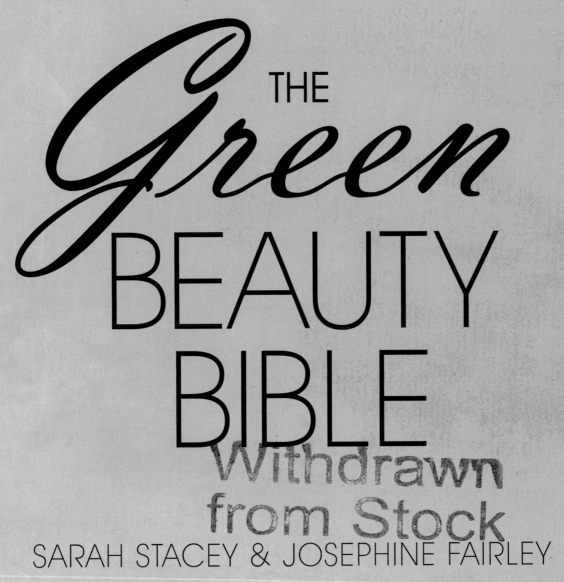

THE *Green* BEAUTY BIBLE

SARAH STACEY & JOSEPHINE FAIRLEY

with illustrations by David Downton

KYLE CATHIE LIMITED

contents

THE *Green* BEAUTY BIBLE

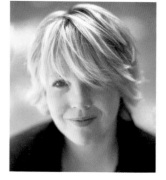
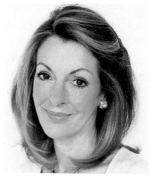

The beauty world is changing – fast. 'Natural', 'pure', 'organic' and 'green' are the new buzzwords. And increasingly, questions to our website (www.beautybible.com) are about how to be 'naturally' gorgeous. Since we published the hardback edition of this book, hundreds of new natural and organic beauty products have landed on our desks – which we have sent out to our thousands of diligent testers, resulting in plenty of new entries...

We believe that it really is possible to look (and feel) your absolute glowing, radiant best in a more sustainable way – and the results from our panellists confirm that. But it's not just about what you massage into your face/body/scalp – although of course that matters. It's about what you put inside your body – and your mind. About how you live: a more natural, healthier way of living and being that is gentler on you – and gentler on the planet's precious resources, too. Since the hardback edition of this book, the world has changed. But just because headlines have been so dominated by coverage of the global financial meltdown, that doesn't mean the world's eco-problems have gone away. On the contrary. It's more important than ever to 'think' before we consume – and that's why we believe *Beauty Bible*'s time has really come.

We don't want you to waste a single penny (or cent) on products that don't deliver. It's a waste of your resources – and the planet's. So our crusade – and it really is a crusade – is to help women make smarter beauty choices. We give real products to real women, with each product trialled by a panel of ten, over a period of months. So naturally (sorry!), that's just what we've done again – recruiting 1050 new testers to try everything from organic 'miracle' creams to suncare, mascara to shampoo, from over 120 brands. Their verdict? That many natural, 'more' natural and organic products perform really well, smell blissful, and deliver the perfect element of pampering. As usual, we let you in on the secrets of the natural products we love, too. (Where we still make beauty compromises, we're not afraid to 'fess up. We're not 'perfect' – but we're trying.)

But do we recommend you clutter your bathroom shelf and make-up bag with all 43 categories we trialled? No way. By the end of this book, we hope we'll have helped you work out what you really need.

(Which is probably less than you think.) Because the idea is also to help you find your own, completely individual allure – and spend less time chasing after beauty rainbows. Which leaves more time to stop and smell the roses. Or walk on the beach. Or cook a scrummy, convivial dinner for friends and family.

Interestingly, many of our volunteers came to this project because they have touchy complexions and, in quite a few cases, rosacea. Those testers have found that a shorter and more natural ingredients list is often kinder to skin. Others have health concerns: some enlightened cancer specialists now suggest to patients that they seek out natural and organic cosmetics, because of the as-yet unknown impact of some chemical ingredients on the immune system. Certainly, for anyone who chooses to eat organic food whenever possible, it makes no sense then to slap a cocktail of synthetic chemicals on the skin.

We understand that questions of 'green' living – not to mention 'green gorgeousness' – can be so complicated your head spins. And we can't pretend to have done a 'life-cycle analysis' on every product featured here, to assess its green cred from cradle to – well, your make-up bag. But many companies out there are working hard to offer more sustainable, natural and 'greener' beauty products. What we've done with this book is to help steer you through an increasingly over-grown jungle, to the natural products that really deliver.

But there's another important 'green' element to this book. Many beauty products are still based principally on petrochemicals – non-renewable, non-sustainable. (Not to mention pore-blocking, in the case of paraffin and mineral oil...) When we say 'oil crisis', it means both a shiny T-zone and the world's oil running out. While boffins and oil barons argue about just how many barrels are left, we don't think it makes sense to slather petrochemicals on our bodies or faces, when we may in time need every last drop for light, heat and other life essentials. Especially when nature has such amazing, bountiful, renewable beautifiers to offer.

We always find it helps to be inspired by people who are 'walking their talk'. So we've tried to do that, and throughout *The Green Beauty Bible* we've also spotlighted some of our heroines – 'green goddesses' – who talk about how they're living a greener lifestyle, and following a more natural beauty regime.

The bottom line is this: it really <u>is</u> possible to be naturally gorgeous. To live healthily, vibrantly, feeling – and looking – alive and beautiful. And we're about to show you how…

Sarah x   Jo

THE DAISY RATING

Is everything in this book 100 per cent natural? No. But (with the help of an industry expert, this time) we've assessed each product featured in these pages. This is how it works:

✿ **ONE DAISY** These are products that are mostly botanical (with a small percentage of petrochemically-derived ingredients).

✿✿ **TWO DAISIES** Botanically-derived with no synthetics.

✿✿✿ **THREE DAISIES** Certified organic by The Soil Association in the UK, or one of the international certifiers such as USDA, Ecocert, etc. Certifiers around the world are currently aiming towards total harmonisation, so although there may be some small variations between standards, the vital point is that the organic claims of manufacturers have been verified by a third party – so you can be sure there's no 'greenwashing'

★ **STAR BUY** Look for these brilliant-value 'beauty steals'

(NB: though we can't list each and every ingredient in this book, you can find all the lists of ingredients on our website. In print that's big enough to read. So you won't go half-blind checking out what's in the jar, bottle or tube. Just check out www.beautybible.com, and go to the 'GREEN BEAUTY' section. You'll find we have also arranged discounts for you on many of the winning products in this book.)

DISCLAIMER: All product names and prices were correct at the time of going to press.

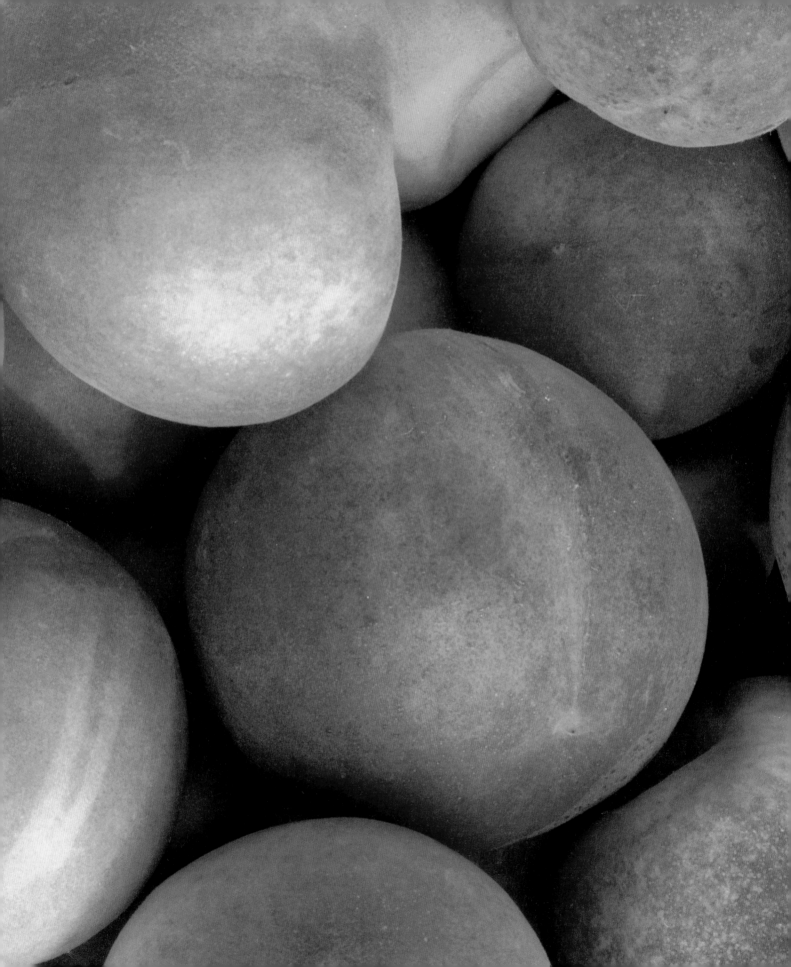

Skin

Your skin is your very own top-to-toe packaging. And just like any other beauty wrapping, it needs to be gorgeous. There is no reason why we shouldn't all – whatever age and stage we are at – feel *bien dans la peau* (comfortable in our skins, as the French put it). So we love the feeling of stroking on ingredients from herbs, flowers and other natural sources that have been used the world over for centuries – and still work brilliantly today.

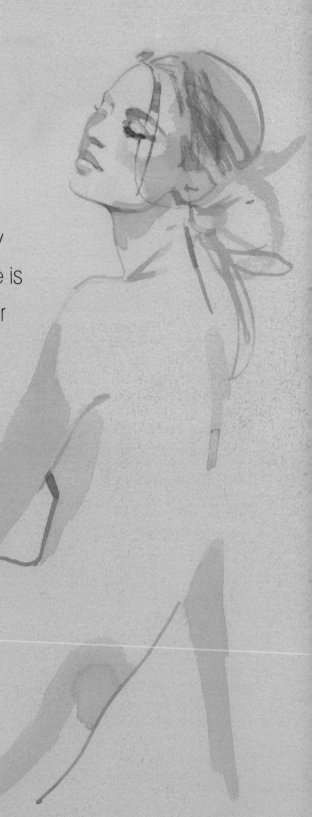

LET'S GET BACK TO
beauty basics

This is beauty industry heresy: your beauty regime is probably way more complicated than it needs to be. We've all come to believe that in order to look our lovely best, bathroom shelves need to groan with an armoury of lotions, potions, problem-solvers and anti-agers. Well, we think it's time to simplify.

One of the reasons our bathrooms become cluttered with products is that we get seduced into buying stuff that just doesn't work – and then feel too guilty to throw it away. That's one of the key reasons we began writing our books: to help women find products that actually do the job, whether that's cleansing, moisturising, zit-zapping, fighting dark circles and puffiness…whatever. More than a decade after our first book, we know our Tried & Tested system is pretty foolproof: if our teams of ten women (all beauty hounds with different wants, needs, looks and ages) like a product and agree it does the trick, chances are that other women will too.

Don't get us wrong: we enjoy beauty products as much as the next woman.

Are you overwhelmed by skincare choices? Is your skin confused – maybe even sensitised – by an ever-changing routine? And is your bathroom cupboard so cluttered that your toes get crushed by bottles making a bid for freedom as you open the door? (You're not the first.) So join us in the beauty regime revolution

(We wouldn't do this if we didn't!). But over the past few years we've come to feel like we're on product-overload: more and more brands, more and more launches targeted at problems we didn't even know we had. We know plenty of other women whose skins are on product-overload too – and are acting confused and rebellious as a result.

So instead of cluttering the bathroom shelf with three cleansers that do the job half-heartedly, or aren't a pleasure to use, we'd like you to have one brilliant cleanser and one fantastic day cream (plus one with an SPF, for when it's sunny – or anti-ageing ingredients if you're past 35). To be honest, you don't actually need a special night cream – an (SPF-free) day moisturiser will

do just fine for overnight skin renewal. Facial oils are terrific – but, again, optional. And it's an oil or a cream at night, unless you're over 50, in which case it's good to use both. As for toners? We don't believe in them. But if you like a fresh sensation, use rosewater (we think you can't beat Neal's Yard Remedies Rosewater or Pukka Rosewater spray). A mask is great for an occasional blitz, if you like to pamper yourself. Ditto exfoliators. As for a neck cream? Well, maybe – but we basically agree with Laura Mercier (see her quote opposite). The real key is to use the thing – and most women just don't.

If you're making more natural choices, there's another reason not to have too many jars and bottles on the go at one time: they may have a shorter shelf-life, due to lower levels of preservatives than synthetic, chemical-laden products.

A simplified regime can actually make life itself less complicated. You can devote more time to the things that matter to you: reading; going for a walk; cooking a great meal, then enjoying it with friends or family; riding horses, in Sarah's case; doing a yoga class, in Jo's. So try the less-is-more approach. Your skin (and the planet) will thank you for it.

Fab idea…

Beauty companies never tell you that many products are similar in formulation but marketed in different ways. Over the years we've found some great double-duty beauty products. A leave-in conditioner can make a great hand cream, at a pinch. We once styled our hair with anti-cellulite gel. If you've got the frizzies, try massaging a little moisturiser or facial oil into your hands and skimming over your hair. Balms are brilliant for skin everywhere, cuticles and flyaway locks. Experiment! (Avoid the eye zone, though, except with special eye products.) You may discover some very clever ways to pare down your regime: do e-mail us at www.beautybible.com and let us know.

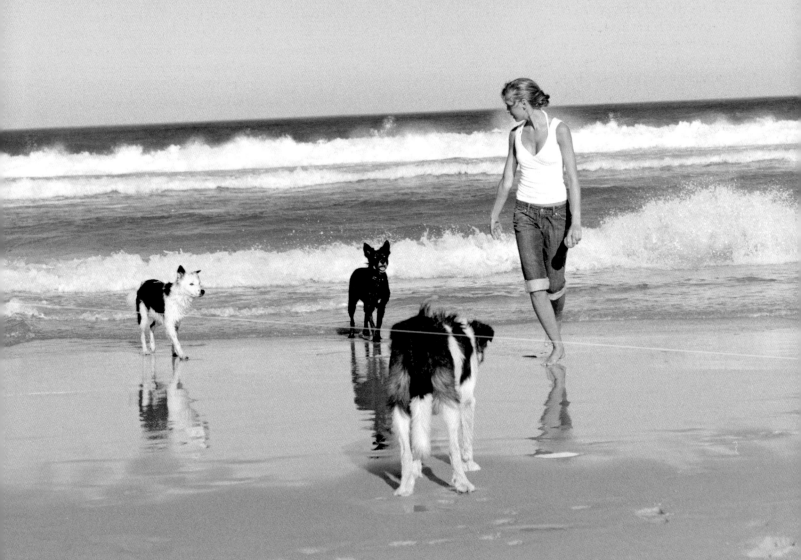

'There are no miracles in this business, just marketing strategies. For example, neck cream. The skin on your neck is basically the same as the skin on your face. You could easily make do with your night cream'

LAURA MERCIER, make-up artist

BOXING CLEVER

You recycle newspapers and wine bottles. But what about your moisturiser jar?

We admit it! We do slightly mourn the sense of wonderment that came when opening extravagant cosmetics packaging. We were as greedy as the next woman for satin boxes, rustly tissue paper and glam carrier bags. Nowadays, we look at pretty over-packaging and see a pile of empty cartons, torn cellophane and wilted tissue paper. Which is sad – but once the packaging genie's out of the (recycled) bottle, there's no going back.

When it comes to over-packaging, the cosmetics industry can be guilty as hell. Some packaging is necessary; there's a lot to fit on a cosmetics label: ingredients, instructions, 'use by' date... They can't cram all that on to a teensy pot of eye cream (which is one reason why cosmetics often come in cardboard outer boxes). But look at the carrier bag, tissue paper, plastic, tube/jar/bottle. Does the product really need it? And do you recycle the box along with the rest of your cardboard? The insert leaflets with your newspapers? Glass bottles can be rinsed and put with your other glass recycling (first remove any plastic components). Aluminium tubes can in many cases be recycled with cans.

We applaud the companies that offer refills, which are highly eco-friendly (and lament the disappearance of The Body Shop's refill service). On our website – www.beautybible.com – you'll find more in-depth info on the brands in this book, and where they are making environmental progress we'll update you on that.

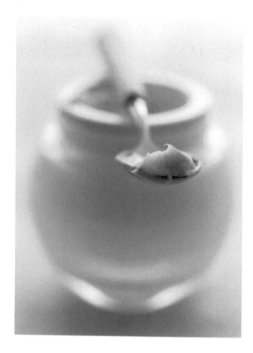

Some companies – natural brand Nude, for instance – are moving towards post-consumer waste packaging. (That means packaging is collected in a recycling programme and made into new products.) Other types of plastic can be recycled, too; somewhere on the packaging there will be a number identifying its type, and you can find out from your local government office whether they offer recycling facilities for that plastic. Origins and REN will take back empty containers for recycling at their counters. Lush sells products, from soap to shampoo bars, by the slice in its shops, and packages them in simple paper bags. By offering these 'solid' products, it also avoids having to transport large amounts of water around the country/globe.

There's no doubt that brands are conscious of reducing the amount of packaging that goes to the dump. Through Liz Earle's mail order service, for instance, you can now specify if you want the products wrapped in tissue paper. And, if you do, the tissue paper comes from a fully sustainable timber source and is also recyclable. We applaud mail order companies that use wood shavings rather than polystyrene – and we're delighted that you can now get recycled as well as recyclable tissue paper.

If you feel strongly about beauty over-packaging, e-mail or write to brands you love and tell them this issue matters to you. They'll get the message faster, and you'll have the warm, rosy glow that comes from having done your bit for Mother Earth. No blusher needed...

Date check

Companies now put the 'use by' date on packaging – usually a symbol that says, for example, '6M', meaning you have six months after opening to use up the product. Do stick by this – especially with natural products, which may be formulated with low (or no) preservative levels. And – common sense, but it can't be repeated often enough – do always wash your hands thoroughly before applying any product, to avoid spreading germs.

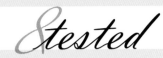

MULTI-PURPOSE BALMS

With a great balm, you can de-junk half your bathroom shelf. The ultimate multi-taskers, they double as make-up remover, moisturiser, cuticle-smoother, hand cream, heel-softener and more. We love, love, love 'em – and here are the top scorers from our 'balmy army' of testers, who tried over two dozen new ones for this paperback alone

★ ❀ ❀ EARTHBOUND ORGANICS ARNICA & GINGER BALM
Score: 8.06/10

This warming concoction of herbs and oils – featuring raw ginger, arnica and hypericum macerated in cold-pressed sunflower and olive oil – is designed to help relieve muscular tension and pain, and for use after sports or physical work. However, our testers gave it good marks as an all-round balm. (NB: not to be used on broken skin.)

Comments: 'Used on numerous occasions for snagged cuticles or slight bumps; over a month, a dry patch on elbow improved and cuticles became easy to push back' • 'a revolution in a cute little tub' • 'very useful product, best used on bumps and bruises, knees and elbows' • 'left a light natural gloss on lips and turned them a healthy pink colour, healed dry patches and softened cuticles, did well on my elbows – very good product' • 'excellent on lips and dry patches!'

❀ ❀ WELEDA SKIN FOOD
Score: 8/10

This 'cult' product has been around since 1926, we're told! – but it's the first time Weleda entered it for our trials, and it excelled. Unlike many 'multi-taskers', this is more like a traditional cream, which is why it's so useful as an overall moisturiser. (It's a favourite of our friend Janey Lee Grace, too, author of *Imperfectly Natural Woman*.) Refreshingly scented with essential oils (orange, lavender), we also recommend it as a fabulous barrier cream in wind-chill weather.

Comments: 'I love this product and the price means I can slap it on – it's the best face mask ever; kept my hands amazing through the winter, softened cuticles nicely, helped heal and protect dry patches' • 'seriously awesome on dry feet and elbows; is rich, smells gorgeous and feels like it's doing real good' • 'AMAZING!!! The first product ever to soothe, improve and clear all my eczema and contact dermatitis'.

★ ❀ ❀ ❀ ESSENTIAL CARE CALENDULA BALM
Score: 7.95/10

This 100 per cent organic pot of wonder gets its healing action from calendula and camomile, in a lubricating base of organic coconut and extra virgin oil, plus shea butter. Devotees have reported great results on psoriasis, but it's recommended for cracked cuticles and chapped skin on fingers, elbows, heels, etc. Essential Care is a commendable UK-based brand founded by a mother-and-daughter team who are deeply committed to creating organic skincare, and are happy to ship worldwide.

Comments: 'Nourishing on the lips; made a significant difference in harsh winter weather' • 'I liked this product and was happy to apply it to my children's skin' • 'calmed a sore lip quickly' • 'very soothing for chapped knuckles; used it on my 12-year-old son's knees before football and it really protected them' • 'melted quickly on the skin' • 'oilier than I usually like, but pleasingly natural and effective'.

❀ ❀ LIZ EARLE NATURALLY ACTIVE SKINCARE SUPERBALM
Score: 7.9/10

The heavenly scent as you open this pot of mega-nourishment (Sarah's all-round fave) comes from its essential oil blend of rosehip, neroli, lavender and camomile, alongside softening vitamin E and shea butter, beeswax and carnauba wax, which protect skin from the elements.

Comments: 'Gave me super-soft, kissable lips' • 'a star product – even works on my frizzy hair!' • 'dry patches instantly moisturised' • 'a little goes a long way' • 'excellent on cuticles' • 'left me with very soft elbows'.

❀ ❀ ❀ NEAL'S YARD REMEDIES WILD ROSE BEAUTY BALM
Score: 7.85/10

Another Soil Association-certified organic multi-tasker, based on retinol-rich rosehip oil – so, in theory, this should also have an age-defying effect, too, if you used it on your face. A Neal's Yard bestseller, try it to rescue skin after long flights or late nights, and for cleansing – in fact, it comes with its own organic muslin cloth.

Comments: 'Softened dry patches and cuticles' • 'lovely rose smell; liked using it as a facial treatment' • 'good to apply at night on hands and nails' • 'I put it on my face and was surprised at the radiance' • 'lovely old-fashioned blue glass jar' • 'worked well as an emergency treatment for chapped or very dry skin, and as a winter cleanser'.

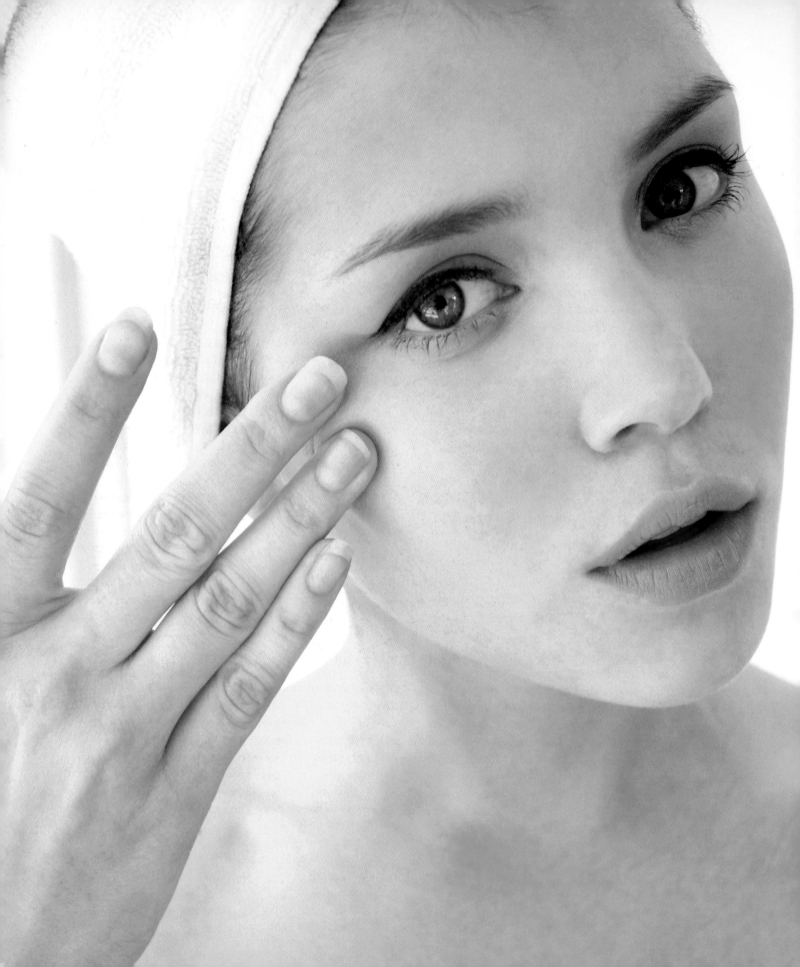

clean sweep

Skincare gurus universally agree: cleansing is the don't-skimp, must-do step in a skincare regime – 'prepping' the complexion for everything else you apply. Otherwise? Your moisturiser, 'miracle' cream or facial oil simply can't get the job done properly

Like most women, we are serious multi-taskers. But one of our favourite multi-tasking activities is turning the action of cleansing into a radiance-boosting, mini-treatment massage. Frankly, it takes a minute before bedtime – and takes off five years. Along with all your make-up and the day's grime. Beat that.

For a specific how-to, we suggest following super-facialist Vaishaly Patel's facial massage technique on page 22. In our experience, though, facial massage works best with balms, milks and cream cleansers, rather than foaming or detergent-based cleansers, which can irritate or over-strip skin if you leave them on for long.

COTTON PICKING

We're unswervingly devoted to wash cloths for our faces. Skincare guru Eve Lom introduced the world to them: swooshed in hot water, then applied to skin, they work with any cleanser – milk, lotion, balm. In fact, if you're using a balm, you have to use a wash cloth; cotton wool will just turn it into a sticky mess. A few tips, though: wash cloths (Jo likes muslin as Eve prescribed originally, Sarah prefers cotton flannels) have to be washed regularly in a washing machine, and dried before reusing, or they can harbour

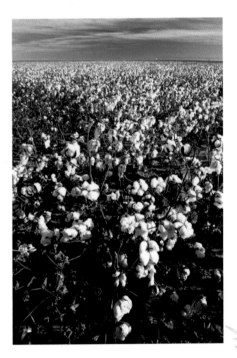

bacteria. (Besides, a dingy grey wash cloth dangling from the towel rail isn't a great style statement in a bathroom.)

We also recommend buying organic flannels or muslin squares (available from www.lizearle.com). Cotton is the most heavily sprayed crop in the world – a process that can poison the land and water

supplies, and which may leave residues on the fibres. There is also a shift towards genetically modified cotton production, which can impact particularly on poor Third World farmers who enter into contracts with the agrichemical/biotech companies. They are forced to buy expensive 'miracle' cotton seeds, often with disappointing results – and as a result, many face ruin.

Organic cotton is now available as cotton pads, buds (great for removing the last traces of mascara), as well as wash cloths: just as soft, just as effective – but this cotton really is as pure as it looks. We say: when it comes to cotton, pick organic every time – and that means for everything from T-shirts to towels.

Tip **There's no need to cleanse from scratch in the morning – it's product overkill. Vaishaly advises: 'For an instant skin boost in the morning, splash cold water on to your face. This is instantly firming, freshening – and brings all the senses (as well as the skin) alive. Follow with moisturiser.'**

'I'm kind to my skin. I remove my make-up as soon as I get home and apply moisturiser. Kindness is a lovely quality to nurture as you get older' IMAN

CLEANSERS

tried & tested

For a cleanser the bottom line is: does it get rid of all the gunk that builds up during the day? Our testers tried more than 20 new 'green' launches for this paperback, resulting in some great new entries in the 'cleanser chart' – which means that, below, you'll find a run-down of the best from over 100 natural and organic cleansers on the beauty market. NB: still leading this category is *Beauty Bible*'s highest-scoring product ever – still unbeaten! – so congrats yet again to Liz Earle Naturally Active Skincare…

★❀ LIZ EARLE NATURALLY ACTIVE SKINCARE CLEANSE & POLISH HOT CLOTH CLEANSER
Score: 9.5/10

The highest-scoring product we've ever had: one woman gave it 11 out of ten and we've never found anyone who didn't like it. From the international brand founded by a former beauty journalist, this creamy cleanser is used with hot water and its own muslin cloth (which also works as an exfoliator). Testers loved the fragrance, from pure essential oils of rosemary, camomile and eucalyptus; it also contains cocoa butter and almond milk. We made it a star buy because it is middle-priced and lasts for months.

Comments: 'My skin felt really clean, fresh and soft after this' • 'left skin feeling velvety and radiant; texture just right – felt rich' • 'loved this product – amazing difference on greasy chin, with noticeably closed pores' • 'took off full Saturday night make-up, including mascara, easily' • 'the muslin cloth was satisfying: good to see all the muck that came off my skin' • 'very uplifting fragrance'.

❀❀ NUDE CLEANSING FACIAL OIL
Score: 9.16/10

Targeted at normal to dry skins, this luxurious, detergent-free oil is enriched with omega-3 and vitamin E oils. After massaging

into skin, a little water transforms it into a milk that can be rinsed away. We applaud Nude's packaging policy: 40 per cent is made from post-industrial recycled plastic.

Comments: 'Fabulous! Skin felt very moisturised and soft' • 'much richer and less drying than my usual cleanser' • 'excellent packaging, with easy lift-off top' • 'love the floral smell' • 'worked on waterproof make-up; no trace on my pillow' • 'easy to use, skin felt velvety'.

❀ REN NO. 1 PURITY CLEANSING BALM
Score: 8.94/10

This new pump-action cleanser marks REN's debut in the cleansing balm category: luxuriously silky, it should be warmed in the palm then massaged over the face, before adding water to emulsify into a rich milk. Testers loved its soothing action – and rose fragrance (becoming a signature for REN…)

Comments: 'Simple, clean packaging and great pump-action dispenser' • 'looks complicated but really simple once I got the hang of it' • 'the texture was just incredible, an absolute pleasure to massage in; incredibly moisturising, much oilier and greasier than any cleanser I'd normally use but I ended up loving it for that' • 'heavenly smell – I can't praise this highly enough' • 'dissolved make-up like an absolute breeze'.

❀ TRILOGY CREAM CLEANSER
Score: 8.7/10

Trilogy, a New Zealand brand that is a personal favourite of ours, is committed to producing skincare free from synthetic fillers, artificial fragrances, mineral oil and parabens. Alongside the rosehip oil (a signature ingredient) are jojoba, almond and carrot oils, plus a dash of orange blossom.

Comments: 'Perfect texture – creamy-rich but not greasy or too thick; easy to dispense and removed waterproof eye make-up; skin felt very moisturised' • 'one of the best products I tested: skin felt clean and soft with no need for toner; a little goes a long way' • 'liked the floral smell – fresh and natural' • 'perfect dispenser and fabulous at cleansing' • 'liked the fact that you can recycle most of the packaging, though the glass bottle is a pain to travel with' • 'took off *all* my make-up, including dark red lipstick and lots of dark eyeshadow'.

❀❀ PURE LOCHSIDE ORGANIC ORANGE CLEANSING OIL
Score: 8.43/10

Testers really enjoyed this product from a small Scottish brand founded by Fiona Tutte, an experienced aromatherapist. Made in small batches – and packaged, unusually, in cute jute bags rather than boxes – this pump-action oil won special praise for its delicious orange fragrance. For best results, use with an organic muslin cleansing cloth.

Comments: 'Worked a treat on my bright blue Dior mascara, which usually takes three morning scrubs!' • 'one application got rid of heavy make-up and waterproof mascara' • 'loved the packaging' • 'the orange smell woke me up' • 'left skin soft and moisturised'.

❀❀ DR HAUSCHKA CLEANSING MILK
Score: 8.4/10

The ingredients in this gentle cleanser are grown organically and biodynamically (in rhythm with the phases of the moon); they include fennel extract, jojoba oil, sweet almond oil and clay, with fermented grains 'to assist in breaking down the impurities in the skin'.

Comments: 'Silky lotion was easily applied and melted off make-up, leaving parched winter skin hydrated, fresh and comfortable' • 'cleansed effectively – gentle but thorough; left skin very moisturised' • 'delicious product, more like a treatment than a cleanser'.

❀❀ VAISHALY CLEANSING BALM
Score: 8.37/10

A 'hero' product created by leading facialist Vaishaly Patel, this melts into skin and is emulsified with water, so it swooshes away. (We still like to use a muslin cloth.) Based on sweet almond and olive oils, plus an

arnica, ginkgo and calendula complex, it's soothing to dry, itchy complexions. Pricy – but a bottle lasts well over six months.

Comments: 'Fantastic at taking off make-up (with muslin cloth), leaving skin like silk. I would buy it' • 'stylish, simple packaging' • 'lovely essential oils, uplifting and relaxing, so it's perfect for morning and night' • 'took off make-up, including waterproof mascara, with no irritation'.

❀ THE ORGANIC PHARMACY CARROT BUTTER CLEANSER
Score: 8.33/10

The Organic Pharmacy was founded by Margo Marrone in 2002, and this award-winning cleanser was a debut product: a solid balm (again, use it with a muslin cloth) enriched with shea and cocoa butters, together with antioxidant carrot, all infused with aromatic camomile, rosemary and lavender essential oils. Several testers commented on its greasy nature – so best for very dry skins.

Comments: 'A real treat: took longer than usual to do the routine but it left my skin feeling great' • 'made skin feel very clean but not at all dry' • 'worked immediately on dry face; easy peasy!' • 'best for extremely dry skin, as left oily film' • 'needed a damp cloth to wipe off properly; pretty nice to use'.

❀ EMMA HARDIE AMAZING FACE CLEANSING SYSTEM
Score: 8.33/10

From the 'natural facelift expert' of TV's *10*

Years Younger, this 'facial in a box' has a cleansing balm (with essential oils of orange, neroli, bergamot and mandarin) which can be 'customised' into an exfoliant by adding the crushed rosehip seeds also in the kit. Testers felt it was quite costly for the length of time it lasted.

Comments: 'My greasy, acne-prone skin really improved using this and stopped feeling tight' • 'both easy to use: I used the balm in the morning and both at night, which left my skin wonderfully clean' • 'ten out of ten, except for the Barbie-pink-and-white packaging!' • 'brilliant booklet with massage tips'.

❀ A'KIN ROSE & GERANIUM PURE CREAMY CLEANSER & TONER IN ONE
Score: 8.33/10

This light, creamy cleanser from an affordable, natural Aussie brand leaves even sensitive skins cleansed and mildly toned, due to the witch hazel in the blend. With vitamin B5, shea butter, plus a naturally cleansing element of Panama bark, this is designed to remove lip, face and eye make-up in one swoosh. Two testers gave it ten out of ten.

Comments: 'I loved this wonderful-smelling product; it's the best cream cleanser I've tried and all natural; a definite improvement in the texture and smoothness of my skin' • 'refreshing and nice smell of roses' • 'I wear a lot of make-up and found it very efficient at removing all of it; left my skin lovely and soft with no tightness' • 'my daughter has very sensitive skin and loved it too'.

We love...

Jo's all-time favourite cleanser is Vaishaly Cleansing Balm: a pump-action, make-up-melting liquid balm. Each pot seems to last for ever – and looks sexy on the bathroom shelf. As well as Sarah's great standby Cleanse and Polish Hot Cloth Cleanser (see opposite), she's loving Gentle Cleansing Milk, in the natural Oliv' range from La Clarée Facial Care.

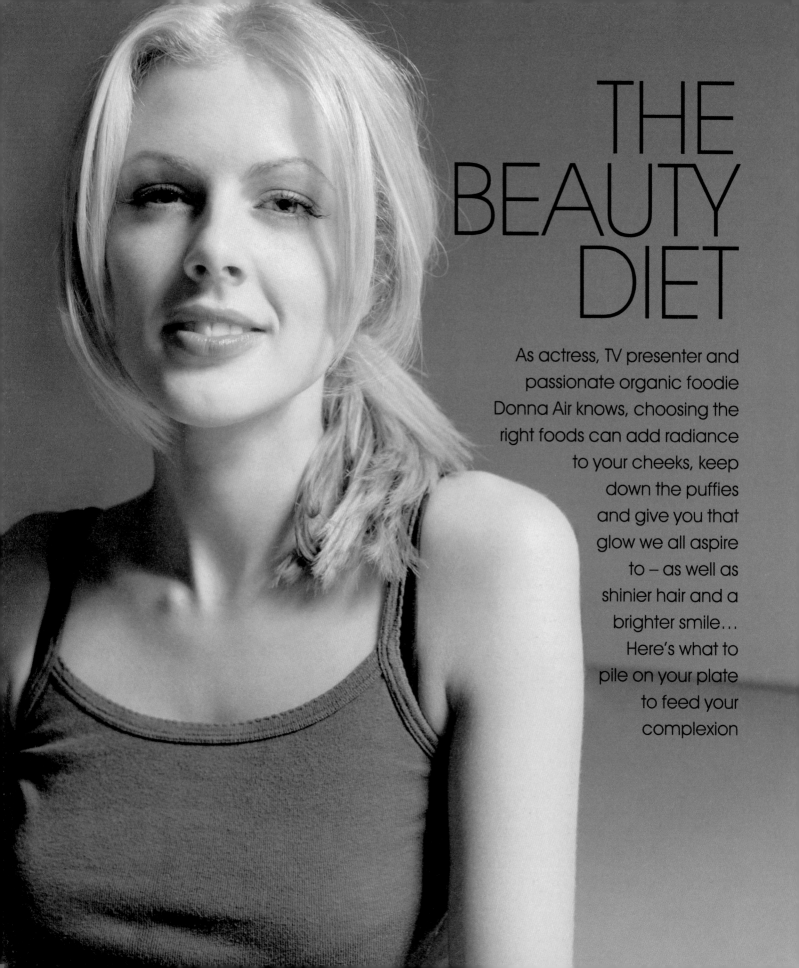

THE BEAUTY DIET

As actress, TV presenter and passionate organic foodie Donna Air knows, choosing the right foods can add radiance to your cheeks, keep down the puffies and give you that glow we all aspire to – as well as shinier hair and a brighter smile… Here's what to pile on your plate to feed your complexion

You can literally feed and water your face. And not only will the right nutrients keep it healthy, they can damp down the inflammation that integrated health expert Dr Andrew Weil of the University of Arizona tells us is the villain in most skin problems. This 'fire within', he says, leads to the skin sensitivity that affects nearly 50 per cent of women today, as well as extreme dryness, lines, wrinkles and puffiness, even flushing and blushing. (For more about skin problems, see pages 26–29.)

Fascinatingly, inflammation is now seen by medical researchers as the underlying culprit in many illnesses, from heart disease to Alzheimer's. 'Normal inflammation is a natural healing response, but what scientists are detecting now is abnormal inflammation,' says Dr Weil. A prime factor in provoking the inflammatory response is the assault on our cells launched by pollutants including the toxic chemicals in food. Other villains are tobacco smoke, UV radiation, other environmental toxins, all manner of household products – and stress. All these factors affect the state of skin just as much as the deeper organs – thus the need to de-stress our complexions.

Sugar is the big enemy, in the view of American dermatologist Dr Frederic Brandt. 'It triggers a process in the body called glycation, where the sugar molecules bind to your protein fibres – those wonderfully springy and resilient collagen and elastin fibres – which are the building blocks of skin. Imagine collagen is your skin's mattress and the elastin fibres are the coils holding it together. The sugar attacks these fibres, making them less elastic and more brittle so they break.' That results in sags, bags, lines and wrinkles. The process of glycation also promotes inflammation. Sweet food and drink is also a disaster for anyone with a gut problem such as irritable bowel syndrome or candida, both of which can dull your skin (not to mention causing bloating and other digestive problems). Simply keeping your sweet tooth in check can help to rejuvenate your skin, 'improving texture, tone and radiance', says Dr Brandt.

The key to good skin, we find, is an inside/outside approach. As well as diet and carefully chosen supplements, your skin will benefit from good products. Regular exercise is a must too: according to Dr Weil, regular aerobic exercise, such as brisk walking (which, of course, helps your bones too), seems to reduce the level of inflammatory proteins in the body. He recommends 30–45 minutes of aerobic exercise, five or more times a week. Lots of sleep and water are the great free beautifiers – and, of course, being happy brings a gorgeous glow to anyone.

The simple advice that we know works…

● Eat foods that are high in skin-plumping, anti-inflammatory omega-3 fatty acids: oily fish (salmon, mackerel, sardines and herrings), walnuts and freshly ground flaxseeds; also eat lots of fresh vegetables and non-citrus fruit (blue- and other berries).
● Consume less animal protein, such as red meat and dairy foods (apart from live natural yogurt). Don't barbecue food (it forms sugary substances, and possibly carcinogens).
● Drink lots of still, pure water – at least eight large glasses daily – plus green or white tea, which is full of antioxidants.
● Avoid sugar in all forms (including too much fruit and fruit juice) and complex carbohydrates, except for vegetables (but not potatoes and parsnips). Complex carbs – bread, rice, pasta, grains – convert to sugar in your bloodstream.
● Consider supplements: as well as eating omega-3 rich food, we take extra essential fatty acids (Essential Oil Formula by Harmony Formula; three to six capsules daily). For anyone with a skin or digestive condition (including children), an eight-week trial of probiotics may help. Dr Weil suggests products with *lactobacillus GG* (such as Culturelle by Allergy Research). Interestingly, research shows that taking probiotics during the last trimester of pregnancy and for six months postnatally may help prevent babies developing eczema, probably by helping to normalise the immune system. Cut down on products made with flour of any kind, avoid processed foods, anything with hydrogenated oils, trans fats or polyunsaturated vegetable oils.
● If you suffer from puffy eyes, look at what you eat the night before: if it's wheat or other grains, try cutting them out for a week and see if the problem goes away. If it does, avoid them as much as possible.

Green food

The billions-of-years-old marine plants called algaes, which include chlorella and spirulina, can really make a marked improvement to skin tone and texture. They're stuffed with nutrients of all kinds, including proteins, vitamins and minerals, essential fats and amino acids, which nourish and also detoxify.

Sarah started taking Sun Chlorella A at quite a low ebb, and watched her tired, drooping face perk and plump up, her skin become noticeably thicker and plushier, and the whites of her eyes start to gleam again. (The other product we recommend is The Really Healthy Company Klamath Blue Green Wild Algae.)

'I would always buy good food rather than designer clothes: it has such a long-term effect on us all' DONNA AIR

DAY CREAMS

Here are the day moisturisers that most impressed our panellists (look out for some new entries). No fancy promises: they are just designed to leave skin nourished, hydrated and comfortable. Simple as that

We've included the highest-scoring products for dry, oily/combination and sensitive complexions, as well as some suits-all-skin-types options – though no certified organic or 100 per cent natural winners.

❀ REN ROSE COMPLEX MOISTURISER
Score: 8.64/10
Targeted at normal skins, a skin-quenching complex with rose petal extracts (picked at high summer, for the highest level of antioxidant polyphenols), rosehip and wild roseberry. Like all REN products, it's free from most chemical nasties but why is a polymer (a plastic-like ingredient) in there?
Comments: 'My blemish-prone oily skin felt soft, and looked smooth and bright; make-up went on very smoothly' • 'beautiful sensual moisturiser – fresh rose smell, rich, creamy texture and instant skin boost' • 'sank in quickly' • 'love the packaging' • 'oily zone contained, skin healthier and even-toned'.

❀ LIZ EARLE NATURALLY ACTIVE SKINCARE SKIN REPAIR LIGHT
Score: 8.56/10
This 'Light' version of the beauty classic Skin Repair was created for normal/oily/problem skin, in a pump dispenser. Key ingredients are skin-saving echinacea, avocado oil and natural-source vitamin E.
Comments: 'Lovely product; perfect for oily skin – the natural products seem to soothe and tame skin, even in hard-water areas' • 'skin was brighter and felt lighter' • 'easy to spread: gave a dewy look; skin felt able to breathe' • 'make-up stayed on longer and looked smoother; made me look radiant'.

❀ ORIGINS A PERFECT WORLD ANTIOXIDANT MOISTURISER WITH WHITE TEA
Score: 8.37/10
Natural goodies alongside white tip tea in this formula include sugarcane extract, murumuru butter, rosehip oil and vitamin C, with an aromatic fragrance of mimosa, orange, bergamot and spearmint.
Comments: 'Skin plumped, smooth and healthier – relative asked if I'd had a face-lift!' • 'loved the orange smell' • 'sank in well' • 'loved everything about this – but no SPF'.

❀❀ NEAL'S YARD REMEDIES ROSE & MALLOW MOISTURISER
Score: 8.11/10
Neal's Yard blend soothing marshmallow, luxurious rose and vitamin-rich carrot and almond in this 35 per cent organic product. Useful as a day cream and at night to rehydrate normal/dry skins.
Comments: 'I work in a lab with very low humidity so my skin's dried out; this cream is the most moisturising so far' • 'my skin felt a lot softer only 24 hours after applying; so many compliments from friends that my skin looks rejuvenated' • 'put the natural glow back in my cheeks' • 'sank in quickly and make-up went on smoothly if I waited a few minutes' • 'I loved the flowery smell but some thought it was a bit overpowering'.

❀❀ NEAL'S YARD REMEDIES FRANKINCENSE HYDRATING CREAM
Score: 8.1/10
Well done to Neal's Yard with two victors in this category! Frankincense – which has spectacular anti-ageing powers – is 'reinforced' with 16 antioxidants and delicate plant oils, rich in omega 3 and 6 fatty acids.
Comments: 'I love this stuff! Instant and noticeable improvement' • 'skin looked brighter, smoother, more toned' • 'light and creamy, sank in very quickly and make-up went on smoothly' • 'definitely makes my skin look younger, dewier – a little jar of magic'.

★ ❀ AVALON ORGANICS LAVENDER DAILY MOISTURIZER
Score: 8.1/10
Created for all skin types to deliver 'weightless hydration', this cream is unscented, so suitable for sensitive skins too. (Though oily skins mostly felt the formula was too rich for them.) Turmeric, arnica and calendula target redness, with antioxidant grapeseed polyphenols, organic white tea and vitamins C and E. Plenty of botanical ingredients, some organically certified (though not as many as we'd like for a company with 'Organics' in its name).
Comments: 'Gave an overall plumpness to face, and calmed my city-living skin' • 'skin smoother and more evenly toned; sensitivity improved too' • 'fantastic job at an amazing price' • 'good base for make-up' • 'lovely product, gorgeous smell – a must-have'.

SPF 15 MOISTURISERS

Precious few of these are available in natural ranges yet – and no new contenders in the latest trials wowed our testers. There still wasn't a huge selection on which to pass judgment, but these were the favourites – and all scored well. We'd like to see more SPF protective daily moisturisers launched, though, please…!

❀ VAISHALY DAY MOISTURISER SPF15
Score: 8.83/10

Super-facialist Vaishaly Patel created this, 'to be absorbed easily, without leaving any residue, stickiness or shine' – and it definitely lives up to that promise, according to our testers. The sinks-in-fast formulation – with a high percentage of organic ingredients (although not, alas, certified) – is a favourite of Jo's, who wears it all summer long. It shields against both UVA and UVB, with an anti-irritation blend of ginkgo and calendula, and is based on sun-blocking, ultra-fine micronised zinc oxide, which protects invisibly, with no telltale whiteness. The version for dry/sensitive skins was the high-scorer here, but it is also available for normal-to-combination complexions (and the company will ship worldwide, so you can enjoy this anywhere under the sun).
Comments: 'This is now my summer standby; it's moisturising enough for my quite dry skin, but absorbs quickly – I don't even have to wait the regulation ten minutes before applying make-up' • 'cream left my skin quite dewy but not oily or greasy; very modern, attractive packaging – I love this product! My skin was much brighter, softer and smoother' • 'I'm a total convert to this and will buy it when my tester product has run out' • 'very light, which I liked, with a subtle, pleasant smell'.

❀ ORIGINS OUT SMART DAILY NATURALLY PROTECTIVE SUNSCREEN
Score: 7.5/10

Origins' suits-all-skin-types face protector boasts an SPF25, so is useful if you're under the sun almost anywhere; the sunscreen is ultra-fine natural titanium dioxide (a mined mineral), which protects against UVA and UVB. It also contains moisture-boosting seaweed extract and antioxidant vitamin C. When we first tested it, we hadn't realised it's very subtly tinted: so the message is: if you're looking for a (more) natural face protector with a tad of skin-tone-evening colour, this is a good botanical-rich choice.
Comments: 'Brilliant product: I can honestly say that my skin is in better condition since I have started using this' • 'absorbed nicely and worked well in scorching Mexican sun' • 'a little goes a long way' • 'squeezy tube is easy to transport' • 'nice light colour that you can wear without foundation if you wish' • 'really like the fact it's a mineral sunscreen, rather than chemical'.

❀ JASON RED ELEMENTS DAILY MOISTURIZING CREME WITH SPF15
Score: 7.25/10

From a leading US brand of skincare that promotes itself all over the globe as 'pure, natural and organic', this is – rather surprisingly – based on chemical sunscreens (rather than physical ones, such as zinc oxide or titanium dioxide), and contains silicones (which explains the glide-on texture). The base, however, is pretty natural, containing vitamin E, aloe and panthenol (vitamin B5). Jason's Red Elements range gets its name from the red tea incorporated to fight free-radical damage, with polypeptides to boost collagen production. This is a richly hydrating cream for normal to dry skin (there is also a Daily Moisturizing Lotion for normal to oily skin). Some testers liked it a lot, though others were less impressed.
Comments: 'Gives a dewiness to skin; it's light (though quite a thick cream) and moisturises without being greasy' • 'this has really grown on me – it's light, delicate, doesn't irritate my skin and has the benefit of SPF15; I'm very impressed' • 'loved this as a moisturiser: skin felt hydrated all day; it wasn't greasy or oily at all, sank in well and provided a good base for make-up'.

We love…

For facial sun protection, Sarah has discovered Kimberly Sayer Ultra Light Organic Facial Moisturizer SPF25 (see page 145) for normal, oily and acne-prone skin. As Jo says, she is a huge fan of Vaishaly Day Moisturiser SPF15 (see above).

the ultimate GREAT-SKIN SECRET

One of the world's best beauty secrets isn't a cream. It isn't a pill. No, it's a way of hands-on caring for your skin on a daily basis that brings more radiance than simply applying products ever can. And best of all? It's free…

We have a radical theory. If you massaged verucca cream, wart ointment or cooking oil into your face using the terrific facial massage technique explained on this page, you could melt away lines and wrinkles and restore skin to vibrancy.

In reality, we're not suggesting for a moment that you ditch your usual skin cream and follow that advice – but it does emphasise our belief that it isn't just the cream you choose that can make a difference to how your skin looks; it's HOW YOU APPLY IT. (Sorry for 'shouty' capitals, but we want you to get this message LOUD AND CLEAR.) We've seen, with our own eyes – and on our own faces – the amazing difference that facial massage can make to a woman's skin. Many women are scared to tug or pull the skin for fear of causing wrinkles; as a result, their skins often look dull. But done properly, you don't pull the skin; you just stimulate it – along with the complex network of blood vessels, muscles and lymph drainage points underneath the surface. What's more, the technique helps deliver nourishment – and without that, skin is more prone to folds and wrinkles.

Now the 'queen' of facial massage, to our minds, is facialist Vaishaly Patel, who is her own best advertisement, by the way. And, as Vaishaly maintains, 'Even just 30 seconds

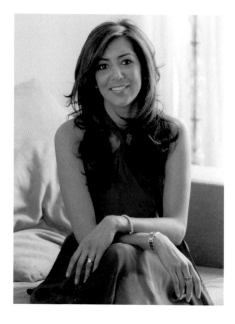

of massage while you're cleansing helps reduce puffiness and jowliness. When you're stressed – and most women are – you hold a lot of tension in your face, especially along the jawline.'

Vaishaly's facial massage

1 Dot a product (preferably a facial oil or moisturiser – cleanser at a pinch; we didn't mean it about the verruca cream!) all over your face.

2 Using the pads of your fingertips, massage the face with firm, circular movements (this boosts the circulation and lymphatic drainage, while helping to disperse any congestion under the surface of the skin). Start from the chin and jawline and work upwards. 'Most women rub in cream working downwards – which is the direction we don't want our faces to go,' explains Vaishaly. 'Don't forget the super-tight muscles on the side of the neck, and work up behind the ears too.'

3 When you reach the eye area, firmly 'sweep' your fingers along the browbone in one, continuous stroke, moving outwards and then underneath the eye towards the nose. This will not stretch the skin as the product you are using will provide lubrication. Repeat two to three times. As well as being relaxing, this technique will help to drain any fluid build-up, boosting blood flow and feeding oxygen to the eye area.

4 Finish off by massaging the forehead, working from the middle of the forehead out towards the temples.

THE ACUPUNCTURE FACE-LIFT

Another 'face-waking' option is facial acupuncture. Like half of Hollywood (the movie babes there are hooked, apparently), we are completely convinced of its face-saving, radiance-boosting power. Facial acupuncture needs to be carried out by trained acupuncturists and is basically a cosmetic application of traditional Oriental acupuncture techniques. 'The skin is a mirror of our inner health, and skin problems such as puffiness, break-outs, dullness or redness all indicate that the body's vital energy, or qi, isn't flowing efficiently,' explains John Yiannis Tsagaris, a doctor of traditional Chinese medicine who gives facial acupuncture treatments designed to combat inner and outer signs of ageing.

'There's no one system, because facial acupuncturists tend to develop their own techniques, which may also include facial massage. By inserting fine needles into the body's energy channels, or meridians, skin functions can be improved.' According to experts, it stimulates skin cells to lay down new collagen fibres under wrinkles, 'filling them in', while also toning and/or relaxing different muscles to combat sagging and restoring glow. Typical results include decreased fine and deep lines, reduction of under-eye bags, firmer eyelids, tighter pores, brighter skin tone and softer, more elastic skin.

For lasting benefits, though, you'd need to schedule a series of treatments. Certainly, facial acupuncture is miraculous for 'tired' faces and Jo finds there's a definite softening of frown – and laugh-lines. (The bonus: though it's called facial acupuncture, the therapist treats the whole body – which is why patients often report their mind feels sharper and they have more energy after a treatment.)

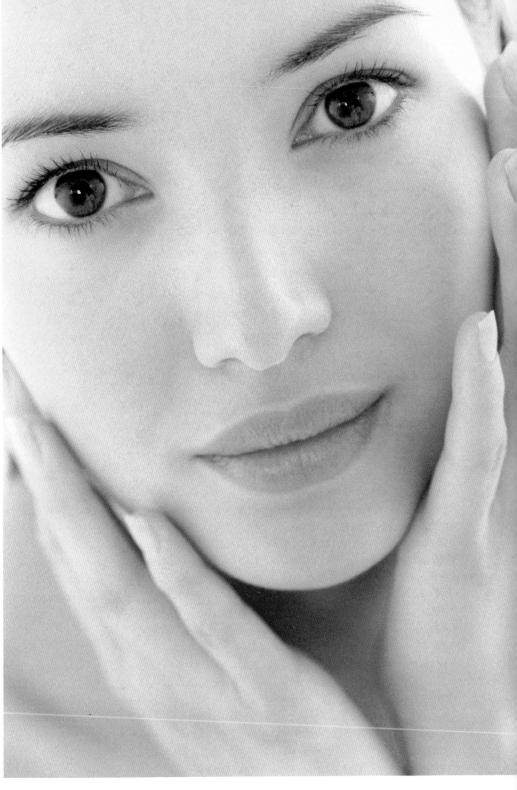

'By inserting fine needles into the body's energy channels, or meridians, skin functions can be improved' JOHN YIANNIS TSAGARIS

CREATING A *skin-friendly* ENVIRONMENT

You're doing everything right for your sensitive skin with skin-calming creams, no perfume – but still your skin's acting touchy. (More than 40 per cent of our testers for this book categorised themselves as 'sensitive-skinned', a clue to how widespread the problem is.) The truth is, it may not just be your beauty regime that's triggering flare-ups: there may be other factors. So try these simple lifestyle shifts, to see if skin 'chills out'. These tips also apply to anyone with skin conditions such as eczema, psoriasis and acne

● Soap is generally way too harsh for faces and we recommend a specific facial cleanser. But if the skin on your body is also sensitive, try using an emollient wash, instead. (For our recommendations on great body washes, see page 119.) If you prefer to stick with soap, seek out a natural version, which retains the glycerine – the natural, moisturising element which is removed from most commercially produced soap bars. An oat-based product can often help calm touchy skin. For an instant bathtime skin-calmer, simply put a handful of oats in a cotton cloth, tie up and hang under a running tap.

● Never use very hot water on sensitive skin: use cool or tepid for washing face and hands, and warm for showering/bathing.

● Use the minimum of washing powder – better still, try Soapods: natural cleansing 'nuts' that you throw in the wash in a special bag, and which does get washing white. NB: we have experimented and find that most clothes get perfectly clean at a temperature of 30°C – far lower than is usually recommended. Try for yourself. (Not if you have eczema, though, and need to exterminate house dust mites.)

● We use cider vinegar in place of fabric conditioner: you don't get that spring-like smell (which is entirely synthetic), but it leaves clothes just as snugglesomely soft. Of course, in warm weather, we dry clothes outside – the greenest option; you can always throw them in the dryer for five minutes at the end to soften them up.

● Switch to household cleaners that don't use harsh chemicals. This may help alleviate allergies, too. Sarah's decades-long eczema disappeared when she started using Ecover and Bio-D. Avoid clothes-washing powders with biological actions, which often end up irritating skin.

● Avoid bubble baths and use bath oils, instead. Try making your own with organic base oil (eg sweet almond) and essential oils.

● Keep the air around you humid: dry air can dry the skin, but air that is too damp can cause mould and house dust mite growth, both of which irritate eczema – so humidity levels should be around 50 per cent. You can buy humidity monitors on the web; if levels dip, place bowls of water around the house, near heat sources – or dry your washing over the radiator, which humidifies brilliantly.

● Keep the temperature down in your house (and workplace, too, if possible): the air won't get so dry – and you'll save money on fuel bills. Pop on an extra woollie (or a chic cashmere/cotton-mix vest) – and jump up and down, or go for a walk to get your circulation moving, instead of staying still and shivering.

● Avoid exposure to passive smoke: it will inflame skin, just as it irritates the rest of your body.

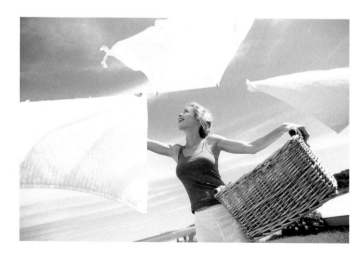

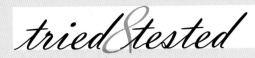

NIGHT CREAMS

A separate night cream is optional, as we've said. But if you want to nourish dry and/or mature skin with rich ingredients, the optimum time is at night. Our testers have now trialled over 50 natural creams designed to be used at night – each for a period of months – and declare these positively dreamy…

✿ KORRES THYME HONEY 24-HOUR MOISTURISING CREAM

Score: 9.03/10

A really ace score for a cream from a Greek brand that targets normal and dry skin, featuring real thyme honey (5 per cent) in the smooth blend (not as sticky as it sounds!)..

Comments: 'Soft, velvety textured, honey-smelling cream; skin was soft and felt smooth with a healthy sheen' • 'wonderful: my skin was less dry, plumper, brighter and softer immediately' • 'great value for money' • 'heaven in a jar' • 'my skin looks and feels like it's had a big drink' • 'it takes time to sink in but it made blemished, dehydrated skin so much better in a short time'.

✿ VAISHALY NIGHT CREAM

Score: 8.6 /10

Top facialist Vaishaly Patel has never liked too-heavy creams, so formulated hers to sink in fast, nourishing skin with active ingredients that include regenerating macadamia and soya bean oils and protective vitamin E, combined with Vaishaly's own arnica, ginkgo and calendula complex to combat irritation.

Comments: 'My skin took on a radiance I hadn't experienced before; the elasticity improved and it looked plumper' • 'helped take away fine lines' • 'directions for massaging into skin very clear' • 'fabulous from first use: skin felt soft and comfortable but not oily; a delight to use, it goes on like a cream but smooths in like a lotion'.

✿✿ WELEDA WILD ROSE NIGHT CREAM

Score: 8.25/10

Weleda purchases more than 400 million roses a year, largely from an organic Fair Trade project in Turkey. Some end up in this winning cream – with revitalising evening primrose, *Sedum purpureum* and myrrh.

Comments: 'My skin was soft, smooth and looked good despite being worn out' • 'smells of roses; a pleasure to put on' • 'my skin looked radiant in the morning' • 'skin looked smoother, less wrinkled' • 'rich, but sinks in easily' • 'skin much brighter'.

✿✿ NEAL'S YARD REMEDIES NOURISHING ORANGE FLOWER NIGHT CREAM

Score: 7.95/10

Ideal for dry skins, this combines EFA-rich oils of sea buckthorn, pomegranate and wild rosehip with vitamin E and orange flower essential oil in a 57 per cent organic product. Testers liked the fact it wasn't over-rich.

Comments: 'An excellent mid-priced night cream; smells delicious, feels nice on the skin and doesn't leave a greasy film' • 'gave my skin a real treat' • 'skin seemed plumper next morning' • 'indulgent and gorgeous' • 'skin felt smoother and looked brighter'.

✿ KORRES OLIVE & RYE NIGHT CREAM

Score: 7.88/10

This intense night cream is rich in vegetable oils, including 'firming' rye active extract for faces which have lost 'bounce-back'; visible results are promised from first application.

Comments: 'reminded me of mayo or creamy pear yoghurt; my skin felt softer and brighter' • 'skin became so radiant that after day two I didn't need foundation, just a little blusher' • 'lots of people said how fresh-faced I look' • 'smell is just gorgeous'.

✿ ANTIPODES AVOCADO PEAR NOURISHING NIGHT CREAM

Score: 7.8/10

This luscious cream incorporates antioxidant vitamins E, A and C, as well as vitamins B1, B2 and D, plus soothing manuka honey, all swirled with pure, fragrant sandalwood oil.

Comments: 'lovely velvety texture, easily absorbed; skin more hydrated, softer and plumper' • 'my skin lapped it up' • 'sank in quickly, skin looked brighter, more supple'.

✿ TAER ICELANDIC 24 HOUR CREAM

Score: 7.64/10

This moisturiser from the cult Icelandic skincare brand meaning 'pure' contains an aromatic blend of herbs that grow in the mineral-rich Icelandic soil.

Comments: 'Skin smoother and softer immediately; over time it seemed to plump out lines and bring a dewy glow' • 'smells gorgeous, even my husband commented' • 'skin looks younger and fresher' • 'also makes a good base for foundation' • 'people have said I look really well'.

HEALING PLANTS FOR

Plants have been recognised for their healing properties for centuries. And the ones featured here – some of which you can grow in your garden or on your kitchen windowsill – pack a potent punch with skin problems, as TV gardener Sarah Raven (who is also a qualified doctor) points out. Cultivating your own first-aid kit couldn't be easier…

Marigold
(*Calendula officinalis*)

Sarah Raven has been growing marigolds in her garden for years. 'They're simple to raise,' she says, 'and are among the most effective healing plants, providing a wonderful cure for cuts, sores and almost any skin lesion. They have antibacterial properties, are a good antiseptic, and contain tannin, which helps to knot together wounds and speed up healing.' All you have to do is press the juice from the fresh flowers and apply directly to the skin. Check out Jo's *Ultimate Natural Beauty Book* for a recipe for marigold salve. What's more, in a recent clinical trial, scientists isolated an active ingredient in marigolds that helps the skin condition psoriasis.

Aloe vera
(*Aloe barbadensis*)

'The healing powers of aloe vera are becoming more widely known,' says Sarah. 'It needs to be grown inside, but it's a hassle-free houseplant that can be grown on a windowsill.' The gel from this spiky succulent, which can be used directly from the leaf or as a ready-prepared product (look for 100 per cent pure aloe gel), has a long history of use for skin problems, from sunburn and cuts, to eczema, rosacea and psoriasis. 'It's brilliant for any kind of skin lesion,' says Sarah. 'My family and I have found that it's particularly effective on sore gums and mouth ulcers.' We have also found aloe to be fantastic for soothing and healing cracked lips.

Celandine
(*Chelidonium majus*)

'Another plant in my healing border is greater celandine,' says Sarah. 'This is an effective treatment for warts. Just pick a stem and it will immediately start to ooze brilliant tangerine yellow sap. Cover your wart every day for three weeks and it will disappear, as my family and I have found to our great delight.'

Camomile
(*Matricaria recutita* and *Chamaemelum nobile*)

This soothing herb, formulated as a topical cream, may help skin problems, but some research suggests it can also cause sensitivity in certain people. Golden camomile (*Chrysanthellum indicum*) has also been seen to be effective in treating skin problems. A 12-week double blind study of 246 people found that a cream containing 1 per cent golden camomile significantly improved the symptoms of moderate rosacea.

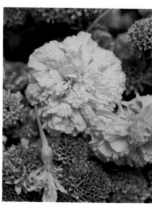
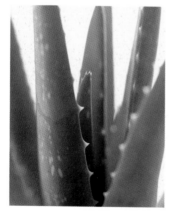
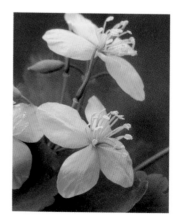
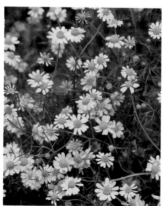

SKIN CONDITIONS

Liquorice
(Glycyrrhiza glabra)

The active substances in liquorice, called glycyrrhizins, are well-known for helping to heal all manner of inflammatory skin conditions, including cold sores, eczema and psoriasis. In one study, a cream with 2 per cent liquorice extract did better than 1 per cent; there are also balms available containing 3 per cent of the active ingredient.

St John's wort
(Hypericum perforatum)

This herb is most often used – very effectively – for the treatment of depression. The active substance, hypericin, also seems to have anti-inflammatory properties and was shown to reduce symptoms in eczema sufferers, albeit in a small trial.

Tea tree
(Melaleuca alternifolia)

In recent years, tea tree oil has become increasingly popular as an antimicrobial agent used against hospital superbugs, such as MRSA. It has also been shown to have anti-inflammatory properties. Many sufferers of the skin condition called molluscum contagiosum – lots of tiny little pearly bumps for which there is virtually no conventional treatment – say that dabbing tea tree oil on the bumps (with a cotton bud) has cured the problem. NB: use it carefully because in some people it may cause dermatitis.

FLOWER REMEDIES

Distilled from plants, flowers and trees, flower remedies (or essences) act as an invisible support tool to support feelings and emotions, according to Somerset GP Dr Andrew Tresidder, who uses them in his practice. We love the whole range, from the Bach Original Flower Remedies (dating back to the 1930s) to Jan de Vries, Australian Bush Flower Essences and smaller brands like Balancing Blooms and T3. We've found that they can help some physical problems too: for instance we put Bach's Rescue Remedy on our computer-tired eyes. Do try them: we can't guarantee the results but flower remedies are now used in hospitals worldwide, with doctors testifying to their effects. We love them and they may work well for you too.

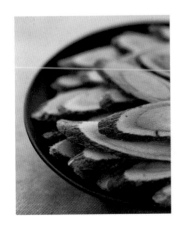
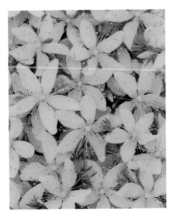
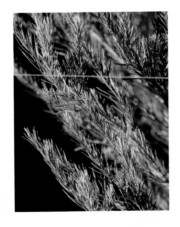

spot the problem

Nobody loves them, but by far the majority of us – both sexes – suffer from spots at some stage, not necessarily in our teens. We wish we could say there's a single cure-all magic bullet, but the truth is that you need to adopt an integrated, consistent approach – and be patient. Here's advice from the experts

● **Avoid milk and products made with it.** Recent large-scale research suggests that drinking two or three glasses of milk daily may seriously exacerbate acne. This is possibly due to the hormones it contains: remember that nearly all milk comes from pregnant animals – which teenage and adult bodies are not designed to deal with. Swap to organic rice, oat or almond milk, fortified with calcium. (Soy milk may suit some, but others are allergic to it.) Instant breakfast drinks, some fizzy drinks, cream cheese and cottage cheese were also significantly associated with acne in the study, but not pizza, chocolate, soda and French fries.

● **Avoid orange and other citrus fruits and juices.** These encourage inflammation of the skin, according to integrated health expert Dr Mosaraf Ali.

● **Consider supplements.** According to pharmacist Shabir Daya, who specialises in natural remedies, the most important one to take is colloidal silver, which acts in the same way as antibiotics. He recommends Source Naturals Ultra Colloidal Silver, 1ml three times daily for ten days; in chronic cases, up the dosage to 5ml. If the spots continue, he suggests a maintenance dose of 1ml daily, preferably with a good probiotic (such as Mega Probiotic-ND by Food Science of

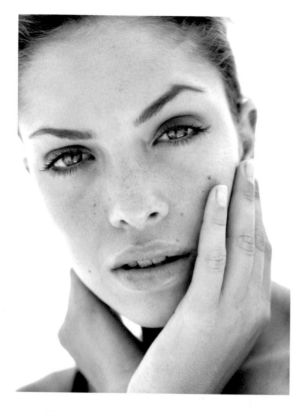

Vermont). Also recommended are vitamin A (try 5000iu daily) and zinc picolinate (try 15–30mg daily).

● **Get out in the sunlight.** This enhances skin healing by helping the body's production of vitamins A and D. NB: in moderation…

● **Try herbs.** If spots occur before a period, or are linked to polycystic ovarian syndrome (PCOS), herbalist Andrew Chevallier

suggests taking chaste berry (also known as *agnus castus*), in the dose recommended by the manufacturer. For men, saw palmetto may help.

● **Avoid stimulants,** such as tea, coffee, alcohol and sugar, as these all upset blood sugar levels, which affect hormones.

● **Herbal teas:** Andrew Chevallier advises infusing equal parts of red clover, cleavers and marigold (as dried herbs) for ten to 15 minutes in a teapot. Drink up to four cups daily, sweetened with honey (try medicinal manuka honey), if you like.

● **Chinese medicine:** integrated health guru Dr Weil suggests consulting a qualified practitioner for chronic skin problems. Mind/body therapies such as clinical hypnosis and meditation can be very effective too.

● **For acne scarring:** apply pure aloe vera gel (or use the goo from the leaf of an aloe plant) and also take two aloe vera capsules twice daily for three to four months. Pure vitamin E oil or rosehip oil can also help; for freshness, pierce a capsule and apply the contents to skin.

● Turn to page 53 for tips on make-up to hide spots.

SPOT ZAPPERS

Zits aren't just for teens. A good third of our testers, all over 25, are still prone to break-outs. We're pleased to announce a new entry in this botanical spot-zapper category, from Aussie brand Jurlique – something else to turn to when an angry red spot threatens to ruin an important date or interview (though some testers still swear by a dot of toothpaste...)

❀ ORIGINS SPOT REMOVER

Score: 7.66/10

This is one of Origins' treatment products for use only as long as a specific condition exists. With salicylic acid (from wintergreen and sweet birch bark), it zeroes in on blemishes, penetrating pores to break up plugs of bacteria-breeding oil, dirt and debris. Oregano and clove bud essential oil act as 'reinforcements', and reduce drying and flaking. It's to be applied at the first signs of a break-out, on to the spot alone. Most testers found it very helpful but a couple of complexions were too sensitive for it.

Comments: 'Within a few hours of applying to a large whitehead, it had reduced significantly; eight hours later I could hardly see it; after another application 24 hours later, I could only see a dry mark; but you have to put it only on the blemish, as it can cause peeling' • 'very pleasant clean fragrance' • 'dries up spots quickly; one went overnight' • 'a very angry red lump was dried out quickly' • 'very good as an anchor for concealer; surprised at its effectiveness'.

❀ AESOP CHAMOMILE CONCENTRATE ANTI-BLEMISH MASQUE

Score: 7.55/10

From an Australian natural beauty brand that we have loved for a long time, this mask targets spots with antibacterial botanicals, iron oxide and montmorillite (a kind of clay). It can be left on skin under concealer or used as a rinse-off overnight treatment.

Comments: 'Used on huge red spots and after three days, the whole area looked less angry' • 'citrussy and fresh – got rid of spots in two days' • 'skin felt silky; easy to use – like a menthol-fragranced mud face pack'.

❀❀ THE BODY SHOP TEA TREE OIL BLEMISH STICK

Score: 7.44/10

This light, translucent gel, packed with tea tree oil, comes with a sponge applicator and has sea algae to help prevent over-drying. It's accessibly priced for those on a budget.

Comments: 'Reduced redness in an aggravated spot' • 'no red mark after the spot had dried up' • 'spot healed entirely in three days – I will buy this' • 'handy to carry around' • 'kept the area clean and fresh'.

❀ JURLIQUE BLEMISH CREAM

Score: 7.16/10

Jurlique got a major makeover a couple of years back, souping up the packaging, tweaking formulations, introducing terrific new lines (and hiking prices). This light cream features blemish-busting calendula, witch hazel, self heal and tea tree oil and is skin-toned to offer some camouflage, though most testers used concealer too.

Comments: 'Did a good job; I was happy using it; helped calm spot and reduced worst redness on day one' • 'spot shrank on days one and two, then dried up on day three' • 'made red lump on my oily nose less noticeable' • 'blended into my skin well'.

In the clear

Stressful events (emotional, mental or physical) can make acne worse, according to doctors. Common triggers include exams, new relationships, the time just before a period, pregnancy, certain cosmetics and medicines. Finding out individual triggers can help, as can knowing that lots of other people have the same problem, so you can swap treatment and camouflage tips. Remember that it does eventually go: Sarah had terrible acne from 12 to 20-something, on her face and back, with a resurgence in her 30s (which improved significantly when she stopped eating sugar). Now she has really good skin, with nary a blemish and no scars, on her face.

FAST FIXES FOR TIRED SKIN

What do you do when your skin looks a tad washed out and you just feel blah? Here are our top tips for instant sparkle. And the great thing is they don't cost a mint – in fact, some are free as air

● Start by breathing: it's the foundation of everything. It calms you down, peps you up – oh, and keeps you living. So, if you want to be more alive, practise this simple, quick technique at least twice daily for five cycles – more is better. Unfold your arms and legs, sit, lie or stand loosely and close your eyes (if possible). With your tongue just behind your top teeth, inhale to a count of four down into your belly; hold for seven (without letting your shoulders rise); exhale through rounded lips for eight. Brilliant for stress control (and one of the basics of tantric sex…).

● If you can, go for a 20-minute walk in the fresh air. If you're stuck indoors, march on the spot, arms swinging, knees coming up, then speed up and down stairs. Try jumping up and down – or even a star jump…

● Sip a glass of warm boiled water, with a squeeze of lemon. Drink at least eight of these daily between meals (so as not to dilute the nutrients in your food).

● Splash your face with alternating hot and cold water; do this several times. And/or: fill a bowl or small basin with warm water, add two drops of rosemary essential oil (or any one which appeals to you), soak a flannel in it and lay it over your face.

● Have a shower and give yourself a top-to-toe scrub (see page 115 for Tried & Tested scrubs). Finish by turning the shower to hot then cold, three times if you can. It's the most amazingly perkifying thing you can do (and truly not as awful as it sounds!).

Easy re-energisers

So tired you can't roll out of bed? Try these pick-me-ups from Margot Lieber of Spa Illuminata in London. You can do them any time….

● Breathe slowly and deeply and, in your mind's eye, see your favourite colour.
● Start with a couple of minutes of 'lazy yoga', lying on your bed and stretching down through your legs and pointing your toes, with your arms stretched above your head. Lift your right foot over your left knee and hold for a moment, then do the same the other side. Repeat.
● Now sit up on the edge of the bed and 'comb' your hair with your fingertips from the hairline back to your nape. Repeat several times, always using slow movements, but you can use quite firm pressure.
● Rub your skull from front to back in zigzag movements; really dig into the area at the back of your head where it meets the neck.
● Next, use your fingers and palms to press on your jawline, temples and all over your skull.
● Move to your forehead and, with your two middle fingers, stroke it firmly with alternate fingers up and down the centre in a flicking motion to ease your mind and relieve stress. (You can practically feel the vertical lines becoming less deep.)
● Pinch your eyebrows with your finger and thumb, working from the nose out. Then pinch your jawline, working upwards.
● If you have time, tap all round the eye area on the bone, round your cheekbones and temples. If you're in a hurry, pinch (gently) and tap your cheeks to bring an instant rosy glow.

● Turbocharge your moisturiser with a squeeze of Bach's Rescue Remedy flower essence, (see page 27).

● Make, or treat, yourself to a fresh juice: try detoxing cucumber and melon or revitalising carrot, apple and ginger. Add a shot of wheatgrass or spirulina if you wish. If you only have a blender at home, whiz up some fresh or frozen berries, all the pinks, purples and reds – they're loaded with vitamins – and add a pot of natural live yoghurt for a real punch.

● Give your cheeks a 'pop' of blusher – make-up artist Bobbi Brown's favourite trick, which miraculously makes your eyes sparkle and your face look alive. Do the concealer bit under your eyes, gloss up your lips, sweep on some mascara – and go-go-go!

● Three quick energisers: rub the rims and the lobes of your ears with your thumb and forefinger; rub and pull your fingers, especially the joints; massage your second little toes, which are linked to the liver. May sound strange but it all works!

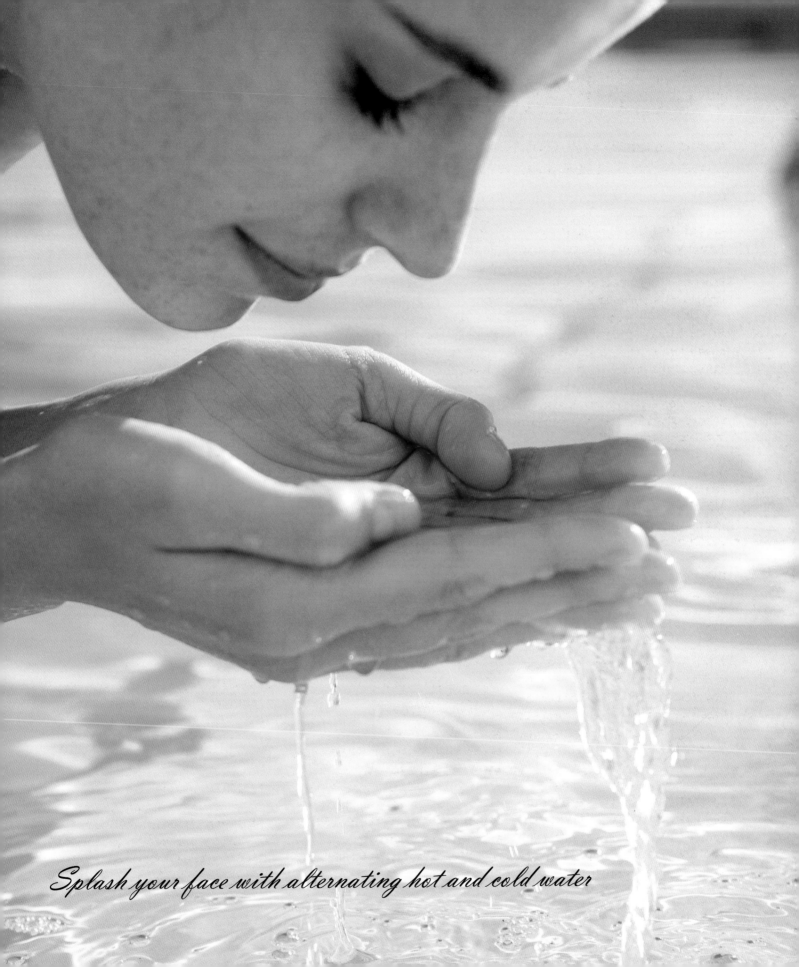

Splash your face with alternating hot and cold water

magic oils

Oils are nature's beauty bounty: concentrated goodness, with a natural affinity for skin. What's more, oils don't need preservatives – making them the ultimate natural beauty choice

Oils from plants, nuts and seeds have been used to beautify skin for literally thousands of years – and are as effective today as when Cleopatra (or, quite likely, her cavewoman ancestors) first discovered their skin-smoothing, age-defying, ultra-softening power. The Ancient Greeks and Egyptians loved olive oil – slurped on to their bodies, as well as on their food. It's naturally rich in vitamin E and, if you were stranded on a desert island, you could survive with a bottle of olive oil as your all-purpose beauty kit. At a pinch, you can use it to remove make-up, nourish skin and hair – and evidence is even emerging that certain elements of olive oil have a slight sun-protective effect. (For more on sun, see pages 140–149.) It says everything that the eternally smooth-skinned Sophia Loren swears by the beauty power of olive oil.

We are long-standing fans of facial oils, which are usually blends of nourishing base oils and fragrant essential oils. But we find that, quite unjustly, fear of oil-slickness often puts many women off. Many oils

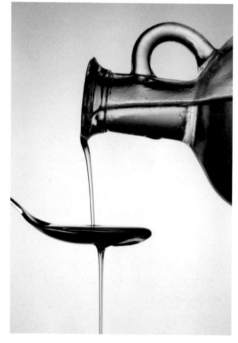

are totally skin-compatible, sinking in fast, sealing in natural moisture by creating an (imperceptible) barrier on the surface, plumping up parched skin and reducing dryness. As leading facialist Amanda Lacey

explains: 'The biggest misconception about using a facial oil is that it gives you spots or makes skin greasy. Actually, many creams are complicated formulations and can plug pores. Plant oils have a finer molecular structure. The body has its own oil-producing sebaceous glands, so oil is something your skin recognises and absorbs more effectively.' For sensitive-skinned women, oils can be an excellent choice because they don't need preservatives, which can trigger skin touchiness; bacteria can't breed in oils – only in water.

In general, oils are most appropriate for night-time use. But if you choose a lightweight one, you can apply it under make-up because it will 'disappear' in minutes, leaving your skin supple and soft. (Don't forget always to leave ten minutes between applying a moisturiser of any kind and cosmetics.) Dry-skinned women (that's us) prefer richer versions, massaged in at night; we can almost hear the sound of our complexions drinking in a luscious, nourishing oil. If you're not a convert, we say: try them.

We love...

Sarah is very impressed with organic Revitalising Face Treatment Oil from Pure Lochside, divinely scented with rose otto. Jo prefers soothing Vaishaly Night Nourisher – which comes in a mess-free, easy-to-use pump – and Care by Stella McCartney Nourishing Elixir, which is from the designer's Ecocert-certified skincare collection.

FACIAL OILS

We really love facial oils so we were delighted that our testers – even those with a tendency to shine – were willing to trial them as part of their skin regime. We dispatched more than 600 bottles, which were trialled over several weeks, notching up some exceptionally high scores

✿✿ LIZ EARLE SUPERSKIN CONCENTRATE

Score: 9.1/10

Liz Earle Naturally Active Skincare repackaged this oil recently, so we sent it out to testers again – who awarded it an even higher score, probably because the classy bottle now gives out just the right amount of oil. It is still the same blend rich in argan oil ('the gold of Morocco'), full of skin-friendly vitamin E, together with rosehip oil. It's 'perfect for tired, lifeless skin and for balancing combination skin,' they say. Just don't apply too much, they warn…

Comments: 'Made a difference immediately and I felt a million dollars!' • 'left my dry, ageing skin silky-soft and night cream after glided on; after a while my skin started to look plump, and fewer lines' • 'oil smelt divine and the pump-action dispenser put it a notch above my usual product' • 'takes a while to sink in, which is fine at night, and leaves a wonderful glow' • 'I followed the massage diagram and my skin still felt wonderfully velvety in the morning, brighter and glowing.'

✿✿ AD SKIN SYNERGY NOURISHING NIGHT TREATMENT

Score: 9.05/10

A few years ago, beauty PR Amanda Denning started her own skincare line, launching it with this nourishing night oil. It was created for all skin types, 'to restore each to optimum condition,' Amanda says. The active ingredients are all organic (though the

overall product isn't certified yet) including rosehip seed oil, rose and Roman camomile, in a base of sweet almond oil, along with coconut oil, evening primrose, grapeseed and jojoba – heaven-scented with essential oils of lavender, palmarosa, ylang-ylang, frankincense, neroli, jasmine, plus vitamin E.

Comments: 'Exceptional! Extreme nourishment for my very dry skin, which was plumper and brighter' • 'vertical lines on my neck and chest became much less noticeable' • 'tones instantly and makes you look as if you have full make-up on!' • 'deeper lines round eyes improved and diminishing lip line plumped out'.

✿✿✿ NEAL'S YARD REMEDIES ORGANIC ORANGE FLOWER FACIAL OIL

Score: 8.75/10

The scent of this neroli (orange blossom) and mandarin blend conjures up a walk through a Spanish orange grove in springtime! To boost cellular regeneration and reduce fine lines, this Soil Association-certified oil is blended with macadamia seed, evening primrose, hemp, pomegranate, sea buckthorn and pomegranate oils, captured in a signature blue bottle, with a dropper dispenser.

Comments: 'My dry, sensitive skin was brighter, clearer, smoother, and felt less tight' • 'made a big difference to fine lines' • 'noticed extra smoothness and plumpness on my skin, fewer fine lines, more bounce and a feeling of ease' • 'sank in beautifully' • 'make-up went on fine after'.

✿✿ BAREFOOT BOTANICALS ROSA FINA SECRET ESSENCE FACE & DECOLLETAGE OIL

Score: 8.75/10

Not long ago, Barefoot repackaged this, and our impressed testers upped its score, enjoying the light, sinks-in-fast blend containing 30 per cent *rosa mosqueta* (a natural source of vitamin A and Omega 3 and 6 fatty acids), plus olive, sea buckthorn, and essential oils of frankincense, *Rosa damascena* and lavender. As the name suggests, perfect for the chest zone too.

Comments: 'Made my skin instantly softer and smoother; fabulous smell of roses' • 'skin definitely more radiant, firmer and plumper' • 'skin felt so good – radiant!' • 'I use this in the day, too; make-up is easier to apply and skin looks gorgeous'.

✿✿ VAISHALY NIGHT NOURISHER FOR NORMAL/COMBINATION SKIN

Score: 8.62/10

Inside these 'designer' chocolate-coloured bottles, by facialist Vaisaly Patel, are high levels of skin-balancing essential oils of lemon, bergamot, orange, coriander and petitgrain, in a base of macadamia, soy bean and rosehip seed oils.

Comments: 'Hubbie noticed my youthful, plump skin – as smooth as glass' • 'soft, silky, healthy-looking skin' • 'enhanced radiance and evened skin tone' • 'this oil has totally transformed my life – it has stopped my monthly eruptions and break-outs'.

feed your face

Even if you do all the right things (cleanse, moisturise, sip water as if it's going out of style), forces beyond your control can sometimes leave skin looking less than gorgeous. (Think: internal factors such as stress and lack of sleep, or external, such as the Sahara-dry atmosphere of a centrally heated house, or cold winter winds.) That's where masks come in – an excellent way to give your face an intense, nourishing dose of what it needs

Masks are the easiest, peasiest beauty creations to make yourself. Even honey or yoghurt, smeared on to the skin straight from the jar/tub, can be hugely skin-brightening or moisturising. But here are a few more sophisticated suggestions for DIY masks. (You can virtually eat them – which is more than you can say for almost anything that comes from a high-street beauty counter.) Remember, too: applying them should be like putting a do-not-disturb sign around your neck: your passport to ten minutes of cloistered tranquillity. (Masks aren't a beauty ritual we want to do in company, thanks…) Leave on for five to ten minutes, then rinse off with warm water, pat skin gently dry and apply moisturiser as usual.

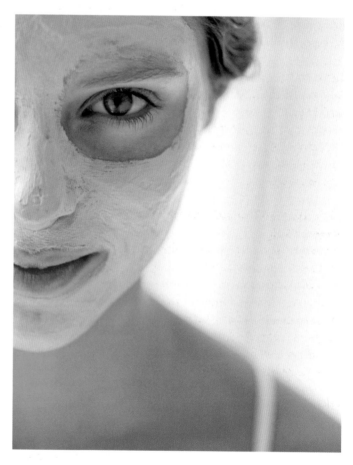

Lemon Face Food for Blemished or Spotty Skin

3 tablespoons fresh, strained lemon juice
1 tablespoon clear runny honey
4 tablespoons green clay (available from The Organic Pharmacy)
A splash of water

Put the lemon juice in a bowl, add the honey and mix until completely dissolved. Slowly add the green clay and mix to a thick paste. If it's too thick to stir easily, add a bit of water. If it's too runny, add a little more clay. The paste should be thick enough to stay in place on the spoon (and your face) without dripping. Apply and rinse off, as suggested above.

Banana and Cornmeal Booster for Normal to Dry Skin

Half a banana
2 teaspoons cornmeal (from health food shops)
1 egg yolk
A little milk (full-fat organic, if possible)

Mash the banana and blend with the cornmeal and egg yolk. Add milk to make a smooth but not runny paste. Then apply and rinse off, as suggested above.

Rich Avocado Facial for Dry Skin

1 tablespoon ripe avocado, mashed
1 teaspoon honey
3 drops cider vinegar
A little sesame oil

Mix the first three ingredients and add enough sesame oil to create a spreadable consistency. Apply as suggested above, then, after washing it off, finish with rosewater and moisturiser.

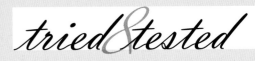

FACE MASKS

Several exciting new botanical-rich contenders earned a place in the ranks, in this section – which is a must-read if your life's too short to make an omelette, let alone whisk up a DIY face mask

✿ KORRES WILD ROSE MASK
Score: 8.68/10

Wild rose turns up again in this instantly brightening, pure white mask, suitable for all skintypes. The secret? Probably that wild rose oil is a rich natural source of vitamin C, said to have a significant repairing action.

Comments: 'Looked like calamine lotion but felt beautiful and left my skin smooth' • 'instant brightening effect and blemishes less noticeable' • 'easiest to use in the bath, as needs leaving for 10–15 minutes' • 'loved the delicate scent of roses'.

✿✿ DR HAUSCHKA SOOTHING MASK
Score: 8.55/10

Our testers found this suitable for even the most sensitive skin conditions, plumping up skin with moisture – thanks to shea butter, macadamia nut and coconut oils. The soothing botanicals include lady's mantle, borage, buckwheat and mullein.

Comments: 'Feels luxurious: brightens skin; made me very relaxed' • 'I adored this mask; my skin was calmer and generally pampered' • 'areas of dryness relieved and skin felt smooth and "glowed"' • 'used weekly, it reduced flare-ups of redness and dry skin'.

✿ KORRES POMEGRANATE CLEANSING MASK
Score: 8.37/10

Clever Korres: two products which outperformed dozens of others – in this case, a mask targeted at oilier skins with sebum-absorbing white argile clay. Pomegranate extract reduces pore size,

while zinc balances oily skin, and offers antibacterial protection.

Comments: 'Pores looked smaller and face more matt, clearer and more glowing; used regularly, skin looks generally clearer' • 'nourished my skin and left it glowing but not oily' • 'somewhat drying but doesn't leave skin taut' • 'gorgeous fragrance' • 'if my skin felt too tender to scrub, I would reach for this'.

★ ✿ LIZ EARLE NATURALLY ACTIVE SKINCARE INTENSIVE NOURISHING TREATMENT
Score: 8.02/10

Moisturising ingredients include borage oil, comfrey extract, shea butter, glycerine and St John's wort oil. It comes with one of Liz's signature muslin cloths.

Comments: 'Skin felt like a soft, ripe peach' • 'skin "plumped up"' • 'useful for backs of hands in winter' • 'skin had blushing bride tone!' • 'skin brighter and pores tighter'.

✿ DR. ANDREW WEIL FOR ORIGINS MEGA-MUSHROOM SKIN-CALMING FACE MASK
Score: 8/10

Masks often irritate, but our testers found this skin-comforting and soothing. (It's said to be clinically proven to reduce redness.) Key botanicals include bamboo leaf extract, ginger, holy basil and turmeric, plus marine algae to revitalise skin, strengthen its barrier and guard against future flare-ups.

Comments: 'Calmed my daughter's stress-related flare-up and redness; left overnight it made her skin feel calmer and

hydrated' • 'skin felt really lovely, radiant and smooth; effects lasted about a week'.

✿✿✿ NEAL'S YARD REMEDIES ORGANIC ROSE FORMULA ANTI-OXIDANT FACIAL MASK
Score: 7.87/10

This is targeted at more mature skins. It's clay-based, but doesn't become ultra-tight, thanks to oils from soya, sunflower, rose and macadamia, plus maple extract.

Comments: 'Skin clearer and brighter, pores smaller' • 'cool and soft when first applied' • 'an amazing product' • 'skin refreshed and rosy' • 'skin felt rejuvenated'.

✿✿ DR HAUSCHKA REJUVENATING MASK
Score: 7.75/10

Dr Hauschka promise this will 'bring life and vitality to pale, dry skin' – and our testers adored it. The mask contains nurturing plant oils such as carrot and borage extract.

Comments: 'Skin soft and refreshed, plus pores smaller' • 'skin texture more refined and nourished' • 'my sensitive skin reacts to most things, but this was wonderful'.

★ ✿✿ WELEDA WILD ROSE INTENSIVE FACIAL MASQUE
Score: 7.75/10

This true beauty steal harnesses the skin-regenerating powers of rose to restore radiance to dull complexions.

Comments: 'Skin smooth, radiant, firm and plump' • 'one of the best I have used' • 'skin softer, hydrated, brighter' • 'inexpensive and pampering – this is an excellent buy'.

ELETTRA ROSSELLINI WIEDEMANN

Manhattan-dweller Elettra Rosselini Wiedemann manages to combine being an international model (one of the 'faces' of Lancôme) with studying bio-medicine and environmental health. A passionate 'green', Elettra persuaded Lancôme to start a series of eco-chic initiatives with Carbonfund.org, a campaigning organisation that helps people reduce their carbon footprint

'I want to understand more about conservation, and

I've been interested in the environment since I was a little girl. I helped on a wildlife refuge in Florida, feeding baby antelope and cheetah, going on trips to see zebras, giraffes and emus, and listening to zoologists telling me how the butterflies' lives were connected with the giraffes – how the whole web of life is interconnected. I wanted to be a vet but my brain can't figure out maths and chemistry. Now I want to understand more about sustainable agriculture and conservation, and somehow bring it all together with my love of travel and meeting people.

We need more green warriors in the beauty business. I asked if Lancôme would sponsor my taking part in Carbonfund.org to offset the environmental impact of my airline travel. Carbonfund.org uses a multi-pronged approach, including tree-planting, community initiatives and green architecture.

There are a million little things you can do to help the environment. I am fanatical about switching lights off, and not keeping appliances on standby. I try to use natural household cleaners such as Seventh Generation, which includes recycled paper towels. I try not to wash clothes after just one day and don't dry-clean at all.

I like to eat healthy food with lots of raw foods and salads – and bangers and mash once in a while! When I was 24, my body changed and I had to really start taking care. I don't drink much and I don't smoke ever. I'm obsessed with yerba maté iced tea – it's my water replacement. I sleep at least seven hours a night, but more for sanity than beauty: if

I get less than that, it's like there's a big glass wall in front of me and it takes 20 seconds to clock what people have said. It really works: I'm stronger, I run faster, I have more endurance – and clear skin.

My style heroine is Audrey Hepburn: I love her femininity, warmth and charm. I try to be as chic as I can, but it always has to be comfortable. I wear high-waist jeans with black turtle-necks, but I also love wearing dresses and boots with heels.

My family is fantastic and such a source of comfort – they love me unconditionally no matter how silly I am. My parents divorced when I was very young but everyone is very mature and very loving. My dad [Jonathan Wiedemann] has three children, and my mum [Isabella Rossellini] adopted my brother Roberto – we all spend Christmas and holidays together. When I'm tired, I go to our beautiful house in Long Island and get spoiled by my mother.

I used to have really bad back pain due to scoliosis [curvature of the spine]. Now my back is fine as long as I am working out five or six times a week – running, yoga, military fitness. It's a great incentive not to be lazy.

I love the turquoise of the ocean. When I see it, my heart wells up into my soul.

When I wake up with a big day ahead, or when I face bad times, I take a deep breath, put a smile on my face and remind myself to be kind – then everything will turn out fine. People respond to what we project on them – being empathetic and understanding repays you a million times over the long term.

somehow bring it all together with my love of travel and meeting people'

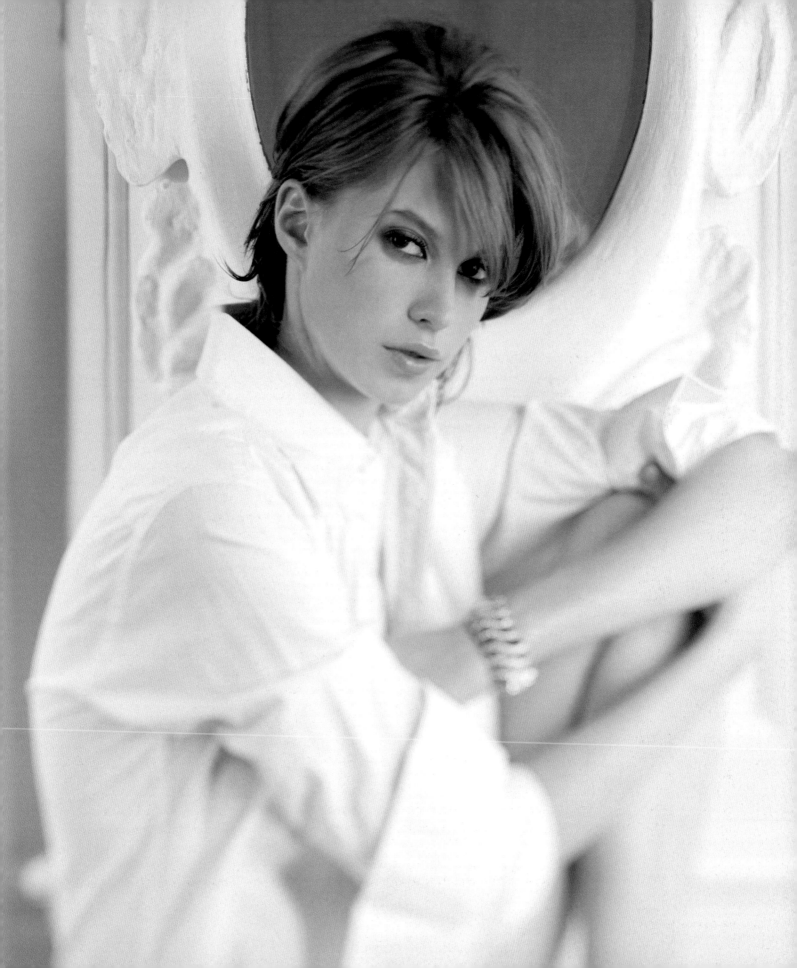

DO THE BRIGHT THING

We are not believers in the new trend for giving your skin harsh microdermabrasion and peel treatments at home. But sometimes, when skin looks dingy and drab, a simple facial scrub can put you on the fast-track back to brightness

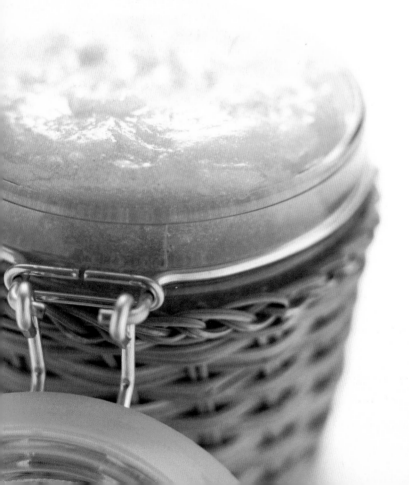

There is one single watch word when it comes to scrubs and exfoliators: gentle. That's why we're extremely cautious about the trend to use ever-harsher treatments to buff and dissolve the top layers of skin, revealing 'new, fresh, young' skin cells underneath (as the ads promise). We know several women – in particular, friends with 'English rose' and black complexions – who've suffered redness and soreness afterwards. Trouble is, the success (or not) of these skin-blitzers is largely down to 'operator skill'. There's a risk, with at-home versions, of thinking 'if a little's good, more must be better'. Not so: facial skin should always be handled with TLC. There's no need to go at it as if you were scrubbing a grubby floor.

Generally, however, we believe that if you're using a wash cloth when you cleanse (thoroughly, of course), that does all the exfoliating you need. (Body scrubs are different, read our rave reviews on page 115.) But of course it depends on your skin, its age, texture, type – and your environment. And there is no doubt that lightly scuffing away the top (dead) skin cells can enhance the effects of your moisturiser – up to four times, some experts claim – by allowing it to sink in further. But do choose gentle products, such as a clay-based scrub (which will also help to draw out impurities).

You can make your own very simply, as we explain below – or try one of the products that impressed our testers, opposite. These all contain gentle, 'rounded' scrub particles. To be on the safe side, anyone with sensitive skin would do well to avoid scrubs made with crushed nut shells or seeds, both of which may irritate the skin. (Though the Spa Facial Polish with minute bits of walnut shells and the Eminence Organic Skin Care Pear & Poppy Seed product, opposite, did work well for most of our testers, rather to our surprise.)

Before you start, there are some simple steps to follow:
- Always cleanse skin perfectly.
- Ideally, warm it with a hot flannel or wash cloth, to soften the dead cells. Apply your scrub in ultra-gentle, light, circular movements, using the fingertips only.
- Avoid any areas of broken skin or red veins, and focus instead on dry patches, or areas where skin cells build up – usually around the nose, and in the chin 'groove'.
- Rinse thoroughly afterwards, pat dry and moisturise.

THE HOME-MADE OPTION

If you'd rather not splash out on one of the treatments opposite, you can create your own gentle exfoliator in a few seconds. Put a handful of oats in a bowl with enough water to moisten, then massage this mixture into your skin, concentrating on areas where dead cells build up (around the nose, cleft of the chin, ears, etc). NB: sugar and salt are often used in body scrubs, but they are too harsh for your face.

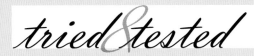

FACIAL SCRUBS

The perfect scrub is gentle but effective. It doesn't scratch, but delicately exfoliates the top layer of (dead) cells so that your skin look fresher and brighter. Our teams of *Beauty Bible* scrubbers trialled another 20-plus entries in this category for the paperback (on top of more than 30 originally), and declared a new victor...

❀ AVEDA TOURMALINE-CHARGED EXFOLIATING CLEANSER
Score: 9.22/10

Is it a cleanser or is it a scrub? To be honest, we're not convinced that any exfoliator should be used daily, but we can't argue with the verdict of our testers – who sent this new entry sky-rocketing to the top of the scrub league. The jojoba exfoliating beads are gentle and rounded, and there's lush mango butter in there for creaminess. It's said to complement their other tourmaline-based products, but our testers used it with non-Aveda products and were still wowed (though one found it a bit too potent).

Comments: 'I struggled to wash it off at first but the results were so good – radiant, clean, smooth skin – that I persevered' • 'nothing has made such a difference to my skin' • 'both my husband and best friend commented on how well I looked' • 'with regular use, skin seems more refined and has a natural shine and radiance' • 'creamy base didn't strip my skin, ideal for very sensitive skins. I absolutely love it' • 'like it being a cleanser and scrub in one; huge bottle lasts ages, so no guilt!'.

❀ ORIGINS MODERN FRICTION
Score: 8.4/10

Origins launched this specifically as a gentle alternative to microdermabrasion products; it's a creamy buffing paste, based on a mix of rice starch, skin-brightening skullcap, cooling and soothing cucumber and aloe leaf – with lemon and bergamot essential oils. Gentle enough to use two or three times a week – but it may sting if it gets in your eyes (and we wish Origins had used an alternative to sodium lauryl sulfate as a surfactant).

Comments: 'Skin looked brighter, fresher, more evenly toned and cleaner, and felt so soft and smooth. After a month, it's wonderful' • 'really does give my skin a more youthful appearance' • 'you don't have to use much' • 'my T-zone isn't so greasy now' • 'has minimised my open pores to a truly astonishing degree'.

❀❀ THE SPA JASMINE & FRANKINCENSE FACIAL POLISH
Score: 8.06/10

This rich, creamy, blissful-smelling exfoliator, created for The Spa (at Pennyhill Park Hotel) by Circaroma, gets its buffing action from tiny particles of walnut shell with jojoba beads, and has high levels of organic ingredients including carrot oil. (We fret a little about very touchy skins using walnut shells, however fine they are.)

Comments: 'I raved about this to my boyfriend and he agreed my skin was soft and smooth' • 'rosy glow on my cheeks and skin felt brill' • 'nice consistency, easily rinsed off with warm water' • 'smelt gorgeously expensive' • 'I'm pleased it's natural – saving the earth while indulging me!'

❀❀❀ ÉMINENCE ORGANIC SKIN CARE PEAR & POPPY SEED

MICRODERM POLISHER
Score: 8.05/10

This 'intense microderm skin polisher' for all skin types features poppy seeds turbocharged by finely crushed walnut shells, plus fruit acid from green apples, and comes as a solid jelly to be mixed with water. Green tea, bioflavonoids, apricot kernel oil and alfalfa act as a counterbalance, providing 'rich nutrition for the newly exfoliated skin', say the Hungarian makers.

Comments: 'My skin felt like new: soft and silky, glowing and smooth – lovely product and ideal gift' • 'skin healthy and glowy using this once or twice weekly' • 'slight redness died down quickly, then skin glowed and moisturiser more easily absorbed' • 'redness reduced and skin feels more supple'.

❀ LIZ EARLE NATURALLY ACTIVE SKINCARE GENTLE FACE EXFOLIATOR
Score: 8.05/10

We both have super-sensitive skins (partly the legacy of trying too many products over the years), but this is gentle enough even for us. It blends moisturising cocoa butter with softly buffing jojoba beads, plus tangy eucalyptus for its antiseptic powers.

Comments: 'My very sensitive and acne-prone skin is now smooth, clear and glowing; it feels much more balanced' • 'wonderful: my skin feels clean and much softer, and looks healthier generally; dry skin, spots and pimples all seem to have lessened' • 'lovely energising smell'.

MIRACLE CREAMS

Years after we began these books in 1995, we're still asked more about this category – what works, what doesn't – than any other. We know, from past experience, that there is such a thing as a miracle – and that botanically-based products out-perform some of the most high-tech options out there. And now – ta-dah! – our testers have identified some new natural miracle-workers, too…

Testers, as per usual protocol, were asked to use the creams on one side of their face for comparison.

❀❀ LOGONA WRINKLE THERAPY FLUID
Score: 8.81/10

From a pioneering German natural brand, this is certified by the BDIH (see page 209), so it carries the European seal that denotes naturalness. A truly fabulous result for this cream, designed to treat elasticity, radiance, suppleness, 'facial fatigue and stress'. Clinical results carried out by Logona show a 33 per cent improvement in moisture and a 30 per cent reduction in the depth of lines and wrinkles. The phyto- (plant) active ingredients helping to achieve that include certified organic jojoba, soy oil and sea buckthorn oil, plus hyaluronic acid, shea butter, grapeseed oil, and extracts of bamboo and quince. It may not be the most sexily-packaged, but with comments like these, who gives a damn?
Comments: 'Like the texture, a cross between a serum and hydrating milk; smells like fresh flowers and strawberries, sinks in quickly, leaving light film on skin; faint sun spots nearly gone and frown line too; this product marks a turning point' • 'a nice treat' • 'skin smoother, softer, more radiant and youthful: bigger wrinkles improving steadily, everyone has noticed' • 'I don't normally gush, but this is a wonder product – I am truly amazed and impressed; I give ten to

infinity marks – and beyond' • 'I'm 39 and it has wiped off 15 years – reducing redness, blemishes and fine lines' • 'visible difference in skin softness and smoothness as well as plumpness' • 'reduced crêpiness on neck'.

❀ LIZ EARLE SUPERSKIN MOISTURISER
Score: 8.62/10

Jo's smiling about this new, impressively-scoring entry – as she's been unswervingly devoted to it since day one of its launch. When Liz's own tester panel trialled this product, 96 per cent of respondents declared it was effective at rejuvenation, after 15 weeks. The *Beauty Bible* trial was only slightly shorter, and our panellists concurred: this rich moisturiser, featuring rich-in-EFA cranberry seed, borage seed and rosehip oils, really does have a time-defying effect, helping to 'plump' and firm.
Comments: 'Wonderfully silky, ultra-smooth texture which sinks readily into the skin and leaves an outstanding base for make-up' • 'skin looks so much brighter and people say I "look well"'; perfect for my dry skin and I love it more each day' • 'could see results immediately: skin looked much calmer and redness reduced, tone more even – soft and smoother, too' • 'fine lines not as noticeable' • 'noticed a large difference in the skin round my jaw area: not so lined and crêpe-y; smile lines not so deep and skin looks plumper' • 'love it! Will definitely continue'.

❀❀ KIMIA EXQUISITE REJUVENATING FACIAL SYSTEM
Score: 8.49/10

Initially, testers didn't love the fact that this is a two-product 'system' to be used daily – 'why can't they fit it in the bottle?' asked one – but rapidly became converted by the visible improvements. Kimia claim 'a unique niche in the world of natural skincare', and this 'system' features a facial serum (with calendula, rose oil, clary sage, rosehip, cranberry seed oil, neroli in sweet almond oil, witch hazel and grapeseed oil), and a 'hydro activator' which contains lady's mantle, 'a plant that produces its own drops of moisture or "celestial water", believed by ancient alchemists to be the catalyst for turning matter into pure gold'. Hmmm, not sure about that. But our testers did declare it a 22-carat jewel of a treatment.
Comments: 'Skin was instantly lovely, soft, smooth and felt well hydrated and plumper; after two weeks my wrinkles and fine lines smoother and less noticeable, skin looked brighter and fresher, less crêpey; bigger wrinkles smoother and plumper – fantastic product: people have complimented me' • 'gave marked improvements and husband says I am looking good' • 'can't live without this now – I'm feeling radiant!' • 'gorgeous smell and texture; I just love this product: skin brighter, really soft, plumped up, reduction in crow's feet; can't be without it'.

✿ ELEMIS LIQUID RADIANCE CELL RENEWAL SYSTEM

Score: 8.41/10

This two-phase product is a luxury 30-day programme to 'detox' the complexion – for visibly more youthful and radiant effects. It contains a 'Phase 1 pH Optimiser', used for 15 days to 'clear the pathway' for the delivery of the 'Phase 2 Vitamin Boost', which you then apply for just over a fortnight. Active botanicals include amino acids, carotenes, encapsulated vitamins B, B5, E and F (from green pistachio, star fruit, olive, carrot, grape and honey), and over 15 antioxidants.

Comments: 'Skin brighter and more even in tone and texture; no dry patches and less sheen; sinks in straight away, leaving skin smooth and soft' • 'skin noticeably better, fine lines more blurred, others softer, pores smaller – great results' • 'evened out my skin tone and skin felt good' • 'I would use this whenever my skin needs an extra boost' • 'noticeable results for minimal effort'.

✿ ÉMINENCE ORGANIC SKIN CARE NASEBERRY TREATMENT CREAM

Score: 8.28/10

Hungarian brand Éminence has been handmaking cosmetics since 1958 and is now more globally available, including being on the spa menu at hotels like the Ritz-Carlton and Hotel de Rome in Berlin. Each product is claimed to contain two kilos of hand-picked fruit, giving 95–98 per cent active antioxidant ingredients, and is rich in alpha-lipoic acid, vitamins A, Ester-C and E, plus co-enzyme Q10. Awarded the Best Organic Face Cream prize in the 2007 Image Beauty Awards in Ireland, it's certified in Hungary and by the USDA (see page 209). This richly hydrating cream gets its skin-brightening action from fruit acids, so may not be suitable for those with touchy complexions.

Comments: 'Sweet smell lingers all day; skin noticeably plumper and smoother within 24 hours; after two weeks, fine lines round mouth less noticeable; at end of testing, skin brighter, softer and smoother, fine lines much improved, some larger ones on forehead beginning to reduce, pores less noticeable – lots of compliments!' • 'very impressed: complexion more luminous, dewy, younger; will definitely buy again' • 'visible results: I love this product; enhanced look of make-up too' • 'I love everything about this product'.

★ ✿ NEAL'S YARD FRANKINCENSE NOURISHING CREAM

Score: 8.25/10

When this now-classic product featured in the original edition of our book *Feel Fab Forever*, not only did Neal's Yard sell out, but as production stepped up to meet demand, it triggered a global shortage of blue glass (for the jars). This natural, essential-oil-based rich cream contains nourishing oils of wheatgerm, jojoba, almond and apricot kernel, with frankincense and myrrh – renowned for their regenerating and moisturising properties. It can be used at night or as a day make-up base – and is also a great 'beauty steal'.

Comments: 'The immediate feeling of plumpness has been replaced by a smooth uplift and youthful tightness, yet skin still feels comfortable, has no dry patches or discomfort' • 'always felt my skin looked colourless and grey until I tested this' • 'after two weeks, I felt able to go out without foundation – I've never been able to before' • 'no adverse reactions on my sensitive skin' • 'noticeable improvement in brightness and translucency'.

✿✿ ✿ ESSENTIAL CARE SUPERFRUIT CONCENTRATE

Score: 8/10

Essential Care – a fast-growing brand founded by an aromatherapist mother and her business-savvy daughter – is a 'super-nutrient combination' of organic avocado, pomegranate, rosehip and sea buckthorn berries, designed to be 'locked in' by applying your usual moisturiser over the top. Great results, but not everyone loved the woodsy scent and natural orange-y colour.

Comments: 'Feels rich, oily and full of nutrients; pleasant enough smell, definitely brighter healthier looking skin; my eye lines loved it and drank it up' • 'loved this product, after one pump of oil at night, my skin was softer and more radiant! – not my usual grey pallor' • 'fine lines less noticeable, lovely to wake up to really soft skin – it really delivers' • 'surprised at the noticeable results: skin plumper smoother and much brighter, fewer blemishes and free of congested pores'.

We love...

We've tried a gazillion age-defying products over the years – so which have wowed us most? Jo says that Liz Earle Superskin Moisturiser is 'the best moisturiser ever, ever, EVER' – and is utterly devoted to the way it plumps her skin and leaves it dewy and velvety. Sarah layers on oil (vital for the glow factor), night and morning, then serum, then moisturiser, to keep her dry skin hydrated – she loves Aromatherapy Associates fabulous Anti-Age range, Oliv' products by La Clarée, and Extra Rich Beauty Elixir by Santaverde.

HOW TO
save your neck

The neck seems to have an ageing process all of its own. To keep yours swan-like, sensual and smooth for as long as possible, make sure your beauty regime doesn't end at the chin

The big reason that most women's neck zones age more rapidly than the rest of the body is simple: downright neglect (or 'neck-glect'!). To prevent the 'necklace lines' multiplying – and plump out existing ones, make sure that your neck is an integral part of your facial regime, moisturised twice daily with your face. Better still, incorporate the neck zone into your body-care regime, too – so it gets twice the dose of TLC. Noella Gabriel, director of treatments and product development for global skincare and spa brand Elemis, suggests applying neck products by stroking them into skin in an upwards direction (always upwards) with the back of the hand – palm pressure is 'too forceful', she says (although we are definitely sinners here...).

As we've said before, an ounce of prevention is better than thousands of pounds of cure when it comes to turning back the clock. The neck and chest often suffer badly from sun exposure: because the skin's so fine, it's more vulnerable to the ravages of UV light than many other body parts – that's why they're prone to age spots and crepiness. Try to keep the area covered up when you're outdoors, with a

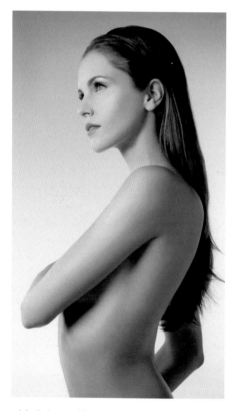

wide-brimmed hat and loose scarves if it's too hot to stay buttoned up. Slather on an SPF15 or higher, with mineral sun-blocking ingredients (zinc oxide and titanium dioxide). Prickly heat is often worst on the neck

and décolletage: Jo suffered agonisingly from this until she switched from chemical sunscreens to physical (ie mineral) sun protection, whereupon she never got it again.

Here are some other lifestyle shifts for neck beautification…

● Try to get used to sleeping on a lower pillow so that your neck is 'stretched out' rather than curled down into your chest: it helps guard against those 'necklace lines'.

● Take up yoga, dance or other stretching activity; it's no coincidence that the quite elderly women we know who have enviably fabulous necks have practised these techniques for years.

● Walk tall at all times. If you want to take years off, there are few better ways than simply elongating your neck.

● If all else fails, read Nora Ephron's wonderful, hilarious book *I Feel Bad about My Neck and Other Thoughts on Being a Woman*. At least you'll get a laugh out of it…

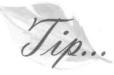

Tip… **Jo keeps a pot of rich moisturiser on her desk, and tries to use it several times a day. She's found that keeping the moisture level of her neck constantly topped up is the best strategy for tackling crepiness – the downside of an English rose complexion. It also really helps to prevent necklace lines, which affect the long-necked like Sarah.**

NECK CREAMS

Regular application of a moisturiser or oil will go a long way to keeping the skin on your neck smooth and supple. But if you are concerned about droop and sag, here are our winning natural neck-savers. Our testers trialled these over a period of two months, using twice daily – and were impressed. We'd have liked some new entries in this category, but no recent launches wowed our tester panel. Our message to the beauty industry: we won't ignore our neck zone if you don't…

★ ❀ LIZ EARLE NATURALLY ACTIVE SKINCARE SKIN REPAIR MOISTURISER
Score: 7.85/10

With the usual high level of active botanicals you would expect from Liz Earle, this is also one of our star buy recommendations. It's actually a facial nourisher, but they were so confident of its performance as a neck cream that they submitted it for this category – and our testers loved it. As a two-in-one product it certainly saves pennies and packaging. Active natural ingredients include echinacea, borage oil, avocado, betacarotene, hop extract and wheatgerm.

Comments: 'My neck, which tends to be crêpey, is smooth and soft – a significant difference' • 'smells divine and has a nice, creamy texture' • 'I'm raving about this – it actually does more than it says on the jar!' • 'cleavage in party frock – achieved with a Wonderbra – wasn't as crêpey' • 'neck looked less like plucked chicken skin – skin had a lovely sheen'.

❀❀ KIMIA PERFECTION NECK & DÉCOLLETÉ SERUM
Score: 7.66/10

This enriched serum from a start-up luxury skincare brand targets the neck and chest area with a 100 per cent botanical blend that includes sweet almond oil, witch hazel, rose oil, avocado seed oil, hemp seed oil and vitamin C, fragranced with a blend of neroli and clary sage. Kimia extravagantly promise to 'combat and even reverse the signs of ageing'. We're not quite sure about that, but we do know our testers loved it. We would suggest using it in the evening.

Comments: 'Skin softer and smoother, less lines; not miraculous but definitely an improvement: tram lines on my décolletage were less and skin looked more hydrated and evenly textured' • 'smells delicious; fine lines definitely reduced, skin glowed and felt smoother; décolletage hugely improved, with fine wrinkles no longer visible and skin tighter and firmer; has boosted my confidence – worth the price and lasts a long time' • 'glorious smell and wonderful texture – skin noticeably less wrinkly and more hydrated: I will buy this again'.

❀ JURLIQUE HERBAL RECOVERY NECK SERUM
Score: 7.55/10

This sinks-in-fast gel has high quantities of organic ingredients, and Jurlique (one of our favourite natural companies) promise us that the soya on which it's based is not genetically engineered. Botanical actives include frankincense and myrrh, ginkgo flavonoids, vitamin C and oils of jojoba, rosehip, avocado and evening primrose.

Comments: 'My neck looks slightly younger, smoother, more hydrated and clearer' • 'definitely less crêpiness' • 'lovely fresh, natural smell; lines are less visible' • 'skin on neck and décolletage noticeably smoother' • 'I'm amazed how much better my skin feels – definite improvement in fine lines'.

Beautify your décolletage

While we're not fans of bust-boosting creams per se, we do suggest extending the moisturising product you use on your neck down your décolletage (aka décolleté) – that's literally the bit beneath your collar. Giving that area lots of TLC will reap anti-ageing dividends many times over by preventing 'lizard' skin. It's easier to do with your night cream, in our experience, rather than applying a day moisturiser down to your bra. Also, soaking in an oily bath with your bosom below the water line can make a real difference.

A WORD FROM ONE OF OUR
beauty heroes

Basically, we worship Bobbi Brown. We love her realistic attitude to beauty and her philosophy that beauty isn't about striving for impossible ideals; it's about looking the best you can. We were so taken with the introduction for her recent book, *Living Beauty* (written as she enters her fifties), that we asked Bobbi if we could quote from it here. We believe it will strike a chord with any woman who believes in a natural approach to beauty

'I don't know why it's not OK to age. I think that a face without lines and planes is an expressionless face – it's a face that lacks warmth and confidence. That's why I'm dismayed at the number of women today who are altering their faces in an attempt to look younger. Visits to the plastic surgeon have become as commonplace as visits to the hair salon.

'Of course it's very easy to feel bad. Open any magazine and you're inundated by pictures of seemingly flawless girls who are barely 20 years old (and in some cases, as young as 14). Models older than 30 are a rarity. Television shows set in Los Angeles and New York glorify the lives of 20-something characters. My advice? Don't compare yourself to these images of youthful perfection – you'll always lose. It's human nature to compare, but at least do it in a realistic way, with women close to your age.

'Too many women of my generation feel bad about the fact that they're no longer young. These women have a laundry list of things they don't like about themselves: wrinkles, baggy eyelids, a too-small upper lip… I could go on for days. These women are so caught up in the negative that they don't have any energy left to focus on the positive.

'I believe there needs to be a fundamental change in the way we think about beauty. I want to get rid of the stigma that surrounds ageing. Getting older should be seen as a process through which a woman can gain more vitality, strength, wisdom and a new sense of her beauty…'

'Too many women of my generation feel bad about the fact that they're no longer young'

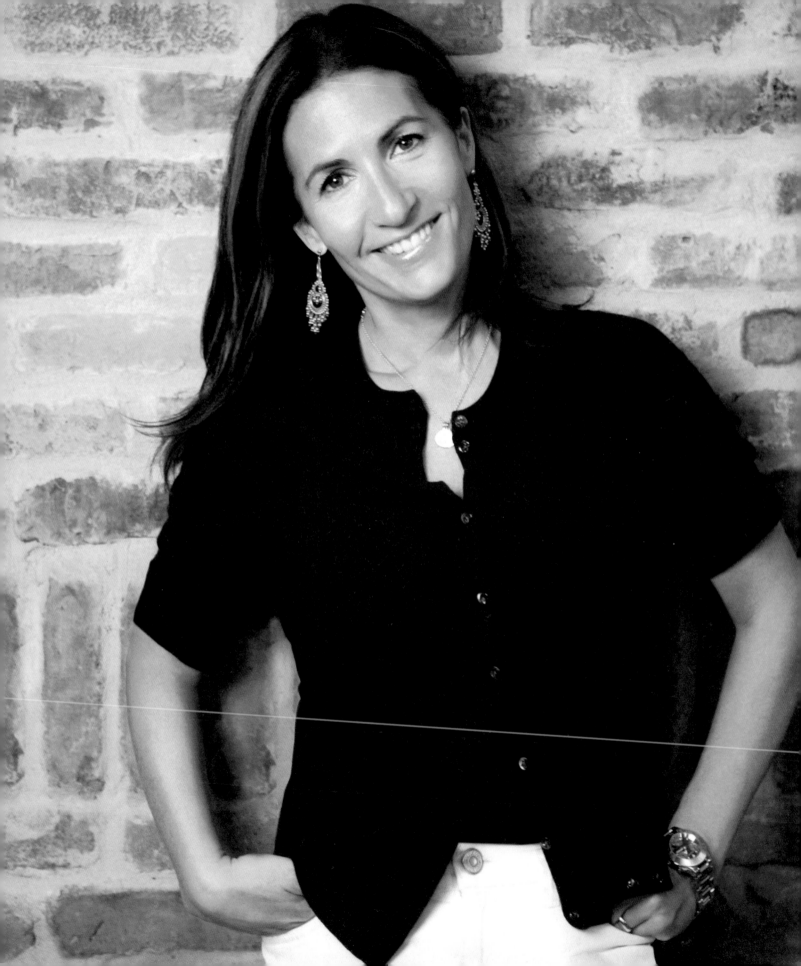

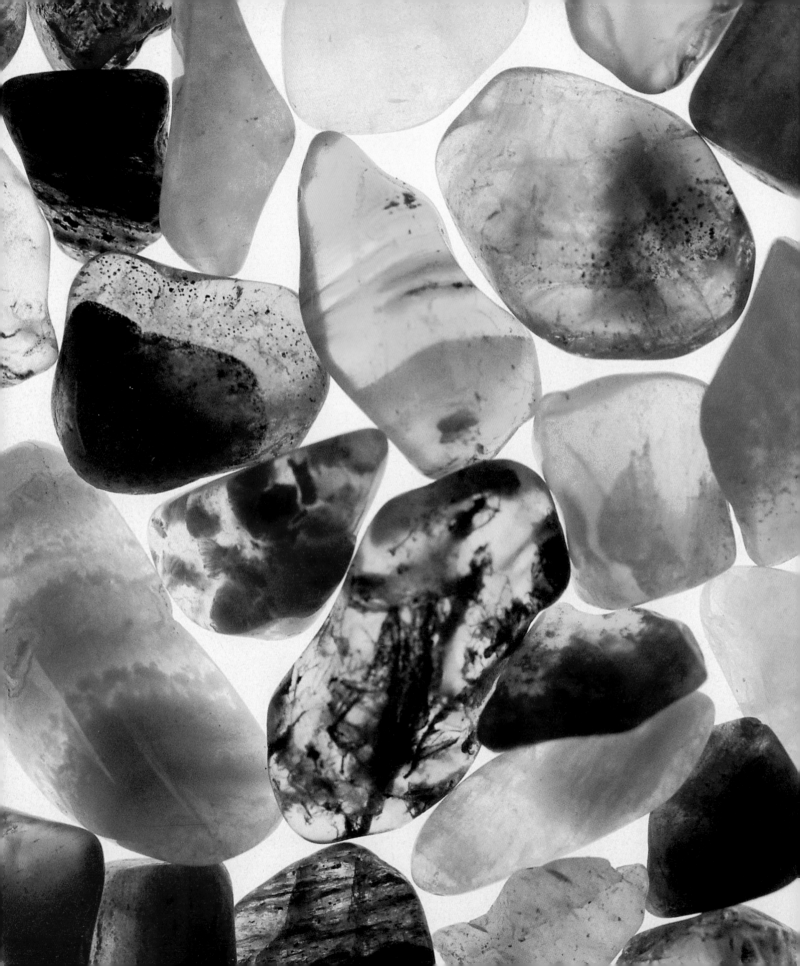

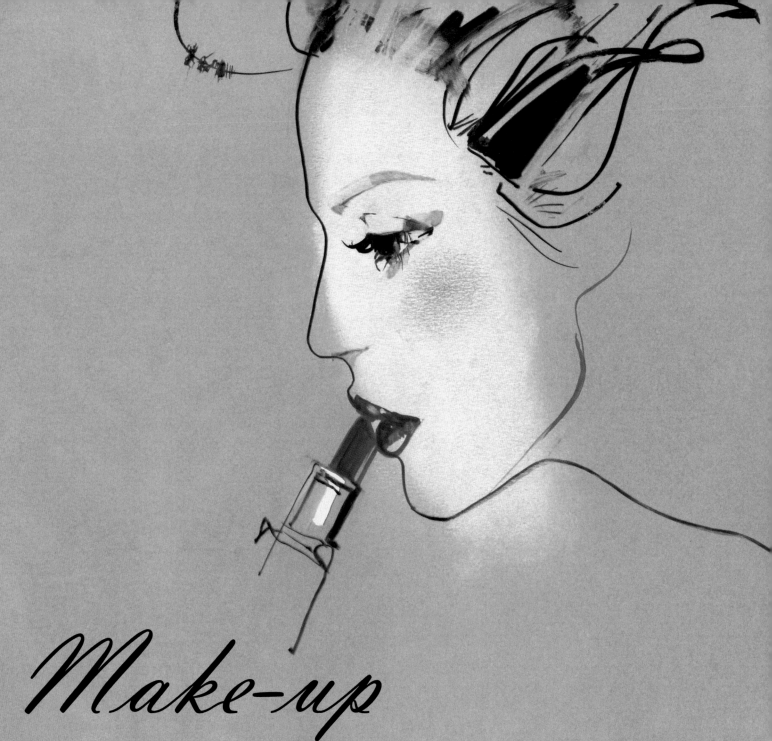

Make-up

Make-up should enhance your looks, not create a mask. It should accent your best features, cover up flaws and leave you looking just like yourself but prettier, smoother, fresher... Natural, in other words. And 'green' cosmetics can give you the natural look both ways.

LESS IS MORE

Like our bathroom cupboards, wardrobes and houses generally, most of us tend to have over-stuffed make-up bags. We say: it's time for a clear-out. What you really need is a handful of products that do the job brilliantly, and that make the most difference to your individual appearance

MAKE-UP FOR DIFFERENT COLOUR TYPES

In this chapter, we look at the more natural make-up options on the beauty counters – the mineral make-up phenomenon, and the increasing number of products from brands that are trying to shrink their carbon footprint by using more natural ingredients, recycled packaging, or – as Aveda do – by using wind power at their manufacturing plants.

But first, let's get something straight. We firmly believe that it's not possible just to shop our way out of the crisis facing the planet – in other words, to just carry on buying as much stuff, but the 'greener' options. So we'd like to make a plea for paring down your beauty regime (and the rest of your life, actually). Almost everyone can get away with a handful of products for daily use – the key is knowing which ones make the most impact on how you look.

To ease you into that 'edit', Hana Sutherland, make-up spokeswoman for mineral make-up brand Inika, has helped us put together a skin-tone-matched guide to help you identify your make-up must-haves – the products you can sweep on for an instant transformation, getting you ready to skip out of the door in a couple of minutes flat, plus the ones that will give you evening glam in a trice. (NB: if you have grey hair, follow the rules for your previous hair colour)

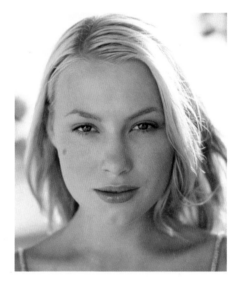

Blondes

These are the everyday essentials that will make the most difference to your looks:

● Brow pencil/powder: look for grey/taupey shades
● Brown (not black) mascara
● Brown/black eyeliner: otherwise eyes disappear
● Concealer: blondes often have good skin, so a touch of concealer may be all you need to even out your skin tone
● Blusher, maybe. Fair complexions fall into two categories – some are prone to flushing, and blusher may just make you look hot, whereas other blondes are washed out and need a 'kick' of colour
● Lipstick is often optional for blondes

For evening, add in:

● Eyeshadow
● Foundation
● Lipstick
● Lip gloss

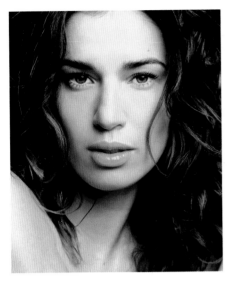

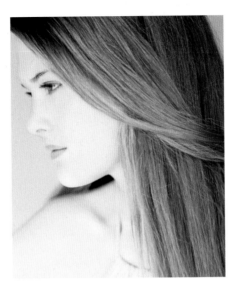

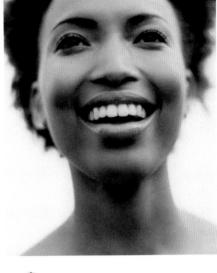

Brunettes

These are the must-haves for brunettes, which will give you instant oomph:

● Concealer: if you have dark shadows or small flaws such as thread veins
● Tinted moisturiser: often all you need, especially in summer
● Foundation: if you need it to even out skin tone
● Powder: or use a mineral make-up that works as powder and foundation in one
● Bronzing powder: this can do double-duty, evening out skin tone and accenting cheeks
● Blusher: soft, peachy blusher looks great on brunettes

For evening, add in:

● Eyeshadow
● Mascara
● Brow pencil
● Tinted lip gloss

Redheads

The essentials to transform you in a flash:

● Brown mascara
● Brow pencil: like blondes, redheads often lack definition around the eyes – so this will make a huge difference
● Bronzer: to prevent a washed-out look
● Blusher: peachy, nutmeg tones work well for redheads

For evening, add in:

● Mineral make-up: this works well on freckled complexions, covering lightly without creating a 'mask' look
● Eyeshadow
● Lipstick
● Lip gloss

Black skin

You're lucky: you need the fewest products on a daily basis because your natural colouring has such impact:

● Eyeshadow
● Bright lipstick: purple shades look wonderful on dark skins

For evenings, add in:

● Mineral foundation in a dark shade
● Highlighter: use a lighter, brighter shade of mineral make-up, or gold powder swept across cheekbones
● Mascara
● Brow pencil
● Lip gloss

'Taking joy in living is a woman's best cosmetic' ROSALIND RUSSELL

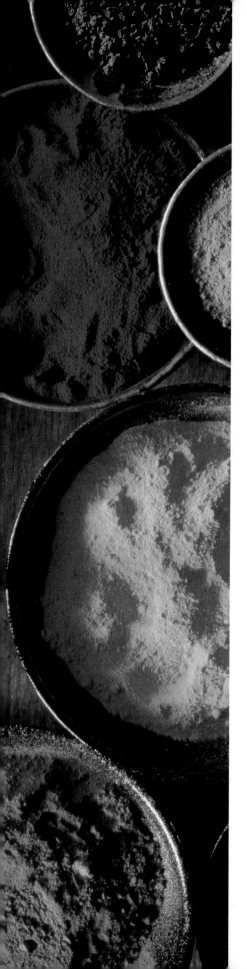

MINERAL MAGIC

Mineral make-up isn't new. (Cleopatra was apparently one of the first aficionados.) But from having been a tiny beauty 'niche' – mostly available only in dermatologists' and cosmetic surgeons' clinics – mineral make-up has gone from beauty buzz to beauty bandwagon. Is mineral make-up – which is mined from the earth – really a better choice? We dug deep, to find out…

Mineral make-up is being touted by the beauty press as the 'natural' alternative to other powders, paints and pencils. You can get mineral base/foundation, blusher, eyeshadow and bronzer, all of which we trialled for this book – alongside other more natural make-up options.

Trouble is, as with so many beauty trends, there are now dozens of companies jumping on the mineral bandwagon. Many traditional foundations and powders are now being given the label 'mineral' when they actually contain much more than pure minerals: preservatives, fillers, petrochemicals etc. (Most foundations have always relied on titanium dioxide – a key mineral in mineral make-up – to create an opaque finish, which is why brands can get away with the 'mineral' label.) On the following pages, you'll find only the purest mineral brands, rather than the recent 'faux mineral' introductions, as we like to call them.

Mineral make-up is literally made from crushed mined minerals: titanium dioxide, mica, iron oxides (which can vary in colour from red to brown, black, orange and yellow), pearl and even gold. These highly sophisticated blends of natural earth minerals and crystals are micro-pulverised to form microscopic flat crystals, which overlap each other on the skin allowing skin to breathe and function normally. And as mineral make-up pioneer Jane Iredale – who launched her line 15 years ago – explains, 'these microscopic crystals allow the pores to stay un-clogged too'. In fact, they are gentle enough to use very soon after cosmetic surgery or chemical peels and laser resurfacing. (For a long time, the only people to market mineral cosmetics were cosmetic surgeons and dermatologists, because they had noted the make-up actually had anti-inflammatory properties.)

Because they're slightly iridescent, these powdered minerals 'bounce' light back off the skin, creating the optical illusion that it's smoother and more flawless by minimising pores and wrinkles. One of the big plus points for older faces is that mineral make-up can have a turn-back-the-clock effect. 'Make-up with light reflecting minerals can help draw attention away from fine lines and wrinkles and soften your whole look,' explains L.A-based make-up artist Robin Siegal.

They are also sun-protective, acting as a mirror on the skin's surface. (Titanium and zinc oxide are key ingredients in sun protection products.) Mineral make-up and powders often emphasise their SPFs, which typically range from 17 to 20. But Dr Jeanette Jacknin, author of Smart Medicine for the Skin (see page 217) advises against relying solely on make-up as sunblock: the SPF of mineral make-up is only effective where it's applied (and you shouldn't ever wear make-up like a mask, from ear-to-ear or hair-line to chin). If you're going to be outdoors, don't be lulled into a false sense of sun security, believing your make-up's going to shield skin as effectively as a cream. It won't.

There are a few slight health question marks, over talc and aluminium – which appear in some mineral make-up, as well as some 'conventional' options. And a few eco question marks over minerals too: the mining industry can contaminate water, wreck habitats and exploit the local workforce. But since these mineral ingredients do appear in most make-up on the shelves, there's really no 'perfect' answer except going bare-faced (and we suspect that as a Beauty Bible reader, that really isn't an option…!)

The how to

Mineral foundation isn't quite like normal 'base', which you dot on then blend until it's seamless. With mineral make-up – which comes in powder form – you literally build and build coverage, layer by layer with a brush, until you're happy with how your skin looks. There are two types of mineral foundation: loose, in a little pot, or contained within the handle of a brush, which dispenses the powder. You can use a normal powder brush with mineral make-up: pick up some of the powder, tap the handle to remove excess, and then use what's called a 'buff and swirl technique': circle the brush on the skin, in a buffing motion. Reapply for greater depth of coverage. (Don't ever dip the brush directly in the powder; there's usually enough just

Tip… **One of the big advantages of mineral make-up is that it blends seamlessly, avoiding a 'tide-mark'. But products still come in different shades – and the best place to test a mineral foundation, according to Jane Iredale, is 'to do it on the jaw-line in daylight. The colour should disappear if it blends perfectly into the skin.' (In other words, it's the same rule as for testing any other foundation.)**

lurking in the pot lid to do your face.) 'So long as you have the right shade, you'll never look over-made-up with mineral make-up', observes Susan Posnick, one of the mineral make-up pioneers. Susan Posnick's Colorflo mineral foundation is the 'brush-handle' type: the powder's inside a cylinder-shaped handle, and is dispensed with a click, then buffed and swirled into skin: again, you go on 'building' till you've got your perfect level of coverage. Same technique, different packaging – which we personally find easier to use, with less risk of spills in a make-up bag.

We love…

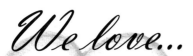

Jo is a very late-in-the-day convert to mineral make-up – and only when make-up artist Susan Posnick demo-ed her own Colorflo, with the perfect, English rose pale shade. Sarah has been a Colorflo fan for years: 'you need practise and a light hand, but it gives a lovely, almost liquid foundation finish as the powder warms on the skin.' Sarah also rates the award-winning Aussie brand Inika.

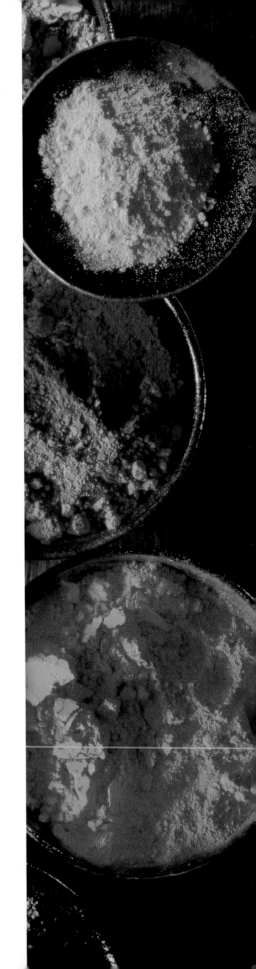

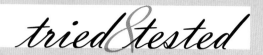

FACE BASES

In this section, you will find our testers' reports on mineral foundations (which did pretty well), natural liquid foundations (which only delivered one recommendation) and concealers (with three options)

Mineral foundations

As we predicted in the first edition of this book, mineral make-up has proved one of the biggest beauty trends this decade, with mainstream brands joining the mineral revolution. Although we put another slew of products through rigorous tests, these smaller brands still outperformed the big-brand options. NB: minerals can't be certified organic.

❀ PHILOSOPHY THE SUPERNATURAL 4-IN-ONE MINERAL MAKEUP

Score: 8.16/10

Philosophy aren't known for their naturalness, but this fairly pricy option contains high levels of mineral pigments in a talc-free formulation. It's described as a 'silk-to-satin SPF foundation' and they promise it leaves the skin 'with a smooth, air-brushed finish'; a big plus is the built-in sponge applicator (though this twists off, if you prefer to use a brush). *Comments:* 'Amazing coverage, all flaws air-brushed out' • 'natural finish, smoothed skin tone, not too powdery' • 'no mess, beautiful coverage; I'm hooked for life!' • 'coped with thread veins' • 'natural dewy finish'.

❀❀ BARE ESCENTUALS SPF15 FOUNDATION

Score: 7.94/10

Bare Escentuals say of this that 'it may look like a powder (in 12 shades), but it feels and applies like a cream', delivering a flawless finish, with an SPF15. Still looks like a powder to us, but definitely worth a try, say our testers. *Comments:* 'With practice I liked this; gave a natural dewy finish' • 'so pleased with this, I have bought other products in the range' • 'light on the face – makes skin feel soft and silky, not powdery'.

❀ BARE ESCENTUALS MINERAL VEIL

Score: 7.93/10

Bare Escentuals say this 'morphs into skin, infusing it with softness and light', gently absorbing oil and heat while minimising the appearance of pores. If you like to use a liquid or cream foundation, this could be used to 'set' that too – and they also recommend you use it over their SPF15 Foundation (see above). Our testers trialled the basic shade, but it's also available in a tinted version. *Comments:* 'Natural finish; great over light foundation' • 'takes any shine off your complexion without being powdery' • 'I would recommend these products to everyone: the powder is the finishing touch'.

❀ JANE IREDALE PUREPRESSED PRESSED MINERALS SPF20

Score: 7.75/10

If you like to make up on the go, this is your best bet, as the minerals are pressed into a compact. Jane Iredale pretty much pioneered this category, so it's no surprise this base scored well. It's described as 'a four-in-one product: concealer, foundation, powder and sunblock' (offering SPF20). NB: some shades contain carmine, from beetles, so it's not necessarily vegan. *Comments:* 'Gave a matt look and evened out skin tone' • 'easy to use; very blendable; finish was natural and comfortable on skin' • 'balanced out redness, very impressed' • 'like a sheer veil of dew – my skin glowed!'

❀❀ LILY LOLO FOUNDATION

Score: 7.3/10

This loose mineral powder is very similar to the Lily Lolo loose powder (see page 55), but with a little shimmer, for a fresh-faced glow;

Brush strokes... To apply mineral foundation as a base all over, you need quite a chunky brush, like the powder brush pictured below. A liquid foundation brush (see picture opposite) helps get it into nooks and crannies. (NB: some mineral formulas have a built-in brush – so, of course, you don't need a separate brush for those.)

powder
polvos
poudre
PALLADIO

there's a choice of 21 shades, from the palest through to shades suitable for black and Asian skin tones. Our testers were assigned a light shade called Blondie.

Comments: 'Took away most of the redness' • 'unbelievably natural finish, with a fabulous glow' • 'with a flush of blush and this, I've finally captured the no make-up make-up!'

❀ ❀ INIKA MINERAL FOUNDATION
Score: 7.27/10

This loose mineral powder-formula base from up-and-coming Aussie all-vegan brand Inika comes in a screw-top plastic container, and should be applied (so they advise) using their special 'kabuki' brush. We sent the shade Unity (there are 12) to fairer-skinned testers.

Comments: 'Brilliant! Like a perfect second skin' • 'blended well, balanced skin tone and looked good as long as my skin was well-hydrated' • 'thrilled with this product, but you need to master the art of application'.

Liquid foundation

For women who prefer a 'conventional' liquid foundation, there are some more natural bases. But of the dozen we trialled, most elicited comments like 'chalky', 'drying', 'doesn't blend well' – probably because it's the synthetic ingredients that make foundation more skin-compatible.

❀ DR HAUSCHKA TRANSLUCENT MAKE-UP
Score: 7.35/10

In a choice of three shades (we tested 01, the palest), this features high-quality plant oils (including avocado and jojoba) and waxes in a lightweight formulation, which help to moisturise and protect the skin. Some websites and salons offer the option of buying a tester, so you can trial before buying.

Comments: 'Blended effortlessly and gave fantastic coverage for such a light formulation' • 'beautiful, sheer, non-powdery finish that matched my English rose skin tone perfectly and lasted all day' • 'blended well with fingers or a foundation brush, smelt like roses – evened my skin tone but didn't look cakey, covered small red veins and spots, evened out pores' • 'mattifying effect'.

Concealers

We wish we could bring you a raft of fabulous natural concealers – but only three from more than a dozen tested proved worthy of inclusion in the make-up bag. Do try them, natural beauty babes – but if you return to your Touche Éclat while waiting for this category to become more sophisticated, we promise we won't tell the green beauty police.

❀ ❀ JANE IREDALE CIRCLE/DELETE UNDER EYE CONCEALER
Score: 7.62/10

These duo palettes in three colourways not only cover dark circles (and other blemishes) but also act as a treatment. That's down to the vitamin K, which is thought to help repair the damaged tiny blood vessels that cause dark circles, also acting as a skin lightener. The base is a skin-nourishing blend of jojoba and avocado. Use a small brush to custom blend the colours on the back of your hand, apply, then pat with your finger to feather the edges.

Comments: 'Blended well and gave a natural finish – love the fact there are two shades you combine to create a perfect third' • 'I used this the morning after a late boozy night – and it definitely made me look better' • 'made a huge angry spot invisible'.

❀ JANE IREDALE DISAPPEAR CONCEALER WITH GREEN TEA EXTRACT (MEDIUM)
Score: 7/10

Jane Iredale, it seems, nearly has this category sewn up. Circle/Delete's best for eyes, this for spots and other blemishes. It has an angled, foam-tipped applicator to dispense the concealer, which is enriched with antioxidant green tea, said to help combat acne bacteria.

Comments: 'Good coverage, with minimum blending required; didn't sit in wrinkles and helped create a smoother appearance' • 'I don't normally use a concealer so had to work on my application technique: the instruction leaflet was a great help' • 'easy to apply with the foam applicator tip on the tube; blended easily into the skin; gave a subtle coverage and didn't leave dry patches' • 'covered thread veins and dark circles, also blemishes, but not effective with wrinkles'.

❀ ❀ DR HAUSCHKA PURE CARE COVER STICK
Score: 6.78/10

This is designed to disguise blemishes and treat them with clarifying ingredients, targeting bacteria with tea tree and manuka oils. Naturally soothing anthyllis and calendula support the skin's healing process. Natural waxes help nurture the skin, while tapioca starch defies shine. This neat, pen-shaped stick comes in two shades (unfortunately there's no shade for darker skins yet). It's certified natural (but not organic) by the BDIH (see page 209).

Comments: 'Made veins look less visible' • 'smooth but thick, so could apply directly to spots' • 'covers spots really well' • 'did help dry up spots' • 'blended well and disguised most imperfections' • 'shiny initially but looked good under foundation'.

PALLADIO

foundation base fond de teint

FACE POWDER

We welcome a couple of high-scoring new entries in this category, but there are still too few options for wannabe-natural beauties who don't want to go down the mineral make-up route, preferring to stick with foundation and powder, to 'set' it. We've given the results for loose and pressed powders here; we suggest loose for at-home use and pressed for on-the-go touch-ups

❀❀ DR HAUSCHKA TRANSLUCENT FACE POWDER COMPACT
Score: 7.83/10

An extremely high score for this lightly rose-fragranced powder, which features a high content of silk, alongside mica and asbestos-free talc. (See opposite for talc health concerns; but in a pressed format – rather than flying-about-loose powder – it's unlikely to present problems.) Said to be fine for even the touchiest skins, it comes in one, universal Translucent shade.

Comments: 'Fabulously fine, divine-smelling powder that gives a lovely softness to my skin' • 'great finish, natural, totally matt: evened skin tone' • 'gave my combination skin a long-lasting finish' • 'set my make-up to perfection'.

❀ JURLIQUE CITRUS SILK FINISHING POWDER
Score: 7.56/10

Attractively packaged (Jurlique have done a great job with redesign, bringing the brand into the 21st century), this silky translucent loose face powder is formulated to help rebalance oiliness, with ingredients that absorb shine. (The tester panel had mixed skin types, but still found it worked well.)
Comments: 'Set my make-up, which allowed it to look fresher for longer, and reduced oiliness so foundation didn't slide off; very effective on shine, and no chalky residue' • 'longlasting matt effect but no dullness' • 'expensive but lasts a long time' • 'very fine silky texture, easy to use and natural finish – un-shine lasted all day, just over moisturiser: lovely product' • 'gorgeous finish and make-up lasted longer than usual – loved the luxury packaging'.

❀ KORRES WILD ROSE COMPACT POWDER BRIGHTENING/FLAWLESS FINISH
Score: 7.4/10

With Origins currently pulled out of the colour cosmetics market, Korres seem to have stolen their crown. 'Brightening/Flawless finish' is the promise on the packaging: it's velvety, enriched with wild rose (a potent source of vitamin C), and is said 'to repair fine lines and brighten uneven skintone'. In five shades, of which our testers trialled the palest (WRP1).
Comments: 'This has converted me to powder; great finish, not too chalky, easy to use, and gave extra coverage where I needed it' • 'fine, silky texture and good mirror, though compact was chunky to

BUNNY-LOVING BRUSHES

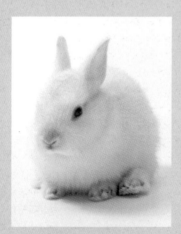

Many of our website readers have written in asking about cruelty-free brushes. Although brush companies are always keen to point out that natural (ie, animal) brush hairs are produced without pain to the animal (by brushing, in the case of goat, squirrel, badger, but sometimes as a by-product of the fur industry, of which we completely disapprove), the good news for animal-lovers is that there are now excellent synthetic brushes (usually Taklon or nylon), which also happen to have a great affinity with the mineral make-up we focus on in this chapter.
Some brands to look for: EcoTools (which won an award for Best Cruelty-Free Make-up Brushes from PETA in 2008), Palladio Cosmetics, Aveda Flaz Sticks, Urban Decay, Good Karma, Hard Candy, Ecco Bella, The Body Shop and Sevi Vegan Cosmetics. Visit www.naturewatch.org for more on *The Compassionate Shopping Guide*, which is supported by Twiggy, who says, 'The way ahead is cruelty-free. It is up to the consumer to make sure that these are the products we buy.'

round' • 'natural finish, easy to use, good coverage' • 'applied with my own brush, rather than the sponge enclosed; silky, fine texture and set my foundation well, so I didn't have to apply – too big for most handbags'.

❀ THE BODY SHOP PRESSED FACE POWDER

Score: 7.12/10

Definitely 'more natural' rather than all-natural this one (full ingredients on our website, www.beautybible.com), but we do feel that in many make-up categories, compromises may still have to be made unless you're a Jane Birkin truly natural babe. On the (big) plus side, this powder contains a touch of community traded marula oil from Namibia and Italian community trade olive oil, which helps give the velvety-smooth finish (but isn't enough to make you shiny, by the way). Available in six shades.
Comments: 'Perfect mirror: definitely a highlight' • 'good coverage – skin "finish" is better, especially if applied over foundation' • 'went on smoothly with no mess: natural finish took the edge off high colour and reduced shine' • 'fine silky texture; make-up was "set" and lasted longer' • 'gave a matt finish to T-zone' • 'perfect for my Oriental complexion: blemishes less noticeable'.

❀ KORRES MULTIVITAMIN COMPACT POWDER

Score: 7.11/10

We're a little surprised to find that this 'natural' powder contained nylon (!) and talc (see our comments about this, above) but, as we say, this category is beauty compromise territory. A pressed powder targeted at oily and combination skins, this Korres compact has a shine-defying action, and contains vitamins E and C.
Comments: 'Excellent lasting texture; natural finish balanced skin tone' • 'small but useful

Talc alert

Talc is a common ingredient in make-up and one of the most contentious ingredients because it can contain potentially carcinogenic asbestos. The American Cancer Prevention Coalition advises against its use. Many natural brands avoid it but some have found a way round the problem. The super-natural German brand Logona, for instance, does use talc, but each batch is certified by an independent lab as asbestos-free. If you're concerned about talc in your make-up or body products, e-mail the company that makes them for their policy on sourcing and testing talc. (Remember that you can look up the ingredients for each product featured in this book on our website, www.beautybible.com)

mirror, worked well on oily areas' • 'lasted six hours without a touch-up' • 'good coverage, and I've had no break-outs' • 'mattified skin without excessive chalky look'.

❀❀ LILY LOLO FLAWLESS SILK FINISHING POWDER

Score: 7/10

This ultra-lightweight powder comes in a shaker pot, in a choice of four shades. The simple formulation includes iron oxides (mined minerals) plus mica for a light-diffusing, imperfection-blurring sheen. We like the funky name and 'vintage-style' graphics – a welcome dash of humour.
Comments: 'Angel dust in a jar – smooth, natural finish lasted for hours with little need to retouch' • 'set make-up perfectly and worked famously with my shiny skin: didn't clog pores or sit heavy' • 'moderated shine so my skin looked healthy not greasy' • 'very smooth and silky texture, set my make-up and evened out my skin' • 'lovely product, providing a glow to the skin'.

❀ AVEDA PRESSED POWDER

Score: 7/10

An ultra-fine, talc-free pressed powder delivering a semi-matt finish, which – so Aveda promise – increases skin's radiance by 20 per cent, thanks to mineral and plant-derived ingredients such as micronised tourmaline and malachite gemstones, murumuru butter (an Amazonian skin-nourisher) and antioxidant resveratrol, from Japanese knotweed. It comes in three versatile shades – our testers trialled 01/ Cream – and is minimally packaged in a 'clam shell', designed to slip into Aveda's refillable Environmental Compacts.
Comments: 'Offered a natural finish and enhanced coverage of foundation' • 'set my make-up and lasted all day' • 'used over a tinted moisturiser, gave lovely natural finish' • 'loved it; nice and silky on my skin, absolutely natural finish lasted all day – just had to top up the shiny nose now and then' • 'I've never used a powder before but it lasted and lasted, so I might change my mind'.

ALICIA SILVERSTONE

When Sarah met animal-adoring eco-activist Alicia in New York City, a big Heinz 57 rescue dog lay peacefully at her feet while uber-stylist John Barrett glammed up her hair. Alicia, a long-time vegan and fan of natural beauty brands such as Burt's Bees, Ecco Bella, John Masters and Kiss My Face, sends daily round-robin e-mails, lobbying about everything from a new home for a special needs boxer pup to protecting a Colorado wildlife refuge from oil drilling. She's truly a green goddess

'It's empowering to know that you're responsible

It's just so lovely to appreciate the trees and birds and animals. Everything you do in the name of the environment not only saves our health, it saves our souls.

We all sit round talking about things we want to change, but unless you change, it ain't going to happen. I used to say, 'What can I do? I'm just one person.' It's a lovely excuse but it's a bunch of BS. Once I made the change [to being green] I saw how powerful one person is.

It's all about respect for life. What I've learnt is that you can make little choices every day that change the world to be a better, happier, lovelier place.

Rather than recycling (which is important), I just keep reusing things. I'll refill and refill and refill a water bottle as long as I can.

The awesome thing about being a vegetarian is that you are taking care of the environment, the animals and your health at the same time. I don't get sick any more, all my allergies went away, my whole life changed. I sleep better, I have more energy, my skin is really clear and my body's in the shape it needs to be in. Now I'm a total health nut. It's empowering to know that you're responsible for how you feel each day because of the way you treat your body. I love living this way – it's so satisfying and inspiring.

I love cooking and one of my favourite things to do with my husband [musician Christopher Jarecki] is open up the refrigerator. On Sunday mornings we go to the farmer's market and get everything that we couldn't get out of our own garden. Then I'll take everything out of the refrigerator while he turns on the basketball game. I start organising what needs to be eaten first: this way you save money, you don't waste food and you get to eat yummy stuff.

My dogs are all vegan, they're the healthiest – they eat greens. If ever you're cooking broccoli, just throw the stalks on the floor: they love them. They eat tomatoes, bananas, avocados – my dogs are fat from eating avocados…

I love yoga. I love pilates. I love walking with my dogs.

I'm pretty open and sensitive, a big baby really. But the good news is that I don't care what anybody says if I don't know and respect them. If my best friend didn't like something, it would kill [me] but superficial nonsense doesn't faze me one bit.

I've gained so much confidence as a woman from figuring out that I don't want to be destructive. I don't want to stomp through the world and be number one. I just want to tread really lightly and not destroy anything. Hopefully I can try to mend some things. That's my goal.

Every time you buy something, just think, 'Where does this go?' It's not difficult. I'm not perfect, I just try really hard. Just do the most you can. It's not all or nothing.

for how you feel each day because of the way you treat your body'

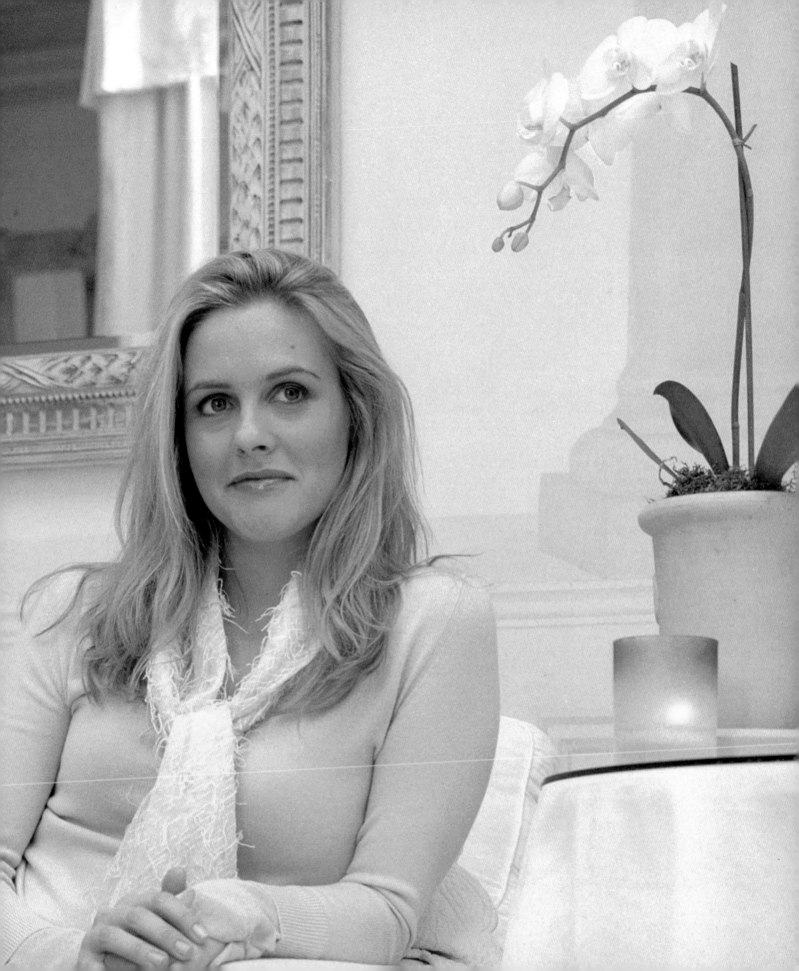

BLUSHERS

Several new blushers were launched in time for our latest trials – and two did well. So we've now tested more than 25 natural options. Our advice is still to be cautious about too much shimmer – stick to matt/velvety tones, with a hint of a glint if you like

✿✿ LOGONA DUO COMPACT BLUSHER
Score: 8/10
From the German brand Logona, this contains two shades of blusher, which you can 'customise'. Our testers trialled Peche 02, which should suit most skin tones. Logona avoid the use of nano-particles and it contains asbestos-free talc, 'not highly refined' (for more about talc, see page 55), and certified natural by the BDIH (see page 209).
Comments: 'Was complimented on my fresh skin' • 'colour long-lasting' • 'blended well and the two colours make it easy to get a shade that works' • 'a great example of how natural products can be just as effective as synthetics' • 'gave natural glow'.

✿✿ SANTÉ BLUSHER
Score: 7.55/10
Alongside the minerals in this blusher – which comes in a cute metal tin – are skin-caring certified organic jojoba and camomile extract, plus olive and essential oils. They say it's suitable for sensitive skins. Santé also avoid the use of any nano-coated or refined ingredients. We trialled 03 Beige Nature.
Comments: 'Easy to apply; matt, long-lasting natural glow' • 'natural-looking, but you can

build up for evening' • 'went on seamlessly; pigment left a natural flush to cheeks' • 'people said I looked well' • 'compares well to big brand blushers'.

✿✿ SUSAN POSNICK COLORME
Score: 7.66/10
Our testers liked this soft rose Peony shade even more than the originally trialled Camelia – and still enjoyed the product's travel-friendly design: a mirrored lid, and snugglesomely soft sponge.
Comments: 'Looked very natural; gave me a nice healthy look' • 'like a dusting of fairy powder, I felt very 1950s screen goddess with this packaging' • 'easy to apply, velvety – and made me look fresh-faced' • 'liked the built-in puff and mirror in the lid; useful for your handbag' • 'natural glowing effect, but you need to moisturise well to get a velvety effect'.

✿✿ NVEY ECO ORGANIC POWDER BLUSH
Score: 7.25/10
Nvey Eco, a new Australian brand, have twice scooped Natural Health Beauty Awards, and did well in a couple of categories for this book. In a stylish black

compact, this soft, seamless-finish blush blends corn silk, camomile, jojoba oil and vitamins A, C and E. Testers tried shade 951 – Plum (shimmer), which suited most well.
Comments: 'Went on smoothly, blended well and looked natural, seamless and glowing! People said how well I looked' • 'you don't need much of this; finish is smooth with a slight shimmer, love the packaging' • 'a lot of pigment so needed blending to soften it, but looked natural and stayed on all day'.

✿✿ ORGANIC GLAM BLUSHER
Score: 7.22/10
This is The Organic Pharmacy's stylishly packaged make-up range. Our testers trialled the Peach shade in this powder blush, which is good for warmer skintones and summer months – though there's also a pink tone for a 'pop' of face-wakening colour.
Comments: 'Great natural-look blush, which went on smoothly and blended well' • 'nice mix of matt and slightly shimmery' • 'made me look healthy and radiant' • 'lasted all day' • 'the shade was very natural' • 'velvety texture and didn't drag at all' • 'natural look and lasted much longer than my usual cream blush' • 'a little went a long way'.

Brush strokes... **This is a perfect blusher brush, but if you only have a foundation brush, use that.**

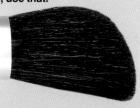

blush rubor blush   PALLADIO

BRONZERS

A dozen or so natural bronzers landed in our 'beauty dungeon' for this trial. In general, our panellists were pretty underwhelmed, with some products scoring dismally. The two highest-scoring products were actually trialled for our previous books, but none of the newcomers out-paced them, and they remain worthy winners

❀❀ DR HAUSCHKA BRONZING POWDER
Score: 8/10

Dr Hauschka tell us their bronzing powder is good for your skin, 'created using a caring combination of medicinal plant extracts', including witch hazel and sage to combat skin impurities. It also has a touch of silk in it, which accounts for the softness.

Comments: 'The best bronzing powder ever – glided on and looked totally natural; gave skin a luminescent glow' • 'worked beautifully with mascara and lip gloss' • 'lovely, fine, silky powder; didn't rub off on to clothes'.

❀❀ INIKA SUNKISSED BRONZER
Score: 7.4/10

Inika like to say that their products are 'made of Australia', because they are created from 'crushed mineral pigments from the very rocks that form our land…' All Inika products are vegan, certified by the Choose Cruelty Free organisation in Australia. This is a dust-on bronzer, so needs to be used with the correct 'kabuki' brush – which should be 'tapped' before whisking on to your face, as you only need a tiny bit of bronzer. (PS: Sarah really likes and uses this product.)

Comments: 'I loved this once I had mastered the technique; it sat on my face perfectly and made me look and feel sun-kissed' • 'made my skin look radiant; easy to apply with the correct brush' • 'I found that blending some Inika Bronzer with my moisturiser gave a very nice, easy-to-apply, tinted moisturiser – my new weekend look!' • 'so easy, though I was a complete novice with bronzer: I dusted it over foundation and loose powder and was hugely impressed at the natural glow'.

❀ KORRES BRONZING POWDER MONOI OIL
Score: 7.1/10

This velvety powder, infused with a touch of moisturising monoi oil, can be built up for a deeper tan, said testers. They loved the black compact, but not the lack of sponge. Has the sweet, exotic scent of monoi.

Comments: 'Very easy to use, natural effect; helped to blend uneven skin tone but didn't really cover blemishes' • 'fine, silky, soft texture; not oily at all' • 'left my skin very glowy with a slight sheen'.

❀ COULEUR CARAMEL TERRA CARAMEL BRONZING POWDER
Score: 6.87/10

One of the the things we like about this French natural make-up brand is the packaging: it's all made of cardboard, and so easily recycled. Couleur Caramel's bronzer comes in four shades – two matt, two pearly – and our testers trialled one of the latter. The principal ingredient is talc (see page 55), and the gentle texture is down to sunflower seed, jojoba, apricot and jojoba oil.

Comments: 'Healthy tanned look; lasted all day' • 'I really liked it; gave some colour to my pale complexion' • 'Ten out of ten! Great for quickly touching up tired make-up' • 'I swirled it on with a big fat brush and it took the shine off my foundation but the reflective light particles gave my skin a glow. I love it!'

❀ AVEDA BRONZING POWDER
Score: 6.87/10

This came fifth in its category, but we included it because we applaud Aveda's efforts to become ever-greener, with all manufacturing now powered by wind. The compact is made of recycled aluminium, and reveals a trio of shimmery shades – beige, tan and bronze – which can be swirled together.

Comments: 'Fine silky texture, which blended well with other make-up and gave a soft, dewy, sun-kissed finish' • 'gave a lovely natural glow' • 'liked the little bit of sparkle for special occasions' • 'nice small compact to fit in your handbag' • 'would definitely take on holiday to use on its own over moisturiser' • 'I prefer to use a brush rather than the pad supplied but, tested in winter-time, it gave my skin a glow and I felt I looked better, not as washed out as usual'.

Brush strokes… **Use your powder brush if you are swooshing bronzer all over your face, or your blusher brush if you are using it as a blusher.**

shadow secrets

It's time to open your eyes to a world of more natural, mineral-based eyeshadows

Steer clear of rainbow shades, and opt for flattering browns,

Many eyeshadows – whether they're marketed as natural or not – contain some mineral pigments. It's the quantity that changes, according to Jane Iredale, a pioneer of mineral make-up; 'conventional make-up is composed of ten per cent or less of pigment. The rest is fillers, preservatives and other make-up ingredients that can sensitise the skin.'

So, in 'conventional' shadows, minerals share palette-space with synthetic pigments (derived from petroleum/coal tar) and/or ingredients such as nylon, aluminium or mineral oil. Coal tar-derived pigments are often prefaced with the letters 'FD&C'; they are derived from bituminous coal, which contains substances including benzene, naphthalene and creosote. As Jane says, these ingredients are frequent triggers for allergic reactions. (Animal tests show almost all to be carcinogenic, too...).

Some of the eyeshadows from natural brands that we trialled look and feel very like conventional shadows; others are 'loose' powder and take a bit more getting used to. Will you have to make beauty compromises if you use more natural eyeshadow? Not necessarily. Loose-powder mineral eyeshadow is impressively long-lasting, although it stays put even better if applied with a special nylon shadow brush. You may well find that mineral eyeshadow powders also crease less than other types, creating a more natural look, which is more flattering for older skins.

Our biggest warning with mineral eyeshadows is this: unless you're about seventeen or a woman of colour, please don't be seduced by the dazzling array of colours. (The earth sparkles gloriously with myriad hues ranging from reds, browns and tans to blues, greens and violets.) Mineral eyeshadows can be based on ingredients such as lapis lazuli (bright blue) or malachite (rich green), which means there are some pretty bold colours out there. It's tempting to be seduced. But we would suggest that you steer clear of rainbow shades, and opt for flattering browns, taupes, greys, slate blues or dusty purples, accented with gold or cream.

Mineral eyeshadows tend to have a (varying) degree of shine. Which means older eye areas need a light touch and canny placement. A whisper of glimmer can be flattering, but if you overdo it, you'll actually draw attention to fine lines and wrinkles. So it may be great for browbones (a touch of pearlised ivory or cream can 'lift' the eyes), and even on lids, if it really is a wisp of shimmer. But after a certain age, keep anything faintly shiny away from the socket, where it will just draw attention to any crêpiness. (Remember that because powders are dry, they need no preservatives.)

Tip...

Mineral make-up brands say their products are so pure, you can sleep in them. We say: listen to your mother (and us), and never fall into bed wearing make-up – mineral or not!

taupes, greys, slate blues or dusty purples, accented with gold or cream

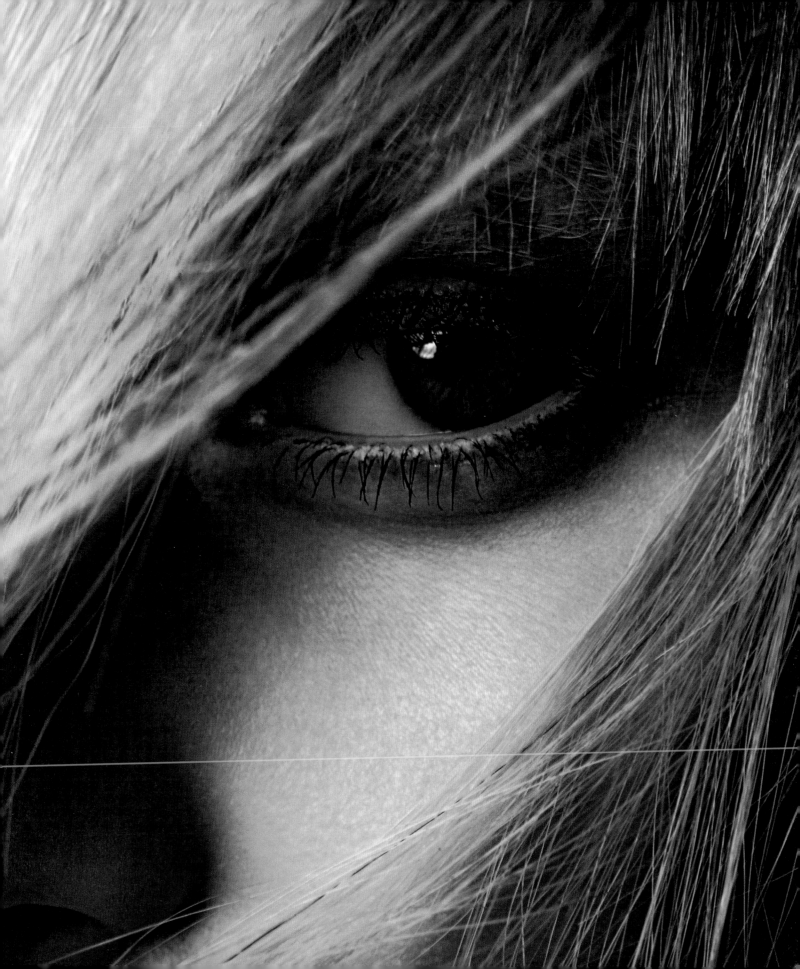

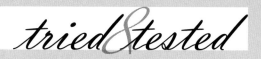

EYESHADOWS

With the trials for this update, we've now tested over 30 eyeshadows from different 'natural' make-up brands. And we're more than sneakily pleased that the results outperformed many 'big name' premium eyeshadows...

We asked for suits-all shades that our testers (whose skin tones range from ivory to black) would find flattering.

⭐ ❀ **PALLADIO HERBAL EYESHADOW**
Score: 8.8/10
This canister of pearlised powder shadow, available in seven shades (we tested matt Beige, shimmery Eggplant and iridescent Silver Sparkle), was popular with testers. It boasts vitamin E, green tea, aloe vera, ginseng and ginkgo biloba in the formulation – but also features parabens and silicones.
Comments: 'Sticky enough to create a strong colour with Beige' • 'Beige very versatile – used lightly or layered for more drama' • 'went on smoothly and blended easily' • 'loved the way Silver Sparkle looked – pale but with depth – lasted and didn't crease' • 'Eggplant is dramatic, with a subtle shimmer'.

❀ ❀ **NVEY ECO ORGANIC EYESHADOW**
Score: 8.56/10
Talc-free shadows come as single mirrored compacts of smooth powder, blended with soothing antioxidant vitamins A, C and E and camomile, corn silk and jojoba, for easy-glide application. Our testers tried 153, Stone/ Neutral Taupe Shimmer. (If you fall in love with the shadows, pro-style combination Eye

Colour System Palettes are also available, featuring a quartet of shades.)
Comments: 'Applied with my own blending brush, this smooth powder stayed put from morning to evening; the finished effect was a little darker than my usual, but I liked it' • 'not drying at all' • 'very easy to apply and blend; could use for eyeliner too' • 'slight shimmer enhanced the effect without being too shiny' • 'lovely, finely milled powder, subtle and flattering, didn't irritate my sensitive eyes'.

❀ ❀ **BARE ESCENTUALS EYESHADOW**
Score: 8.16/10
Bare Escentuals promise that 'these stay-true colours last all day since they don't contain binders or waxes and are so pure you can even sleep in them!' From a choice of 18 shades, our testers were assigned Blush.
Comments: 'Wow! Went on as smooth as gossamer, with a sophisticated effect' • 'easy to apply with a brush; slight shimmer worked well for day and night' • 'didn't irritate my sensitive eyes – I am converted'.

❀ **KORRES EYESHADOW**
Score: 8.07/10
Korres might seem more natural than they are – the ingredients list of this eyeshadow contains a few synthetics. Still, they are more

natural than most, so worthy of inclusion. This shadow comes in 12 shimmering and three matt shades. We tested Matte 35M brown.
Comments: 'Liked eye-enhancing gold/ brown colour; had a beautiful sheen and went on smoothly' • 'better than some mainstream brands; nice, even colour which highlighted the eye without screaming' • 'colour rich with a hint of shimmer; lasted well and felt silky'.

❀ ❀ **SANTÉ EYE SHADOW POWDER**
Score: 7.75/10
This aluminium palette contains a trio of shades, 'rich in certified organic jojoba and camomile extract, olive and essential oils that care for sensitive skin,' according to this truly natural company. With a brush inside the lid (testers preferred their own), the shadow contains certified asbestos-free talc. Our testers liked 71 Terra, a palette with bone (shimmery), taupe (gentle sheen) and a matt chocolatey shade. NB: we'd caution against the blue and green palettes!
Comments: 'I used the dark brown shade with a brush as eyeliner on the top lid, which looked smoky and pretty' • 'good for daytime and stayed on well' • 'colours went on smoothly, lasted well' • 'the trio can be blended to give a range of brown tones' • 'the aluminium tin is a nice change from plastic'.

Brush strokes... **For perfect placement – particularly if you love a smoky look – invest in these two brushes: the Eyeshadow Placement Brush to apply your base colour and the Contour Brush for precision application.**

PALLADIO

PALLADIO

EYE PENCILS

Since the hardback edition of this book, there's been a rush of new make-up brands to the marketplace – but only one launch out-paced our earlier choices, which all remain rivals to synthetically-based formulations. We continue to love eye pencils' multi-tasking powers, as quick-draw eyeshadows or smudged into lashes to create the illusion of length. And (after dark) swooshed on generously for Bardot-esque sultriness...

★ ❀ KORRES SOFT EYELINER PENCIL
Score: 8.52/10

Korres – a fast-growing Greek brand – have two winners in this category, each pencil based on a blend of waxes and pigments with a couple of synthetic ingredients. (As with all products in this book, you can see the full ingredients list at www.beautybible.com; we have also put together great deals on most of the winning products.) Super-soft and easy to blend, it's gentle enough to be used inside the eye like a classic kohl pencil, they say. (While most testers loved it, one was very unimpressed.) It comes in six shades.

Comments: 'Fantastic – easy to use and loved the smoky effect, but too soft to draw a thin line' • 'went on smoothly with no dragging' • 'smudged perfectly to soften colour' • 'the easiest I've ever used; very simple to remove and doesn't come off on fabric or make my eyes itch, as others have'.

❀ ORGANIC GLAM MINERAL EYE PENCIL
Score: 7.87/10

For anyone seduced by chic packaging, these sleek black pencils are as stylish as anything you'll find in a marbled beauty hall – but in this case, free from hydrogenated fats, artificial fragrances or preservatives. Choose from Black (our testers trialled this), Navy (our preference) or Dark Brown, from the make-up range created by the UK's Organic Pharmacy. (No sharpener, though, and one tester found it difficult to take off.)

Comments: 'A joy to use, simple, quick, gentle – the best eye pencil I've ever used' • 'easy to smudge with fingers' • 'soft texture went on absolutely fine and blended to a nice shadow' • 'I'm delighted to find an organic eyeliner – despite the panda eyes in the rain!' • 'a really great eyeliner, though I would have liked a sponge tip to smudge with' • 'didn't irritate my sensitive eyes; impressed that it costs the average for a good eyeliner'.

★ ❀ ❀ SANTÉ KAJAL EYE LINER
Score: 7.71/10

Santé say they created this pencil to have a 'skin-friendly texture', using refined earth pigments, natural waxes, bisabolol (a soothing camomile-derived ingredient) and aloe extract. They acknowledge that it's quite smudgy, though, and suggest 'setting' it with a powder shadow in the same shade to make it budge-proof (which has always been our tip, too.) Available in five shades.

Comments: 'Easy to apply: either soft and smudgy or a more distinct line' • 'I wear lenses and was impressed that it doesn't irritate or migrate into my eye, or end up down my face' • 'I prefer natural products like this as the skin round my eyes is very sensitive' • 'easy to achieve the results I wanted'.

❀ ❀ KORRES EYELINER PENCIL
Score: 7.7/10

Although we asked for this in black (the shade we requested from all brands for this category), Korres sent us a pretty khaki/gold (of the 14 shades on offer) and our testers loved it. This pencil is less smudgy, so your best bet if you like a more precise line.

Comments: 'Superb texture, like soft butter, so you hardly feel it going on; I used it mainly to line the upper lid with lashings of mascara and loved the look!' • 'great texture; quite soft and didn't drag' • 'lovely colour for brown eyes' • 'very smudgeable, which I really like' • 'super to find a natural product for the eye area; loved the pretty shade'.

❀ ❀ LOGONA KAJAL EYELINER PENCIL
Score: 7.4/10

All Logona products are certified by the BDIH (see page 209), carrying that 'natural seal of approval'. Available in six shades, these pencils are made by Faber Castell – one of the most famous pencil factories in the world – with a creamy formulation that allows for easy application. Logona promise that as the pencils don't contain water, they will last for ever. (We say: if you don't lose them first!)

Comments: 'The best eyeliner I have used in a long time: goes on very easily and evenly and you can make it very precise – stays on well' • 'velvety, thick texture that was just right to smudge' • 'I really liked this and it made me more experimental with smoky-eye looks' • 'very soft and easy to apply precisely if you have a steady hand: I really loved this pencil'.

MASCARAS

Our tester panellists diligently swept their way through quite a few new entries to this category – and were mostly disappointed. (Think: smudging, flaking…) But of the 35 of so natural mascaras we have now trialled – largely made up of plant waxes, oils, vitamins and iron oxides – these fared pretty well. They are not waterproof – so remember to powder up under your lower lashes, particularly if you have a tendency to watery eyes

Because conventional formulas rely on high-tech ingredients (such as plastic-like polymers) for curling and 'false lash' effect, we really can't expect those sorts of 'miracles' from a natural version. And alas for water babes, because synthetic ingredients are needed to 'raincoat' lashes, you won't find a natural waterproof mascara – at least not yet – so if you're a blonde swimming fanatic (like Jo), you'll have to stick with mainstream formulations. We know this is one area where readers may want to make a 'beauty compromise'.

❀❀ KORRES PRO-VITAMIN B5 AND RICE BRAN MASCARA
Score: 7.37/10

Korres tell us that the Provitamin B5 in this mascara works to strengthen eyelashes – but our testers were simply trialling its promised ability to volumise, lengthen and define, while adding colour. (You can choose from four shades: we'd suggest Black_02 or Brown_03, not being big fans of coloured mascara – though our testers really liked the blue/black they trialled.) Good to have a new contender to replace Origins, after they (sob, sob) withdrew from make-up.
Comments: 'Looked really natural, like normal lashes, not at all dry, just enhanced in a nice subtle way' • 'the dark bluey-black I tested was actually really good for making

my eyes stand out, but wasn't as harsh as my normal black' • 'definitely no clumping, made lashes quite glossy and healthy looking, a bit longer; well-designed wand. I would buy this' • 'very wearable natural look for day – and it stayed put in driving rain'.

❀❀ LIVING NATURE CONDITIONING MASCARA
Score: 6.88/10

A lash-conditioning offering from this New Zealand-based company, containing castor oil and carnauba wax, as well as manuka honey, 'to moisturise and nourish for soft, sleek lashes'. Testers said it took slightly longer than mainstream brands to dry.
Comments: 'Looked glossy and natural – good for a daytime look' • 'made my lashes slightly longer; no clumps or dryness; strong yet natural-looking colour' • 'went on easily and lengthened lashes' • 'could tell it didn't have artificial polymers' • 'nice natural finish; excellent wand design for accessing lashes at corners of eyes' • 'glossy, silky finish'.

❀❀ DR HAUSCHKA VOLUME MASCARA
Score: 6.72/10

A more recent launch from Dr Hauschka, for those who want some va-va-voom for their lashes, this special lash-building brush is designed to prevent lashes from clumping. It's fast-drying, and said to be suitable for contact lens wearers. PS: Dr Hauschka

mascaras include carmine from crushed beetles; more on this on page 51.
Comments: 'Looked glossy and lustrous, lashes longer and curlier but very natural' • 'didn't volumise as much as I'd expected, but was very good: easy to remove and doesn't irritate my sensitive eyes' • 'my lashes looked a bit longer, thicker and curlier' • 'I liked it – though not when the heavens opened…'

❀❀ DR HAUSCHKA MASCARA
Score: 6.45/10

Personally, we love this second entry from Dr Hauschka – their original mascara formulation, which has a heavenly scent of roses (thanks to the rose oil and wax in the ingredients). It is formulated to strengthen and condition lashes while giving definition and length, and is suitable for contact lens wearers and those with sensitive eyes. It doesn't contain preservatives, so Dr Hauschka recommend using it within six months of opening (but that applies to all mascaras).
Comments: 'No clumping whatsoever – unbelievable! Extremely natural finish, with one coat – just looked like naturally dark lashes; fabulous wand' • 'glossy finish; perfect everyday mascara' • 'made my lashes look darker and thicker' • 'excellent wand – the best I've come across: mascara went right to base of lashes, and it was easy to get at inside and outside corners too'.

EYE MAKE-UP REMOVERS

We'll be frank: natural eye make-up removers aren't up to the task of removing industrial-strength make-up – but they are more than adequate if you're wearing natural cosmetics, without the 'fixatives' of marbled-beauty-hall brands. (Though, to continue with our policy of honesty, we say: you can probably get away with your regular cleanser.) Nevertheless, we welcome a new entry in this category. The more, the merrier

✿ KORRES JASMINE EYE MAKE-UP REMOVER

Score: 8.51/10

From Greek brand Korres, this is formulated to be free from mineral oil, silicones, propylene glycol and ethanolamine (an ingredient shortened to MEA on labels, which can be irritating at the very least, not to mention slightly confusing). Although not pure as the driven snow, it is rich in wheat proteins, pro-vitamin B5, soothing cucumber and calendula, as well as the jasmine in its name. It leaves no oily residue, and Korres tell us it should be suitable even for contact lens wearers.

Comments: 'Brilliant – liquid with no oil (I wear contact lenses and oily eye make-up removers leave a film on the lens); easily took off mascara, eyeshadow – the lot – and no panda eyes in the morning' • 'this had a definite conditioning effect on my eyelashes' • 'removed waterproof mascara – just took a little longer' • 'left skin clean and cool and didn't exacerbate my eczema' • 'smelt beautiful – lovely product to use'.

✿✿ LIVING NATURE KUMERAHOU EYE MAKE-UP REMOVER

Score: 7.27/10

No, we hadn't a clue what 'kumerahou' was, either, until Living Nature told us that it's an indigenous New Zealand shrub with a natural cleansing action – which fits right into this Antipodean company's policy of sourcing native botanicals for their range. Your eyes may also be soothed by the calendula and camomile in the formula. (Some testers loved this, but one pair of sensitive peepers did not.)

Comments: 'Perfectly gentle, I don't wear a lot of eye make-up but it took that off quickly and easily, plus lipstick' • 'I appreciated the fact it wasn't greasy – which can be as difficult to remove as the make-up' • 'if you hold the moistened cotton wool over your eyes for a few moments, make-up comes off easily; no traces of make-up on my face cloth or my pillow' • 'I am totally keen! I think natural products should be mandatory for such a delicate area'.

✿ LIZ EARLE NATURALLY ACTIVE SKINCARE EYEBRIGHT SOOTHING EYE LOTION

Score: 7.12/10

This mild herbal lotion scored well in our Tried & Tested Treats for Tired & Puffy Eyes (see page 79); in this category, different testers found it works well for removing eye make-up too. It's designed to do double-duty but several testers emphasised that it's best suited for light make-up rather than Goth. Alongside eyebright herb, find glycerine, pro-vitamin B5, cornflower, aloe vera and witch hazel, designed to cool and soothe while sweeping away eye make-up.

Comments: 'Gentle, non-greasy liquid, so there were no problems with irritation, and it worked well on light make-up; skin felt refreshed' • 'cool liquid that was gentle on my eyes; very effective on eye make-up – but I wear contact lenses, so I use natural products' • 'I couldn't believe how effective this was: so gentle that when my small niece had conjunctivitis it was the only thing that stopped her rubbing her eyes' • 'there were no black smudges on the pillows; eyes felt refreshed and soothed'.

✿ JURLIQUE REPLENISHING CLEANSING LOTION

Score: 6.83/10

This product from one of our favourite Australian brands is intended as an all-over make-up remover, but our testers tried it specifically for the removal of eye make-up. One of the founders of this natural skincare company used to work with Dr Hauschka in Germany, and the products contain herbs that have been grown on Jurlique's farm. In this formula, you'll find rosewood and lavender, plus antioxidant green tea, red wine grape seeds, vitamin E and turmeric.

Comments: 'No rubbing was required with this product, even for waterproof mascara' • 'skin felt moisturised, plump, soft and rehydrated' • 'I loved the lavender/herbal scent' • 'rich, creamy texture – the skin round my eyes felt very smooth'.

lip service

We each eat, chew and lick our way through the equivalent of as many as four lipsticks in a lifetime. (Or maybe much, much more: some experts say it's a staggering two tubes each year.) So make sure that what you're slathering on your lips is truly good enough to eat

While the debate rages about how much of a moisturiser or a toner is absorbed into the skin, there is no debate about where your lip products are ending up: the same place as your breakfast, lunch and dinner. 'Conventional' lipsticks may contain paraffin, saccharin, mineral oil and synthetic colours, as well as that nostalgic 'mummy's lipstick' fragrance, which can be very drying to the lips.

So to us, it makes sense to 'go natural' with lip balms, sticks, glosses and liners – even if you don't switch your foundation, blusher or mascara. It doesn't make much sense to be buying organic lettuce, strawberries and champagne, only to be munching your way through chemical lip products. If you wouldn't be happy to spread it on your toast, why slick it on your lips?

Let's start with balms. Even if you don't wear lippy, chances are that you rely on lip balm to keep yours comfortable – and kissable! It's often said that lip balm is addictive, but there's no conclusive proof of that. It's the lip-cocooning sensation of a balm that we (and whoever kisses us...) find so irresistible. And, we promise, it's just as easy to get hooked on a natural product.

Conventional lip balms are based on petroleum (*petrolatum*), because it's a great barrier. But the advantage of natural, sustainably produced ingredients is that they offer skin-caring benefits above and beyond a protective barrier function. Plant-derived oils such as avocado and jojoba, shea and

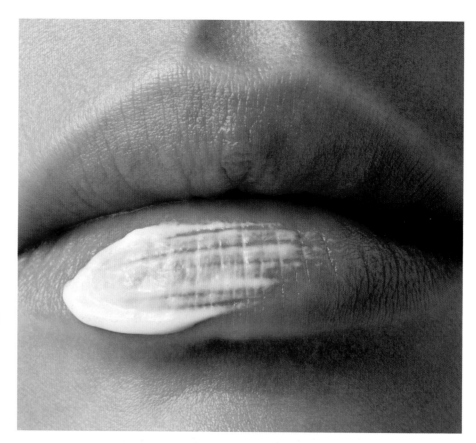

cocoa butter, as well as hemp seed, are rich in essential fatty acids that can actually nourish the very fine lip skin. To create a solid texture, these oils and butters are usually blended with beeswax, which magically helps liquids 'set'. Herbal ingredients such as marigold (see page 26) may be added, for healing. If you're going to be outside a lot, pick a formulation with an SPF – one based on titanium dioxide or zinc oxide, rather than

chemical sun screens (see page 140).

Remember, too, that dry, chapped lips are a response to dry conditions in your body, as well as in your surroundings. So to keep your lips silky smooth, be sure to stay hydrated – it's back to that eight big glasses of water a day, again. Keep your internal reservoir topped up, and you may not find you need to reach for the 'comfort blanket' of your lip balm quite so often.

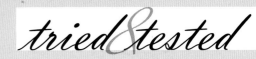
tried&tested

LIP SAVERS

Our testers slicked and licked their way through another dozen or so natural lip balms for this paperback (a total of more than 50) and declared a new number one choice... (NB: could we just also mention our very own, all-natural Beauty Bible Lip Balm – which is getting some rave reviews...)

✽✽✽ ESSENTIAL CARE LIP SILK
Score: 9/10
A Soil Association-certified wonder which went straight to the top of the lip-saver charts when we trialled it (and is recommended by beauty eds galore). The ingredients lists just shea butter, castor oil, beeswax, coconut oil, calendula extract, rosemary extract and orange essential oil – 100 per cent organic (and literally good enough to eat).
Comments: 'Practical, dinky twist-up tube, lovely on the lips; not sticky, just soft and soothing' • 'applied at the first sign of chapping, this does the business' • 'I work in a dry office, so lip balm's essential' • 'looks easily as nice as the lip gloss I tested, gives a soft sexy shine and great kissability...though further research needed'.

★✽ AVEDA LIP SAVER
Score: 8.5/10
This relies on beeswax and other natural waxes to seal in moisture. The waterproof formula comes in a twist-up stick and has a refreshing zing of cinnamon leaf, clove and anise oils. It also offers an SPF15 (chemical) sunscreen and antioxidants.
Comments: 'Loved the honey taste and smell – my lips felt wonderful' • 'dramatic moisturisation: didn't need to reapply for 24 hours' • 'lips felt plumper, especially if dabbed on at night' • 'lipstick lasts longer with this as a base' • 'liked the clear formulation with waxy protective texture'.

★✽✽ JOHN MASTERS ORGANICS LIP CALM
Score: 8.43/10
You'll find this in Jo's handbag (and winter coat pockets): a twist-up stick of hydration, subtly infused with vanilla, lime, tangerine and ylang-ylang. With extra virgin olive oil, shea butter, jojoba, kukui and wheatgerm, it also makes a great 'slick' over lipstick.
Comments: 'By far the best natural lip salve I've tried' • 'nice to have in your handbag' • 'lips felt less dry, even when it was really cold' • 'prevented sore, chapped lips'.

✽✽ LAVERA LAVERÉ LIP EXPERT
Score: 8.38/10
OK, this is actually a cream. However, it scored so highly as a lip treatment that we thought you should be reminded about it.
Comments: 'Since using this, my lips have been smooth and plump' • 'dry, chapped lips are more supple and moisturised' • 'vertical lines above my top lip improved dramatically' • 'made top lip look bee-stung'.

✽✽✽ BALM BALM FRAGRANCE FREE LIP BALM
Score: 8.05/10
Balm Balm's products are multi-functional – you can also use this teeny pot of Soil Association-certified goodness on your face, heels – wherever. And this fragrance-free version is gentle, with just five ingredients (all of them organic): shea butter, sunflower oil, beeswax, calendula oil and jojoba oil.
Comments: 'Gives a natural-looking sheen' • 'eased dry skin on elbows too' • 'I like one product that can do everything' • 'lasted well' • 'even made nails look healthy and shiny'.

✽ KORRES GUAVA LIP BUTTER
Score: 8/10
Korres chose guava fruit for this balm because it's rich in vitamins C and B. In a pot, its base is shea butter and rice wax; Korres offer tinted versions, which our testers praised – but scored behind this. Worth checking out the whole range, we'd say.
Comments: 'Brilliant – tackled sore lips immediately; great flavour, creamy and sweet' • 'super tube – no wastage' • 'my lips felt great' • 'made my lips fabulously shiny'.

★✽✽✽ NEAL'S YARD REMEDIES ORGANIC LIP FORMULA
Score: 7.87/10
If you want something on your lips that's literally good enough to eat, this product was one of the first to be certified organic. It offers soothing calendula, comfrey and lavender, with skin-toning lemon and myrrh, in a protective and vitamin-rich soya oil, wheatgerm, sunflower and beeswax base.
Comments: 'Lips in better condition; lovely citrus aroma and a good base for lipstick' • 'my builder son says it's brilliant for his chapped lips' • 'I've thrown out all my other lip balms' • 'quality at a reasonable price'.

kiss kiss...

Not so long ago, going natural meant doing without rich colour and high gloss. But no longer. Botanically-based lipsticks come in fabulous (flattering) shades

Generally, you won't find fire-engine red or fuchsia in natural lipstick ranges. We say: that's a good thing. Lipstick should flatter and enhance your natural colouring – not stop traffic at 40 paces. Just as the most flattering hair colour is only a couple of shades lighter or darker than your natural hair-colouring, so it is with lipstick and gloss (especially during the daytime). So choose shades that are just a touch deeper – or paler – than your own natural lip tone.

The more natural lipsticks and glosses that we have trialled get their colour from mined minerals, and from plant pigments such as alkanet, chlorophyll powder and betacarotene. Essential oils are generally used in place of chemical fragrances, not least because ingredients such as rosemary extract are powerful natural preservatives.

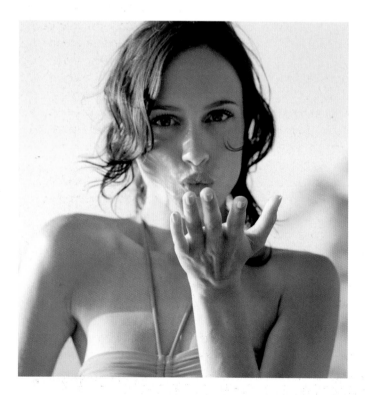

DON'T BE MIS-LEAD

We often get panicky, round-robin e-mails saying many lipsticks contain lead. Rub lipstick on your hand, they say, then scratch the traces with a gold ring – 'if it goes grey, your lipstick has lead in it'.

Recent research released by the Campaign for Safe Cosmetics (CSC) in America indicates that there may be truth in the rumour that some mainstream-brand lippies contain tiny amounts of lead. Tests conducted on 33 lipsticks bought in five US states showed that while 11 had no detectable level of lead, over half did contain detectable levels, some exceeding the Food and Drug Administration (FDA) guideline for lead in 'candy'.

According to Dr Christopher Flower, director general of the Cosmetic, Toiletry & Perfumery Association in London: 'The European Cosmetics Directive specifically prohibits the presence of lead in any cosmetic product. [Though hair dye is an exception to this, for more see page 108.] But, with today's increasingly sophisticated analytical methods, tiny amounts of many substances can now be detected almost anywhere. For this reason and the impossibility of removing every final trace from everything, the Cosmetics Directive allows traces of prohibited substances provided they are technically unavoidable, could not reasonably be removed during or after manufacture, and that the product remains safe. If levels are avoidable, then avoidance is required.'

In the US, it's the same story. Some colouring agents permitted by the FDA contain miniscule amounts of lead, but the FDA say it is such a small amount that it won't be harmful. The CSC say the discovery is 'part of a disturbing pattern of lax safety standards'. Their argument is that lip products should be regulated in the same way as sweets. We agree.

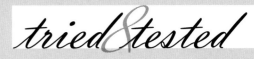

LIPSTICKS

Warning, warning: we've now tried dozens of natural lipsticks, and most fall short of our (simple) requirements: we'd like a lip-friendly formula in a pretty shade, which stays put for more than three seconds flat. One new entry now tops this selection – but our message to the beauty industry: when it comes to lipsticks in general – must try harder! (There were some truly dire results for many others…)

The key ingredients that tint the lipsticks featured here come from plants, vegetables, fruits and mineral pigments, rather than synthetic dyes. And while the range of shades is never going to rival those from Chanel or Revlon, there are still some divinely flattering colours. (Most of the companies have shade selections on their websites.) Our testers were all assigned 'suits-all-skin-tones' colours – generally, rosy-nude. They weren't wowed by most of the natural contenders in this category – getting on for two dozen of them – but short-listed these.

✿ NVEY ECO ORGANIC LIPSTICK
Score: 7.43/10
This lippie, which scored quite considerably more than its nearest rival (Aveda), is from an Australian natural beauty range that's colonising the globe with its more-stylish-than-most packaging and more-than-acceptable formulations. Here: a swivel-up shiny-black-packaged lipstick, (we trialled shade 362 Warm Pink – Slight Shimmer), which slicks on a high level of pigments, in an organic castor oil base that also delivers a softening slick of safflower, beeswax and vitamin E. (Almost balm-style properties, then – but in a lippy.)
Comments: 'Very nice feel, not too greasy or sticky but moisturising and easy to apply; stayed on while I had a drink but had gone by the end of the meal' • 'looked natural but the slight shimmer gave it a bit more of an "evening" look' • 'very pretty natural colour and creamy texture, a good shape and easy to apply; really moisturising but didn't sit heavy on my lips' • 'lasted through most of the evening and didn't leave huge marks on my glass' • 'I felt very feminine wearing this – it was noticeably pretty, very conditioning and made lips a statement without looking over-made-up'.

✿ AVEDA LIP TINT SPF15
Score: 7.06/10
This teeny swivel-up tube is more of a tinted botanical lip-conditioner – and it's sun-protective, with an SPF15. (If you want a dense, full-on lipstick, this isn't your baby; but if you like a sheerer finish, it's fab.) It has a physical UVA/UVB barrier, along with a patented moisture complex to protect and condition, that includes organically grown berries, plus antioxidant algae extract, avocado and mango butter, and jojoba oil. Oils of wintergreen, orange and spearmint give the product a refreshing zing. We tested Copper, from the range of seven shades.
Comments: 'Gorgeous – not my normal colour, but so flattering that I will buy it from now on' • 'easy to apply, lovely colour, softened my lips and I like the added benefit of an SPF' • 'ideal summer lipstick' • 'my lips are usually quite lined, but this product seems to have changed the texture'.

✿ BARE ESCENTUALS LIPSTICK
Score: 6.83/10
The rich pigments in Bare Escentuals make-up come from mined minerals – and you can select from 14 shades (we trialled Wearable Nude). Bare Escentuals claim this gives a 'luxurious aromatherapy treat' for your lips, and the formulation is rich in lip-caring aloe and shea butter.
Comments: 'Like this natural shade as a day lipstick (would choose a more dramatic shade for evening); it's creamy without being too rich, very comfortable, didn't dry lips out, and gives a discreet sheen – I would buy it again' • 'very moisturising, keeps lips soft without being sticky or heavy; has good staying power, packaging looked like a good classic product, and I liked the fact it had no scent or flavour' • 'easy to apply precisely; creamy formula makes lips plump, smooth and younger-looking' • 'I like the texture and the philosophy of using a natural product'.

Brush strokes… **This is the brush you need to apply lipstick. It'll help extend your lipstick's life, too: when you get to the end of the tube, the brush can reach down into the base to extract the last smidgen, so nothing goes to waste.**

elegantouch

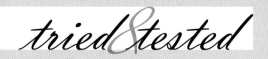

LIP GLOSS

Lip glosses have become an essential part of almost every woman's make-up kit – for the instant feel-good factor – and we're pleased to welcome a new entry for gloss-lovers, recently discovered by our lip-slicking testers

❀ BARE ESCENTUALS LIP GLOSS

Score: 7.87/10

Bare Escentuals have been creating mineral make-up since 1976 – long before it became the current 'beauty buzz'. The range has now expanded hugely, with countless options including this lip gloss, which gets its colour from powdered minerals and is designed to be 'non-gloopy', while still delivering shine, moisture and 'sensuality'. In 12 shades, of which our testers trialled Wearable Nude – a universally wearable buff.

Comments: 'Lovely and glossy – felt instantly comfortable on the lips and not at all sticky; colour is very sheer, which I wanted; just adds a natural wash of glossy niceness!' • 'easy to apply with the wand applicator – no mess' • 'made lips look slightly fuller, but in a very natural way' • 'really liked this: easy to wear when I wanted to look slightly more "made up" but still very natural' • 'lasted a long time, even when drinking tea, etc' • 'great for everyday use, not overly glossy – liked it a lot'.

❀ KORRES CHERRY LIP GLOSS

Score: 7.4/10

Why cherry? It's not just the colour (actually, this gloss comes in 10 shades, from baby pink to deep bronze, although cherry does help with the brightness of the colour, so they tell us). No: Korres – the Greek skincare and make-up brand – have infused this gloss with cherry and jojoba oils: apparently, cherry oil (from the stone of the fruit) is particularly high in antioxidants, and is deeply moisturising

and easily absorbed by the skin. Korres isn't an all-natural brand – we'd file them under pretty-natural-prettifiers – but their range does avoid mineral oil, silicones, propylene glycol and ethanolamine, and is trying hard.

Comments: 'Not shimmery or wet look just glossy! Actually this product has changed me from wearing lipstick to natural colour lip gloss, sometimes over lips filled in with lipliner…' • 'easy to apply with the sponge tip applicator, even without a mirror' • 'my lips looked instantly plumped up and fuller' • 'loved this lip gloss, made my lips feel instantly smoother, and looked bigger and so sexy. It's really a treatment as well' • 'now my fave lipgloss and I will definitely buy more in every colour!'.

❀ THE ORGANIC PHARMACY ULTRA-GLOSSY LIP PLUMP

Score: 7.31/10

This gets its lip-quenching action from castor oil, alongside shea butter, vitamin E and beeswax, and comes in a choice of five shades, including a sheer Crystal Sparkle which adds a slick of glimmer to any lipstick. A slanted tube sweeps the light-reflective formula on to lips, creating the 'illusion' of plumpness, so Organic Pharmacy promise – hence the name. Confusingly, some testers thought it was very sticky (which glosses mostly are) while others said the opposite…

Comments: 'Fabulous: The Organic Pharmacy deserve a medal for formulating a lip balm that can easily compete with any from the top fashion houses without putting

any nasties in it!' • 'shimmery and glossy, with a good amount of colour; it's not particularly sheer, but looks very natural and pretty' • 'juicy looking, glossy and sticky, just like mainstream ones' • 'loved the feel, and you don't need to apply it precisely so no mirror required; I did a double take after putting it on because my lips did look plumper – not like Ms Jolie but certainly different' • 'one to try for a temporary trout-pout effect' • 'it did disappear after a meal, but left a lovely light moisturising sheen on the lips, which was a bonus' • 'very glossy natural shade, which enhanced my own natural lip colour'.

❀ AVEDA LIP SHINE

Score: 7.05/10

This wet-look gloss is packed with nourishing fruit and vegetable extracts (including beetroot), together with an organic 'berry lipid' moisture complex based on vitamin E, cranberry, bilberry and blueberry. In seven shades – we tested Thyme Bud – it delivers a breath-freshening zing of peppermint, cinnamon, anise and basil. A big favourite of both of ours.

Comments: 'Very good moisturising effect – in fact, I'd use this instead of lip balm' • 'the only gloss out of the ones that I tested that didn't make my lips tingle or sting' • 'lovely sheer colour' • 'lasted right the way through a Big Mac meal' • 'if I'm going to end up eating lip gloss along with my food, I'd rather it be natural than petroleum jelly!'

LIP LINER PENCILS

If you want your lipstick to stay put, it's best to create a strong base with a lip pencil: use it to outline lips and fill them in. The pencils in this category performed creditably well – but no new entries beat our original line-up

★ ✿✿ **LOGONA LIPLINER PENCIL**
Score: 7.7/10
Available in three shades (a rather witchy burgundy and a surprisingly Barbie-ish pink), we'd say the shade our beauty sleuths trialled – Nutmeg – is the only safe bet for this lip liner. A proper, high-quality, wooden pencil, this contains no known allergens or sensitisers; it offers palm kernel and jojoba oil among the lip-enriching ingredients, with the colour derived from minerals.
Comments: 'Very easy to apply, quite matt texture but not drying; gave a natural effect, which I liked just with clear gloss; made colour last longer when combined with lipstick' • 'easy to be precise, no sharpener but sharpened easily with ordinary pencil sharpener' • 'doesn't drag, easier to use than my current mainstream brand, looks good and definitely made lipstick last longer; also made a good lip stain' • 'would definitely consider swapping to this natural product' • 'got a good, even line and I am no expert; remarkably soft for a lip pencil – would definitely recommend this'.

✿ **BARE ESCENTUALS LIP LINER**
Score: 7.7/10
From one of the early natural make-up lines, this range is based on crushed mineral pigments – with waxes in this case to give their lip liner a soft texture. Designed to be long-lasting, these creamy crayon lip liners are available only in what Bare Escentuals

describe as 'universally wearable, classic shades' – our testers' shade was Wearable Nude, which suits most and matches the Lip Gloss, opposite.
Comments: 'This is a great product – has a smooth, creamy texture that glides on effortlessly. It can be very precise – or create a full pouty lip outline, if you prefer' • 'wonderful lip base: my lipstick lasted almost all day without reapplying, so creamy my lips felt moisturised' • 'nude colour goes with any shade – a real desert island must-have' • 'made neutral lipstick look much better – more noticeable and "finished"'.

★ ✿✿ **KORRES LIPLINER PENCIL**
Score: 7.16/10
An easy-to-apply pencil available in five shades – our testers trialled Neutral Light, which is the same colour as most lips. Korres promise 'excellent colour consistency is ensured through the high percentage of fine pigments', which are basically finely milled minerals.
Comments: 'Quite creamy, but not too soft to apply easily; nice light colour for a realistic outline; good outline or base for lipstick – liked the colour on its own for "played down" lips' • 'easy to apply, went on smoothly – a good product' • 'testing this product has encouraged me to use a lip liner when I wear lipstick: it is very effective' • 'as a base for lipstick – over my lips, not just lining them – it made my lipstick last much longer, through a meal and the

whole evening' • 'goes on smoothly – even better if held near a lightbulb first to soften! A very good colour for my lips, so the outline was realistic and also good as a base for lipstick/gloss'.

✿✿ **DR HAUSCHKA NOVUM LIPLINER**
Score: 7.05/10
You have a choice of two fairly neutral-toned shades for this wooden pencil from Dr Hauschka's much-loved Novum range (which features somewhat more sophisticated, still-natural formulations than their original make-up collection): our testers trialled Novum 06. The rose wax in its ingredients keep it soft and easy to apply, and it also features nourishing anthyllis extract (also known as kidney vetch), to keep lips conditioned and supple.
Comments: 'Very easy to apply with no dragging, and gave a precise lip outline; liked this as a lipstick colour on its own, and it also helped keep my lipstick on longer when I used it as a base' • 'easy to apply after "blunting" as instructed; gave a definite line that stopped the "bleeding" effect of my (older) lips; works really well as a lipstick alone – stays on for hours – though you really need gloss over the top to moisturise' • 'went on very smoothly, probably down to the rose wax, easy to guide – though I am hopeless with a lip liner' • 'it worked really well as a base coat to keep my lipstick on all day – even when my lipstick had gone, the liner was still there'.

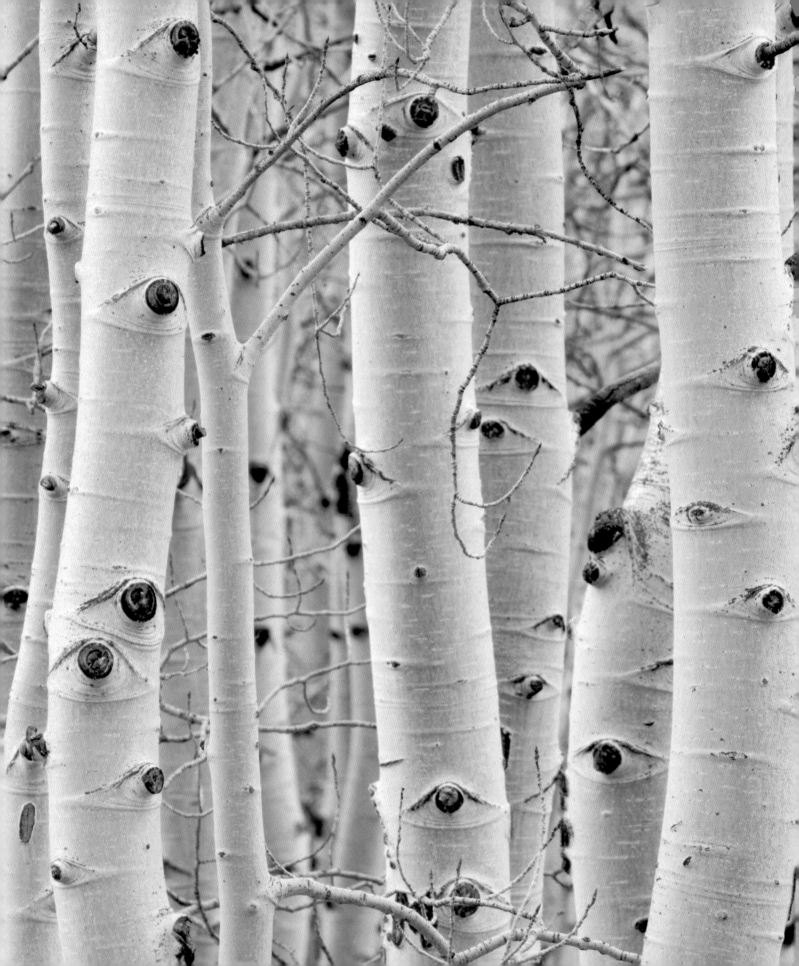

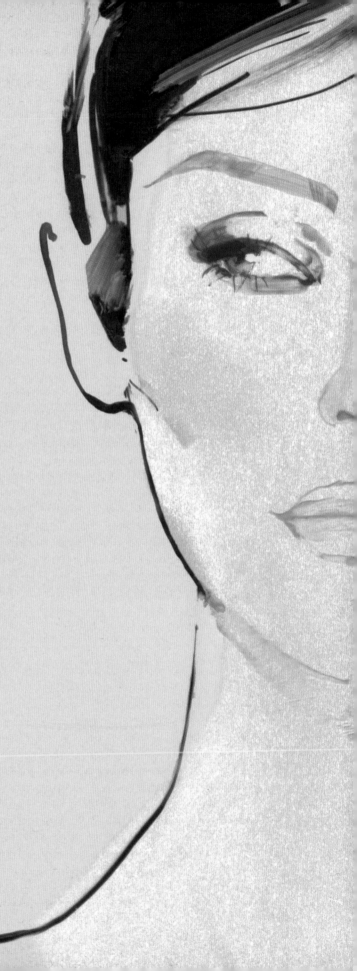

Eyes

Where do you focus when you look at someone's face? Try it now – we bet it's their eyes. And just the same is happening when people look at you. As well as working very hard, our eyes have their own language, which reveals the state of our minds, bodies and souls. So it's vital to cherish them in every way.
PS We love the graceful aspen trees opposite and their 'kohl-rimmed eyes' that follow you gently as you wander past.

SMILE WITH YOUR EYES

It may seem such an old cliché to say that the eyes are the mirror of the soul but, like many clichés, it's more true than we could imagine. If your soul sings, your eyes smile – and everyone notices, consciously or unconsciously

According to psychiatrist Dr David Servan-Schreiber, watching the way people smile – with their eyes or not – is a simple test of whether they are really happy to see us or not. A forced smile – the sort we 'put on' at social situations where we really aren't feeling warm and at ease – mobilises only the muscles round the mouth, showing our teeth (not for nothing do we describe it as 'the smile on the face of the tiger'). A 'real' smile, however, also uses the muscles round our eyes.

The order for smiling with your eyes comes from the deepest and most ancient region of your brain, known as the limbic system, which we can't control with our cognitive brain. As Dr Servan-Schreiber says: 'That explains why the eyes never lie – their folds tell us whether the smile is genuine. A warm smile, a real one, lets us know intuitively that the person we are talking to is, at that exact moment, in a state of harmony with what he or she thinks and feels.' In other words, they are happy to be there with us.

Few people get weak eyes from looking on the bright side

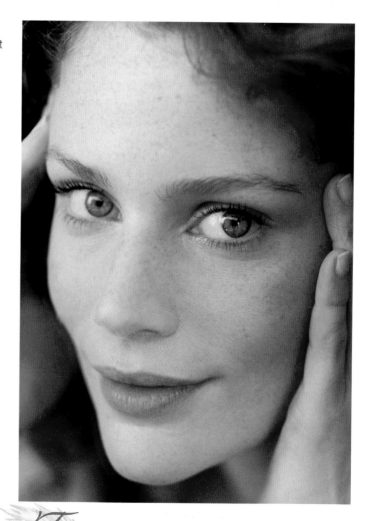

Of course, people who watch us smile are getting the same intuitive messages. If you aren't quite smiling with your eyes, can we recommend you read Dr Servan-Schreiber's book *Healing Without Freud or Prozac*? It's on our very short list of books that can change your life. As well as giving an account of his personal journey searching out natural ways to relieve stress, anxiety and depression, it gives simple ways that we can all help ourselves – and others – to be happier. The key one? Be loving and kind. If you are, no matter what else is going on, people who look into your eyes will see 'the sweet soul shining through them', as one poet put it – and that's real beauty in our book.

It's no accident, by the way, that the cliché about horses is that you should look for one with a 'kind' or 'soft' eye. One horse that Sarah rescued had what a friend who was with her at the time called 'dead eye', as if he had chosen to blank out an unkind world. PS He is now bouncing around, with soft, kind, smiling eyes…

Tip… • Do use an eye cream if you wish, but remember that the biggest favour you can do your eyes is to invest in wraparound sunglasses, which shield the fragile skin around the eyes from sun damage. Avoid thin-armed glasses and go with the Jackie O look every time. (And we say it again in our sun chapter: it's that important!)

EYE CREAMS

We always select testers who are over 35 (and up and up) to try eye creams – because mid-30s onwards is when fine lines and wrinkles really start to show up. They're asked to try them on one eye, for comparison, and were convinced enough to award impressively high scores to these greener products. (NB: we trialled lots of new anti-ageing eye treatments for this book, but none out-ranked the originals – which are, of course, as effective as ever.)

✿ A'KIN GINKGO & CHAMOMILE REVITALISING NIGHT EYE CREME

Score: 8.35/10

Eye creams can cost an arm and a leg – so we're delighted this (unfragranced) winner is from an accessibly-priced Australian range (A'kin means 'being similar to the way the skin behaves naturally'). This is one of a duo – A'kin would also like you to use their White Tea & Cornflower Soothing & Relaxing Eye Day Gel – but our testers got fantastic results from this product alone, with its fusion of cornflower, alpha-lipoic acid, omega-3, -6 and -9 essential fatty acids, and ginkgo.

Comments: 'I liked everything about this – using it was lovely' • 'sank in easily – fine lines less noticeable' • 'positive comments from others' • 'did not irritate my sensitive eyes' • 'shadows round eyes less prominent, helped reduce dark circles' • 'reduction in puffiness and fine lines smoothed'.

✿ TRILOGY EYE CONTOUR CREAM

Score: 7.7/10

Soothing, cooling aloe vera gel helps revive tired eyes, while rosehip, carrot, evening primrose, almond and vitamin E oils get to work longer-term, targeting signs of ageing. We could just as easily have trialled this fragrance-free formula as a Treat for Tired & Puffy Eyes (see 79), but it rose to the bigger anti-ageing challenge brilliantly.

Comments: 'Lids are smoother – noticeably easier to apply eyeshadow' • 'very gentle to use – like wrapping eyes in warm towels' • 'puffy eyes all but vanished after one night – great quick fix for tired eyes' • 'fine lines are less visible and weeks of stress at work with a couple of late nights haven't taken their usual toll' • 'doesn't irritate my sensitive skin'.

★ ✿ LIZ EARLE NATURALLY ACTIVE SKINCARE DAILY EYE REPAIR

Score: 7.68/10

Another affordable bestseller from Liz Earle, this intensive cream contains concentrated botanicals including echinacea and vitamin E, with light-reflective pigments (to brighten the under-eye area *à la* Touche Éclat), and an SPF10 non-chemical sunscreen – to help protect this fragile zone.

Comments: 'Amazed to see a visible difference: fine lines reduced on the eye I used this on' • 'instantly blurred lines, worked very well on puffiness, camouflaged dark circles' • 'sank in quickly' • 'a good base for concealer' • 'this should be marketed as eye and lip treatment: noticeable improvement in both areas – lifting and firming; I looked more radiant and people commented'.

✿ ✿ BAREFOOT BOTANICALS INTENSIVE EYE SERUM

Score: 7.6/10

Barefoot Botanicals' products recently had a long-overdue design makeover with many formulations being reworked, but this top-selling product stays the same: firming, line-smoothing natural ingredients in a light serum specifically formulated to banish shadows, fine lines and all kinds of under-eye baggage, all based on the range's key ingredient – age-defying rosehip oil.

Comments: 'My eyes looked fresher in the morning when I first used it, someone said I looked bright-eyed and bushy-tailed!' • 'gorgeous rose fragrance, lovely glass bottle' • 'eyes feel refreshed and it cooled and soothed puffiness' • 'very hydrating and smoothing for the winter-dry skin round my eyes; used it to treat the rest of my face too'.

✿ TAER ICELANDIC EYE CONTOUR

Score: 7.57/10

The entire Icelandic Taer range is packaged in soft-green glass bottles that just don't look like anyone else's. Cooling and hydrating – thanks to azulene and bisabolol (found in German camomile) – this also features omega-3-rich hemp and evening primrose oils, to nourish, plus Taer's unique 'calming complex', to fight the effects of environmental stress and pollution.

Comments: 'Smoothed and rejuvenated the whole area, even my boyfriend noticed the reduction in crow's feet' • 'sank in immediately' • 'people said how bright my eyes were' • 'skin much smoother and younger looking – love this, and recommend it to everyone!'

eyes bright

Judging by the number of times we've been asked over the years, eye problems affect lots of you, particularly puffy eyes and dark circles, hotly followed by dry itchy eyes. Here's our advice

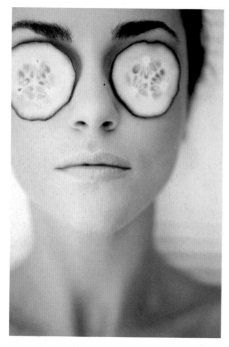

WHY YOU SHOULDN'T DYE YOUR LASHES

We have one thing to say about dyeing your eyelashes: please don't. Jo acquired an eye infection from having it done at a reputable salon. Hair dye is commonly used to dye lashes, despite the fact that the manufacturers warn in the strongest terms against getting the product near your eyes because of the risk of injury, allergic reaction or blindness. There are now specific lash dyes on the market, but they contain basically the same ingredients as hair dye. Some may contain coal tar too.

PROBLEM

Dark circles and/or puffy eyes and eye bags

SOLUTION If you're short of sleep, get more and better slumber (see page 204 for help on this). It might sound obvious but it should help. Dark circles and eye bags are often linked to food allergies or intolerance, so if more sleep makes no difference, cut out wheat – bread, pasta, cakes, biscuits, etc – entirely for a week and see if that helps. (Sarah's eyes can be practically invisible under the bags in the morning if she's had pasta or sandwiches the day before.) If it doesn't, try avoiding all cow's milk products. There could well be other foodie culprits, so for details of an elimination diet, read *Solve Your Food Intolerance* by Dr John Hunter. Also, do stick to fresh food, preferably organic; processed and/or conventionally grown foods may contain additives that you are sensitive to. Cut down on alcohol, sugar and sugary foods, and salt (often hidden in processed foods), and drink lots of still pure water to flush out toxins.

For an immediate rescue strategy, stroke ice cubes over your eyes. If you have time to lie down briefly – or somewhere to lean your head right back – brew a pot of camomile tea with two teabags (look for German camomile, *Chamomilla recutita*) and lay the slightly cooled, slightly squeezed bags on your eyes. Slices of cucumber are also very soothing, and raw potato contains

an enzyme that helps de-puff skin – lay slices straight on your eyes, or grate some potato and pop in a clean cotton hankie.

Camouflage dark circles with a little concealer (see page 53 for Tried & Tested results), patted on thinly with your ring fingers: don't rub, pull or drag the skin. If you use cream around your eyes, be sure not to get it too near: products should be applied on the bone of the eye socket – from there they travel to the skin nearer the eye on their own.

Eye products and cosmetics may be another cause of problems: if you suspect a culprit, bin it immediately – don't go on hoping it will be all right or the problems may continue and be much harder to solve. Remember that even natural ingredients can cause problems – Sarah's eyes flare up if the herb eyebright gets near them.

Puffy eyes respond brilliantly to an instant 'bag-draining' detox in the shape of a run or a vigorous session on the treadmill, followed by a sauna or Turkish bath – or the low-tech solution: steam your face over a bowl of very hot water, with some essential oil such as rosemary to perk you up.

PROBLEM

Red, bloodshot eyes

SOLUTION Sleeeeep! And clean up your diet. If you've excluded conjunctivitis (visit your doctor to make sure) and the veins in your eyes are always on show, the likeliest villain is lack of sleep. However, we have also noticed an amazing difference with a bit of light detoxing (see page 189 for more) and green food supplements, such as algae, chlorella and spirulina. You could also try Japanese detoxing foot patches based on wood vinegar (such as Patch-it! by Nutriworks, available from Victoria Health). After five to seven days, we have noticed brighter eyes, with whiter whites – and better skin, too. They can also help you sleep well.

PROBLEM
Tired, itchy, dry eyes

SOLUTION Firstly, the mucous membrane round eyes needs to be lubricated like every other part of your body, so drink more water – eight large glasses of pure still water between meals. Also make sure you eat plenty of essential fatty acids and follow the suggestions for an anti-inflammatory diet on page 19.

Secondly, dry environments will dry your eyes, so if you work in an office, put a bowl of water and/or an ioniser on your desk; if you have a centrally heated house, put a bowl of water by all the radiators. For instant help, try the camomile teabag trick (see left), or treat your poor sore eyes to a squirt of Clarymist, a gentle, soy-based product that you spray on your eyelids (and it doesn't make your make-up run). It's said to help 80 per cent of cases of dry eyes, where the cause is tear evaporation, compared to other gels and drops, which are only effective in 20 per cent. NB: if you have contact lenses, you should check in with your optometrist: there are now lenses that may help.

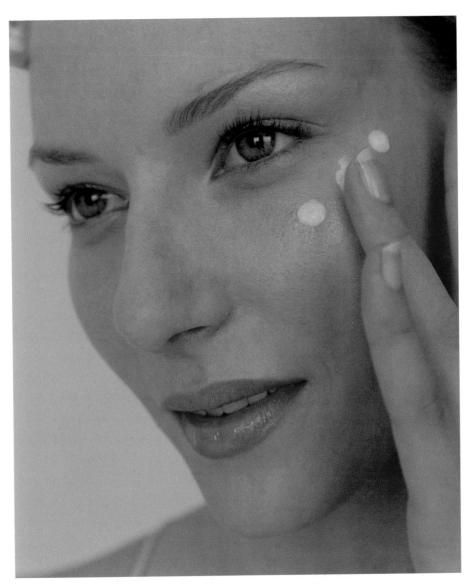

We love...

For tired, sore or itchy eyes, Sarah absolutely loves heaven-scented Pukka Organic Rosewater spray, distilled from the flowers of *Rosa damascena*, grown at high altitude. (A friend with rosacea swears by it for reducing the flushing; it's hefty-ish to carry in your handbag but she says it saved her face on a hot trip.) Scientist Dr Linda Fellows also recommends spraying Rescue Remedy flower essence on your lids and round tired eyes – another tip which Sarah loves. Herbal Eye Drops by Vizulize, which contain soothing chamomile and antioxidant blueberry, help too.

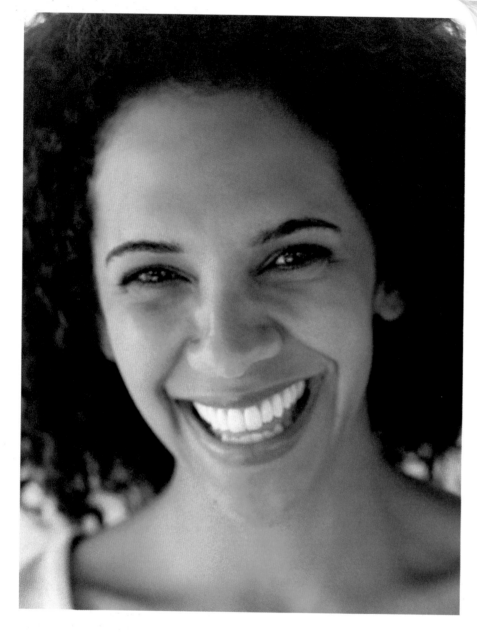

Your eyes thrive on nutrients called lutein (in green veg) and zeaxanthin (in orange and yellow ones), which can help reduce your risk of age-related macular degeneration, the commonest cause of loss of vision. So eat lots of green leafy vegetables, particularly spinach and kale – the richest sources of lutein – plus orange peppers, which are full of zeaxanthin; sweetcorn has a nice lot, too. Jo also swears by a (delicious) mix of dried red fruits with her muesli – cherries, cranberries and, particularly, bilberries: bilberry extract has been shown to improve normal and night vision.

PROBLEM

Computer vision syndrome

SOLUTION Long hours at the screen can lead to all sorts of problems. The symptoms of computer vision syndrome include sore, tired, burning, itchy, watery or dry eyes, blurred or double vision, headaches and a sore neck. You may also have trouble when you try to move your focus between the

monitor and papers on your desk. Some people notice increased light sensitivity or see fringes of colour, or after images, when they look away from the screen.

The first thing to do, according to integrated health expert Dr Andrew Weil, is to ensure that your computer is in the best position.

● Make sure you are sitting straight in front of it, about an arm's length away.

● The top of the screen should be at eye

level or below so that you're looking down slightly (you can get a sore neck if the screen is too high or too low).

● Your keyboard should be directly in front of the monitor.

● Your reference papers and books should be placed at the same level, angle and distance from your eyes.

● To minimise glare from bright lights, put your light source at a right angle to the monitor.

● To reduce eye strain, take periodic breaks from the screen and focus on more distant objects. Try to schedule a five-minute break every hour. Stand up and move around or just lean back and close your eyes for a few minutes.

● Make an effort to blink frequently. If your eyes are dry, you're probably blinking less than normal when you look at the screen. If that doesn't help, get some artificial tears, which are available over the counter at any chemist.

● Try taking bilberry extract (see above).

● Have an eye check every two years, annually if you have glaucoma in the family.

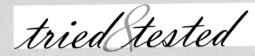

TREATS FOR TIRED & PUFFY EYES

We've lost count of the women who've asked us if there really are products that put the sparkle back, while depuffing eye bags and/or fading dark circles. The good news? According to our testers – who've added some new discoveries to the original list – yes, there are!

★ ✿ LIZ EARLE NATURALLY ACTIVE SKINCARE EYEBRIGHT SOOTHING EYE LOTION

Score: 7.85/10

This actually appears twice in this book – you'll find it did well in the eye make-up remover Tried & Tested. Here, testers were asked to comment on the power of this ultra-lightweight lotion to soothe, calm and de-puff. It gets its name from one of the key ingredients – the eyebright herb, renowned from the wise woman tradition onwards for its ability to tone and reduce puffiness around the eyes. Liz Earle's team recommend using it on cotton wool pads, soaked in the lotion as a revitalising eye compress to relieve even bloodshot eyes.

Comments: 'Eyes definitely clearer, brighter, and more refreshed – excellent at reducing puffiness, but I don't think you could apply over make-up without disturbing it' • 'excellent at perking up tired eyes, particularly after a long day slaving over a computer screen' • 'slight effect on dark circles, but may be down to brighter-looking eyes' • 'a fab pick-me-up for mornings when eyes are really sore and tired; helped with moisturising dry under-eyes' • 'loved this product and plan on stockpiling it after my baby is born in preparation for all those sleepless nights'.

✿ ✿ DR HAUSCHKA EYE SOLACE

Score: 7.76/10

This product also features eyebright, alongside fennel extract, woundwort, camomile and rose essential oil in a cooling lotion that our testers unanimously found super-refreshing.

Comments: 'Rested my eyes and took away the strained feeling at the end of the day' • 'very cooling and refreshing: red tired eyes much clearer' • 'excellent before and after a big night out' • 'great for a pampering lazy day' • 'eyes felt "alive" again'.

✿ AVEDA TOURMALINE CHARGED EYE CREME

Score: 7.65/10

Another product that stars twice: it was also highly rated by testers as an age-defying eye cream. Finely powdered tourmaline (a semi-precious gem) is blended with pennywort (to reduce puffiness), vitamins C and E and tomato extract lycopene, to reinforce skin around the eyes. Light-diffusing silica brightens dark circles, while cucumber cools and soothes; the signature smell is based on essential oils of lavender, geranium, rose, patchouli, lemon, lime and petitgrain.

Comments: 'Rich cream that moisturises and has the desired effect as an eye reviver, particularly after late nights' • 'made a dramatic difference to my dark eyelids and evened up skin tone round my eyes' • 'tube lasted for ages' • 'subtle brightening effect, very refreshing on my computer- and contact lens-strained eyes; minimised morning puffiness; lovely soothing effect' • 'claims to "bring radiance to the tired eye area", and it delivers' • 'excellent base for make-up under my eyes and on the upper eyelid' • 'certainly improves the appearance of dark circles'.

✿ ✿ KORRES MATERIA HERBA MOISTURISING EYE CREAM

Score: 7.19/10

Korres recently launched a sub-range called Materia Herba, which is even more natural than the rest of their range – and ups the organically-sourced content of the products. This is said to boost hydration by 53 per cent within two hours, and although it's actually designed specifically for dark circles, our testers found it good for their tired peepers.

Comments: 'Skin certainly looked plumper after applying this thick cream, and about 30 minutes later the eye area felt more toned, which took away the tired look…skin felt soft and plump all day' • 'only need to dab lightly, and you can put it over make-up' • 'obvious instant effects and over time eye area has improved' • 'lovely cream that did everything I want'.

✿ GREEN PEOPLE EYE GEL

Score: 7.1/10

For day use, this goes-a-long-way gel features an edible seaweed ('Spiny Holdback Bush' – love that!), with a cooling, refreshing action, together with camomile and plant proteins. Good under eye make-up, too, Green People promise.

Comments: 'Eyes look brighter and feel lovely and cool; very effective on puffy eyes and dark circles' • 'wonderful, very pleasant to use, and very effective; puffiness less visible, dark circles visibly lighter and eyes much brighter' • 'non-greasy, thick gel, very user friendly and fits easily into any bag'.

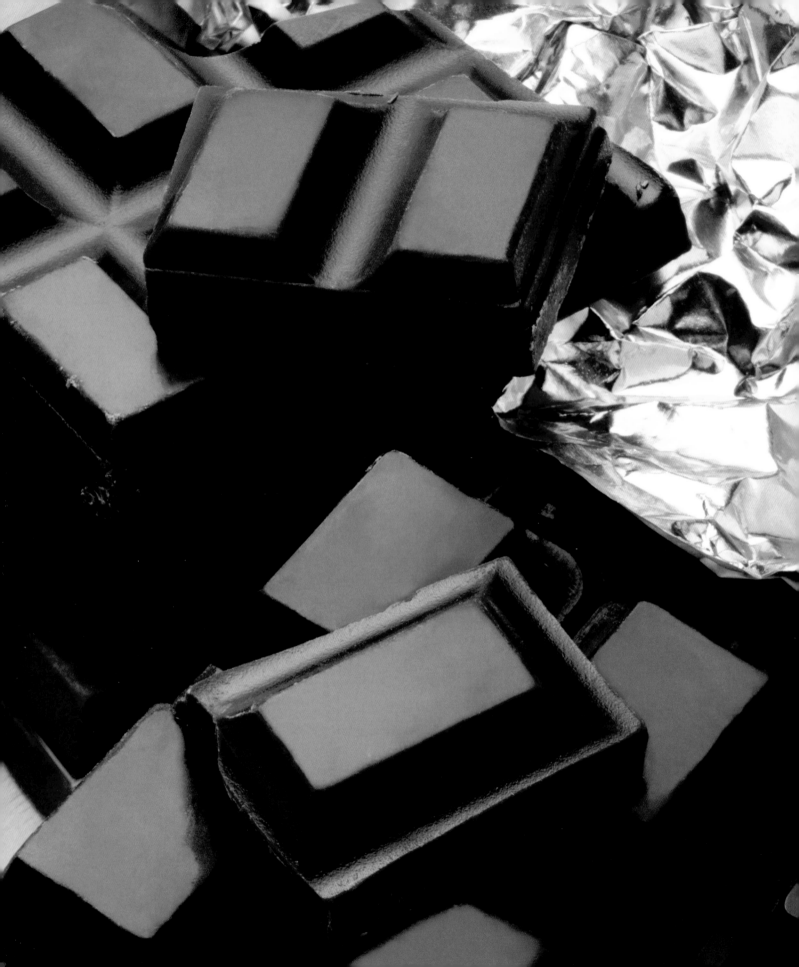

Teeth

Your pearly-whites are vital in every way, but often overlooked. You may not want to flash unlikely-looking Hollywood nippers at the world, but it's worth looking after your teeth and gums (just think of the alternative). And taking heed of natural treats for teeth could mean biting into strawberries dripping in dark chocolate…

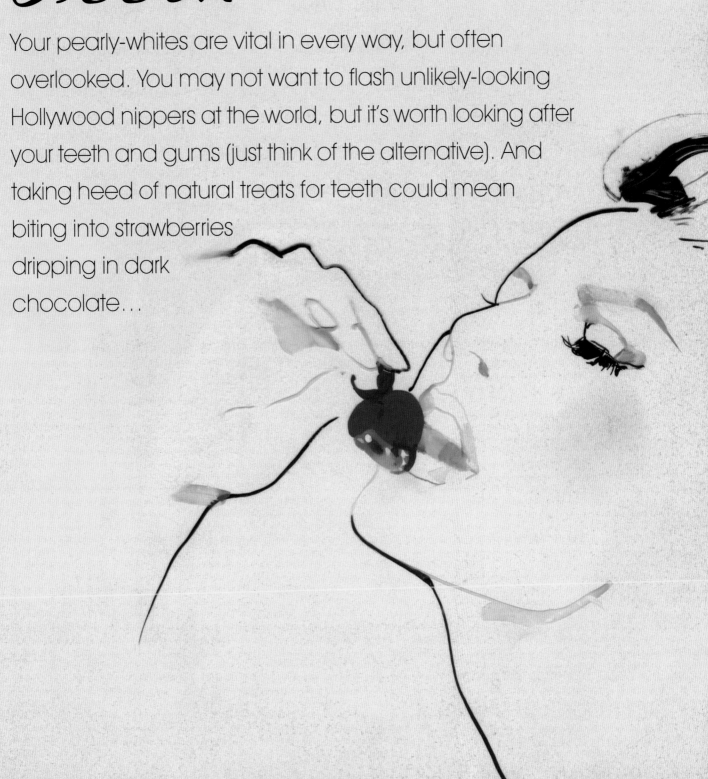

perfect smiles

Over the past decade, the concept of holistic dentistry, where dentists consider your wellbeing generally, has started to become popular. We suspect it surfaced as more became known about the possible dangers of mercury amalgam fillings and also fluoride added to toothpaste and to the water supply. But first things first, all dentists agree that it starts with daily TLC…

The lovely thing about caring for your teeth is that it's not rocket science and day-to-day care is not costly. To keep your teeth and gums in mint condition, you should brush your teeth twice a day for two minutes each time, floss daily and avoid sugar in any form between meals, says Dr Hap Gill, a leading private dentist in London. But beware, most people brush too hard. 'It's a giveaway if the toothbrush head looks like a loo brush within a few days or weeks,' says Dr Gill. 'Hold the brush like a pencil and go round and round in little circles on the chewing surfaces of your teeth. The brush should be at a 45-degree angle towards your gum so the tufts are pressed into it.'

With the choice available, you might think you need a degree to choose the right toothbrush, so here's the lowdown…

● Choose a smallish manual brush with a medium texture, or soft if you've ever been told you brush too hard. We use toothbrushes with replaceable heads; it saves on the plastic handle (plastic comes from petrochemicals and is not recyclable). So hoorah for the Preserve range of toothbrushes for adults and children from Massachusetts company Recycline, with handles made of 100 per cent recycled polypropylene, plus packaging from renewable wood sources and 100 per cent recycled paper printed with soy inks. We also like Soladey-2, an ionic toothbrush from Japan with a titanium ionic conducting rod running through the bristle head into the handle, which (by a complex process we won't go into here) claims to kill bacteria in your mouth and also to remove intractable stains in weeks. Ionic toothbrushes claim to prevent plaque (which causes tooth decay) naturally, by breaking it down at a molecular level and there is some research to back this up. However, although manufacturers claim they work just as well without toothpaste, Dr Gill strongly advises using it.

● For the energy conservationists among you (ie, your energy), electric brushes work well because they have the optimum size and texture and most of the work is done for you. Dr Gill likes Braun's Oral-B Professional Care 5000 and the Oral-B Triumph with SmartGuide.

● Many dentists now agree that toothbrushes should be changed often because they harbour viruses and bacteria. If you're in good health, change the brush (or the head, see left) every four to eight weeks. If you're not well, change it at the first sign of infection, then every few days.

● To ensure a clean, fresh brush, back-to-nature girls can simply swill their brush in a glass of (pure) water with a couple of drops of tea tree oil. Techie types could invest in a toothbrush steriliser but some are quite complicated. We can manage VioClean's UV (as in ultraviolet) Toothbrush Steriliser, which looks like a pencil box: you rinse your brush and pop it in the box. Shut the lid and the ultraviolet is activated for about six minutes. *Très* simple!

● Tongue cleaners (aka scrapers) are important, too, particularly for anyone with bad breath. Try the bargain-priced – and effective – PitRok Tongue Cleaner or the more expensive (but also more aesthetically pleasing) Fushi Ayurvedic Tongue Cleaner.

● And finally, do floss; we like Desert Essence Dental Floss or the wider Dental Tape with antiseptic tea tree oil.

Fab idea…

The Natural Toothbrush, a stout 'twig' from the root of the araak tree, is rich in toothsome nutrients, said to whiten and strengthen tooth enamel. It's curiously satisfactory to use, leaving your teeth smooth and gums fresh. Because you cut off the end and peel back another layer every time you use it, there's no need to worry about germs. And if there's no shop open (or araak tree around), and you're without a dab of toothpaste, try baking soda or salt.

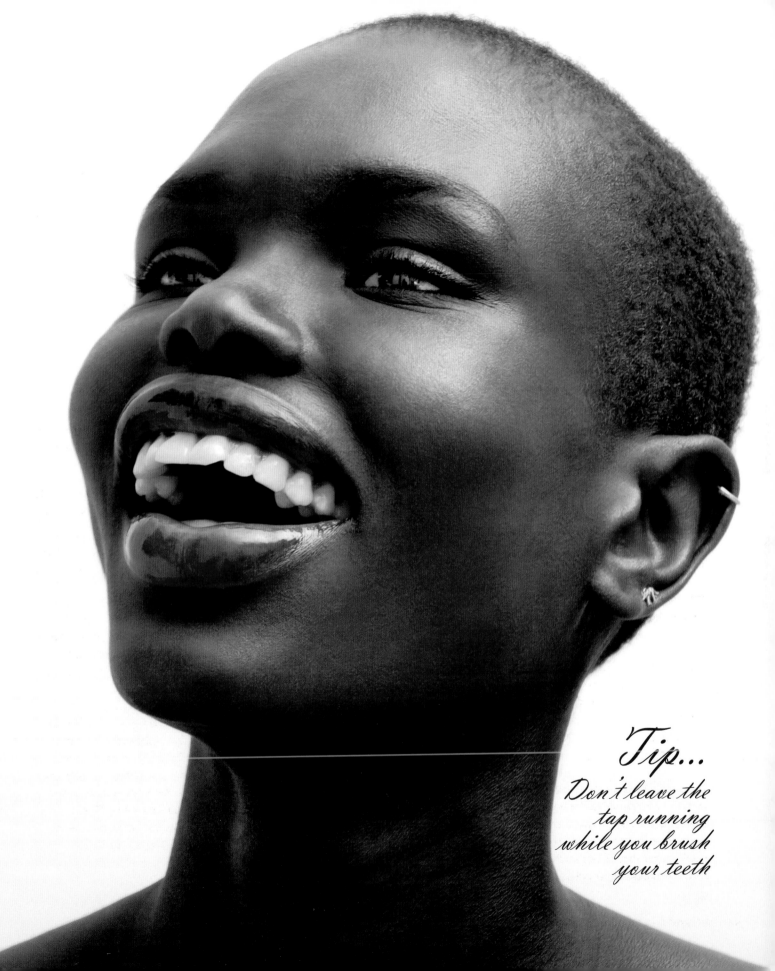

Tip...
Don't leave the
tap running
while you brush
your teeth

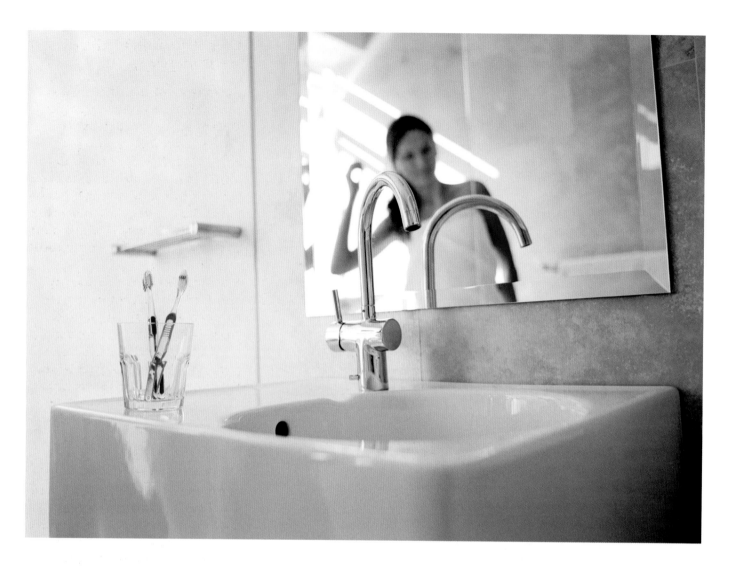

Toothpaste truths

There have been mutterings in the dental world for years about the chemical nasties in big-brand toothpastes. Remember, you use toothpaste twice a day, every day. It comes into direct contact with the mucous membrane in your mouth, so more substances are absorbed than in shampoo, for instance, which is mostly rinsed away. So we went shopping, scooped up all the big-brand toothpastes we could find in a local high street chemist and scoured the ingredients lists. Then we asked Professor Samuel Epstein of the University of Illinois at Chicago School of Public Health to comment on some of the main ones.

Apart from the fluoride that most pastes contain (see opposite), Professor Epstein identified three groups of ingredients which, he believes, are of concern.

● **Sodium lauryl sulfate (SLS)** A harsh detergent, used mainly as a foaming agent, SLS is a well-known irritant and can be a factor in mouth ulcers (see page 88). It is particularly unsuitable for children and anyone with an allergic problem such as skin sensitivity, asthma or hayfever.

● **PEG (polyethylene glycol) 6, 12 and 32** These compounds, mainly used as emulsifiers, are cancer-causing chemicals. Although the ethoxylate carcinogens can be removed during the manufacturing process by 'vacuum stripping', these ingredients should then be labelled as 'highly purified' or 'ethylene oxide free' – phrases that weren't on the products we bought.

● **Saccharin** This artificial sweetener, put in to make toothpaste more palatable, has been recognised as carcinogenic for more than 25 years, according to Professor Epstein.

The fluoride controversy

Fluoride, which is in 95 per cent of toothpastes (find it on the label as sodium fluoride and/or sodium monofluorophosphate), is a highly contentious issue. Pro-fluoride dentists say that the reduction in tooth decay in the past 20 years can be attributed to using these toothpastes (and in some areas fluoridation of the water supply). But one recognised problem is that swallowing too much fluoride while children's teeth are growing (up to seven years) is likely to lead to permanent brown mottling, which may lead to structural damage. This condition – called dental fluorosis – has been shown to affect nearly half of children who drink fluoridated water.

Although there are clearly benefits in using topical fluoride (a 24 per cent reduction in caries), researchers admit there has been little or no investigation into the side effects of using a highly toxic product. Some experts claim that fluoride, a by-product of fertiliser manufacture, can impair the way your immune systems works, and that even low doses may provoke stomach problems and headaches. It may be that eating a healthy diet, with much less sugar and acidic foods and drinks, would produce the same benefits as fluoride.

In America, there is a warning on every tube of fluoride toothpaste: 'In case of accidental ingestion, seek professional assistance or contact a poison centre immediately.' Dr Joseph Mercola (a campaigning American physician) says there is enough fluoride in a typical tube of toothpaste to kill two small children if they consumed the whole tube at once: 'This really isn't rocket science,' he writes on his website. 'If it kills you in large doses, doesn't it stand to reason that in smaller doses it probably is not a wise choice?'

Fluoridating the water supply is mass medication without our permission. A recent review by the US Environmental Protection Agency (EPA) found that the safe limit for added fluoride in water is zero, saying that fluoride can weaken bone and increase the risk of fractures, disrupt your hormones (it's linked to thyroid problems) and may affect brain function and behaviour. A UK expert committee (the York Review) stated that, so far, the scientific evidence worldwide does not prove either benefit or safety.

Tip... Chew on a clove to relieve toothache: clove oil kills the pain naturally

Our favourite natural toothpastes

We like the WalaVita holistic dental-care range (with the same parent company as Dr Hauschka). Lemon & Salt Toothpaste makes your mouth feel incredibly clean and fresh; the slightly salty taste stimulates saliva, which helps rinse out your mouth and helps oral hygiene. Neem & Mint Toothpaste (not suitable for children) has a gentler taste and also contains essential oils of clove and camomile. There's a super-refreshing Sage Mouthwash too.

The cheaper Weleda range, also truly natural, includes a Salt Toothpaste, plus a peppermint-free Calendula version for anyone taking homoeopathic medicines. There's also a Ratanhia Toothpaste (a gum-strengthening herb), and gentle Plant Gel Toothpaste with camomile, which is a good one to start with if you're switching from a conventional brand. Oh, and there's a Children's Tooth Gel, too, formulated especially for milk teeth.

NB: in the first edition of this book, we said we wanted to find a really natural toothpaste with xylitol, the natural sweetener that actually strengthens teeth and helps prevent decay, as well as supporting bones. Well, we have. It's Xyliwhite by NOW foods, a fluoride-free toothpaste gel with xylitol.

Bright green whiteners

Home tooth-whitening kits use hydrogen peroxide, which may aggravate gum disease and cause sensitive teeth, or even chemical burns to the mouth. Recently, the UK Trading Standards Institute found that, in 18 out of 20 home kits, the levels of hydrogen peroxide were up to 230 times higher than the permitted amount. We use Dental Miracle, an all-natural green powder with orris root, juniper berry, peppermint, calendula and acacia gum, for making teeth bright and clean, and breath fresh.

FOODS TO KEEP YOUR TEETH AND MOUTH HEALTHY

We know that some foods, notably sugar, do dreadful things to your teeth, likewise the acid in citrus fruit, vinegar and fruit teas. So it makes sense that there might be some that are good for your teeth and mouth too. Here are five of the top tooth-food fairies!

Cheese is excellent for neutralising acids quickly. When you eat or drink anything sugary, the bacteria in your mouth turn the sugar into acids, which sit on your teeth and cause decay. Saliva can neutralise these acids but it takes two hours; cheese speeds up the process. Try eating a small cube of cheese at the end of every meal. If you do want to eat something sweet, eat it all in one go rather than spreading it out over hours; that way, the acid sits on the teeth for two hours rather than many more.

Very dark chocolate Cacao mass extract (CM), the main ingredient in chocolate, contains some anti-caries substances. These are negated by the sugar in most choccie bars but if you choose very dark (75–85 per cent) chocolate, you should get much of the benefit with little of the risk. Remember: to enjoy chocolate best, let a square melt on your tongue.

Quality water

Tap water contains a cocktail of chemicals you may not really want to drink. If you do not have a purified water system in your home, try at least to filter your drinking and cooking water. Jo's husband Craig Sams, currently chairman of The Soil Association, recommends the Pozzani Reverse Osmosis systems. He also suggests investing in Pozzani's TDS (Total Dissolved Solids) meter, which tells you when you need to change the filter.

Strawberries, plums and pears contain xylitol, a compound that helps prevent bacteria sticking to teeth. You can also use xylitol as a natural sweetener in place of sugar (for this, it's mainly derived from corn cobs). Brands we like are Perfect Sweet and ZyloSweet. Xylitol doesn't raise insulin levels so is suitable for diabetics, is proven to help fight tooth decay and is good for bones. It also helps to alkalise the digestive system and, because it leaves a sweet aftertaste on your tongue, doesn't set up sugar-type cravings.

Wine A regular (small) glass of red or white helps prevent tooth decay, gum disease and sore throats, according to Italian scientists, who say that wine has germ-killing ingredients. (They used supermarket valpolicella and pinot nero, so it doesn't have to be vintage.)

Yoghurt Research shows that eating a small pot of natural live yogurt with 'good' bacteria, such as *lactobacilli*, for two weeks can get rid of bad breath by neutralising the 'bad' bugs that produced the noxious fumes.

Fab idea... For a guilt-free treat, dip strawberries in melted dark chocolate

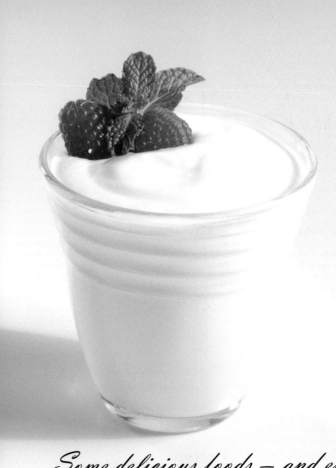
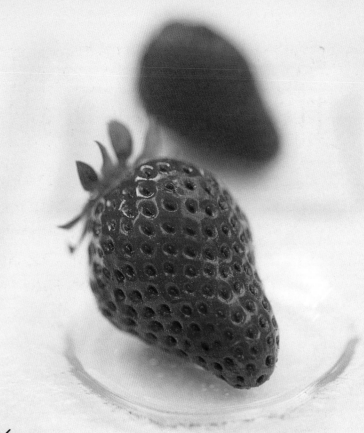

Some delicious foods — and even red wine — are positively good for your teeth, say dentists

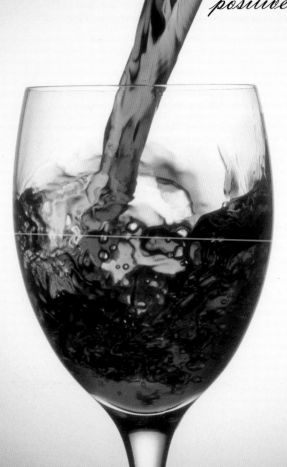
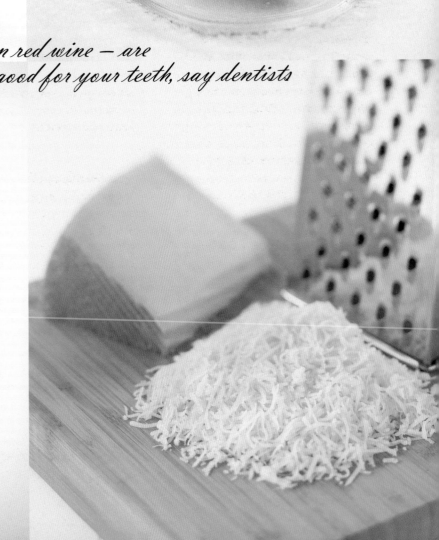

natural ways to
TREAT MOUTH ULCERS

Mouth ulcers are very common and often extremely painful because the ulcer is actually an exposed nerve in the sensitive lining of your mouth. They aren't contagious (unlike cold sores), but lots of people don't want to go out and be social with mouth ulcers, because they feel so painful. But there are effective natural ways of treating them

No one knows exactly why mouth ulcers erupt but there are several possible causes.

● SLS (sodium lauryl sulfate), a common agent in toothpaste: research shows that people prone to ulcers can recover completely by using SLS-free toothpaste.
● Too vigorous tooth brushing.
● Hormonal flurries, including periods, pregnancy and menopause.
● Low immune system/stress.
● Infection, both fungal and viral, including oral thrush.
● Gut problems, including irritable bowel syndrome and ulcerative colitis, can cause outbreaks. Dr Hap Gill refers patients with recurring mouth ulcers for blood tests to see if there is a gastrointestinal condition or anaemia.
● Deficiency in B vitamins, particularly vitamin B12.
● Food allergies or intolerances: many people are intolerant or allergic to gluten, the protein found in grains, including wheat and barley. This is now known to be a common trigger of mouth ulcers, others include spicy foods, tomatoes and even dairy foods. Nutritionist Dr Marilyn Glenville (www.marilynglenville.com) says this is an important connection, which is often overlooked.
● Dental braces.

The mercury menace

Sarah has been investigating mercury in dental fillings since the mid-1990s for newspapers and television (at the instigation of several dentists) and is appalled at what she has found – and the extent of the denial by the dental establishment. We're amazed that a substance that is known to be a potent neurotoxin – and that dentists can only handle with gloves and keep in sealed containers – is used in our mouths (although some countries are now phasing it out).

The issue is this: some people – one estimate is three per cent of the population – are susceptible to the effect of mercury, which may leech out of fillings. So some experts believe these fillings should not be used in anyone, particularly pregnant women, as research shows the mercury could reach the baby. You can have mercury replaced with 'biocompatible' materials (such as white composites), but you need to be careful as the mercury vapour can escape at this point. Consult a dentist who is experienced in amalgam removal and ask him/her to explain the protocol for protecting you from inhaling mercury vapour – and the nutritional measures you should follow beforehand, such as taking antioxidants and charcoal tablets. (For more information, visit www.mercuryfreedentistry.org.uk)

Remedies

● Use an SLS-free toothpaste (see page 85).
● Try to identify problem foods and avoid them completely, suggests Marilyn Glenville.
● Take a good vitamin B complex supplement, such as Solgar Megasorb B-Complex.
● Try Gengigel, which comes as a gel or mouthwash and contains hyaluronic acid plus xylitol. It takes up the moisture in the ulcer and squeezes it out, according to Dr Gill.

● Infuse some camomile tea, let it cool, then swoosh around your mouth before swallowing.
● You could also try remedies containing echinacea, myrrh or liquorice with the glycyrrhizic acid removed (DGL or deglycyrrhizinated liquorice).
● If your ulcers are no better after around two weeks, go to your dentist so you can rule out a serious underlying condition.

TOOTH TIPS FOR PREGNANT MUMS

Looking after your teeth is vitally important for pregnant women. We asked top London dentist Dr Hap Gill, who runs a pregnancy advisory service, to advise

More than half of pregnant women are affected by dental problems, but they get little advice even though they can seriously affect the health of the baby, according to Dr Gill. 'Hormonal changes during pregnancy can significantly affect the health of teeth and gums, as well as stress, trauma, infection and vitamin deficiencies.' Eating really well is vital, he emphasises, and it's worth considering a good multivitamin and mineral supplement.

Even women who have perfect oral health can suddenly have problems in pregnancy, says Dr Gill. 'Two huge factors, which are often overlooked, are morning sickness and gastric reflux. Acid from the stomach can totally dismantle even a well-cared-for mouth. It's like giving your teeth an acid

bath and can turn them from a rock-like consistency to chalk. Sugar cravings add to the problem.' If you have prolonged morning sickness or reflux, his advice is to rinse out your mouth with lots of water immediately after, and not to brush teeth for an hour. This is a high-risk category for tooth decay so do visit your dentist regularly.

Inflammation of the gums (gingivitis) is common. Gums become red and swollen, may bleed easily and feel sensitive or sore. Pregnancy gingivitis usually starts around the second month and reaches its peak around the eighth. As hormones start to fall in the ninth month, inflammation usually subsides.

If pregnancy gingivitis is neglected, however, it can lead to a chronic infection (periodontitis), which may result in premature

birth and low birth weight. It can also cause tooth loss in the mother. It's vital to brush teeth twice daily and become a world champion flosser. 'A pregnant woman often sees blood when she brushes her teeth – an early sign of gum disease – then gets scared and stops brushing,' says Dr Gill. 'But blood is nature's way of telling you: "Clean here." If you don't brush, bacteria are left between your teeth, which can cause plaque and tartar.' It's important to see a hygienist regularly to remove deposits. Rinsing with warm salt water can help soothe inflamed tissues.

During her pregnancy, actress Anna Friel suffered bleeding, warty sores on her gums between her teeth. 'Doctors kept telling me it was fine, but a gum specialist said I had to get them cut out so the infection didn't get to the baby,' she said. Dr Gill says these pyogenic granulomas affect about one per cent of pregnant women, and are an exaggerated response by the immune system to plaque and tartar build-up between teeth.

Ulcers and blood blisters can also affect women during pregnancy, due to a range of causes including sharp foods or harsh brushing, which can tear the salivary ducts of the gums. Blood and saliva can then leak into the gums and cause swelling. If any problem continues for more than two weeks, it is essential to see your dentist or doctor. Anyone who is near a baby or toddler should make sure their mouths are in good shape as they can pass on the organisms that cause problems through vapour from breath or by kissing.

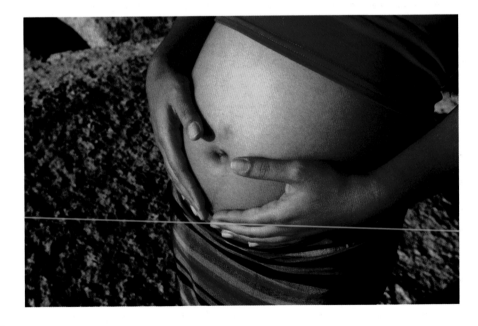

Tip... Help beat bad breath by chewing fresh mint or parsley

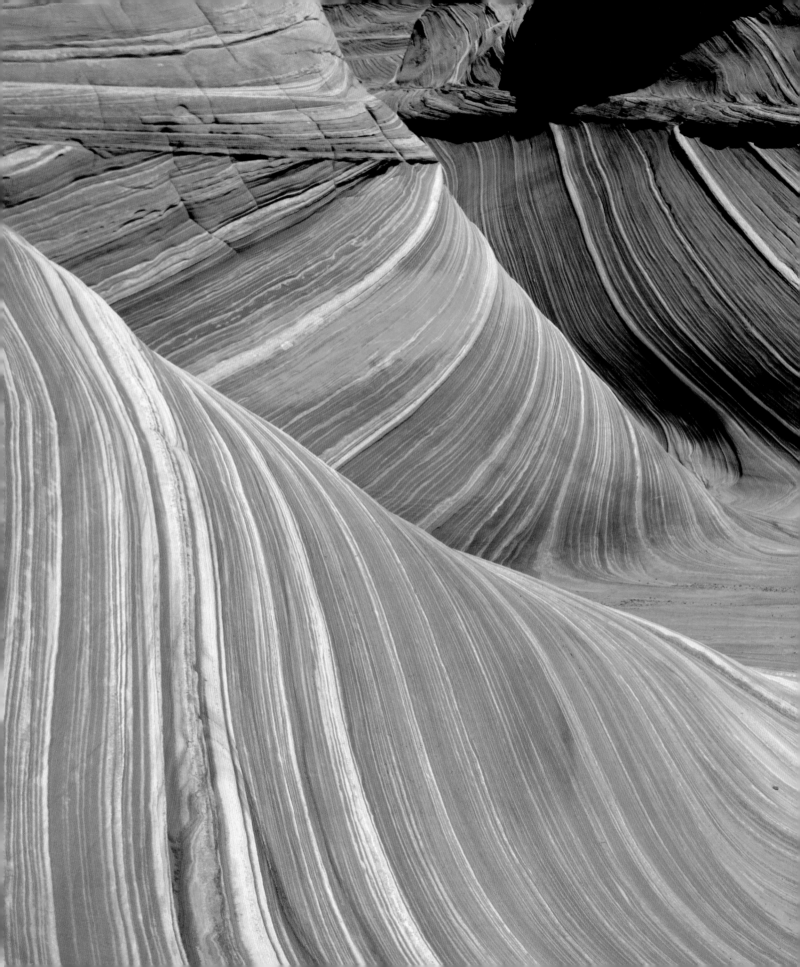

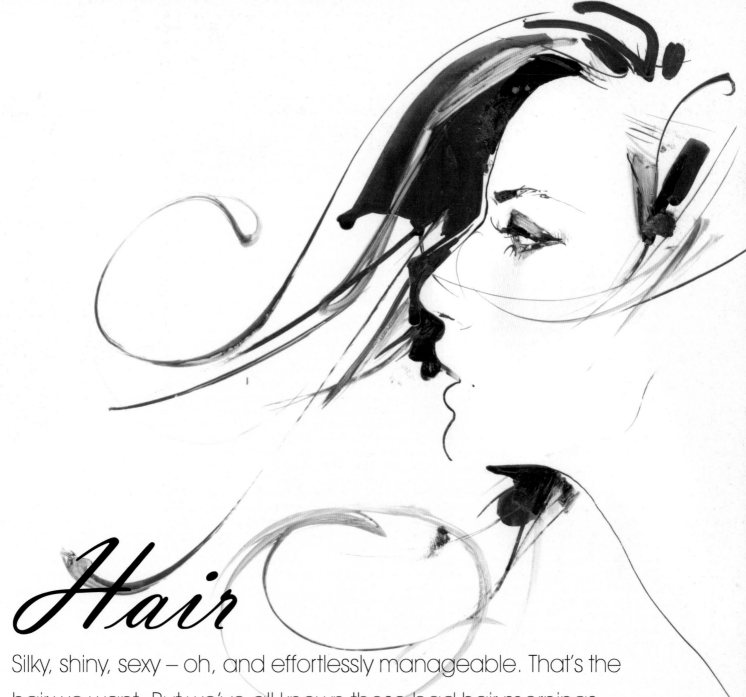

Hair

Silky, shiny, sexy – oh, and effortlessly manageable. That's the hair we want. But we've all known those bad hair mornings when the only solution seems to be to pull a cloche hat down to your nose. In this chapter, we give you the solutions: how to nourish your tresses to glossy, bouncy perfection, de-stress your scalp and work with the nature of your hair.

NATURALLY GORGEOUS HAIR
the healthy way

In a perfect world, you'd look in the mirror every morning and be thrilled with your hair. But in reality, you're not about to make your hair into a second career

Like us, you probably have better things to do than spend 45 minutes scorching your curls into submission with a blow-dryer – or, conversely, forcing body into limp locks. Even just ten minutes a day spent hairstyling adds up to 60 hours a year. That's more than a working week! No wonder most women we know complain that they don't have enough time to do the things they want to do!

The answer isn't rocket science. If you want to minimise the amount of time you spend on your hair, explains John Masters (the world's first 'organic hairdresser', whose Manhattan salon is a must-stop for all eco-beauties, see page 104), 'You basically have to go with what nature gave you. The reason women end up spending so long on their hair is simple: they fight nature. If you have curly hair, find a way of styling it that enables you to live with the wave. If you have straight hair, just think about all the women who spend hour upon hour each month trying to achieve what you are naturally blessed with.'

Otherwise, John adds, you will spend a fortune on products – not to mention on electricity bills as you plug blow-dryers, straightening irons or curling tongs into the power grid. And all that time, lost for ever… So, as with most things in beautyland, we'll be so bold as to suggest a little acceptance. A good hairdresser can give you a low-maintenance cut, which allows you to style your hair – whatever your natural hair type – with the minimum of time and product, yet still look great. Our years of experience have told us: the best investment you can possibly make is in a fantastic haircut. The very, very best you can afford; it's worth it, every time. We are both utterly devoted to John Frieda, where all stylists are encouraged to do life drawing and sculpture, to they can really look at bone structure – and so give a haircut that flatters the individual, and isn't just inspired by whichever celebrity happens to be on the cover of *Vanity Fair*.

You may have to learn to let your curls be curls. Or live with your poker-straight hair. But trust us: with a great cut, gentle, shine-boosting products and hair-friendly nutrition (see page 94), life can still be one long Happy Hair Day.

'The secret of a good fringe is to cut it yourself in one go, with kitchen scissors. Hold a knot in front of the eyebrows' 'FRINGE QUEEN' JANE BIRKIN

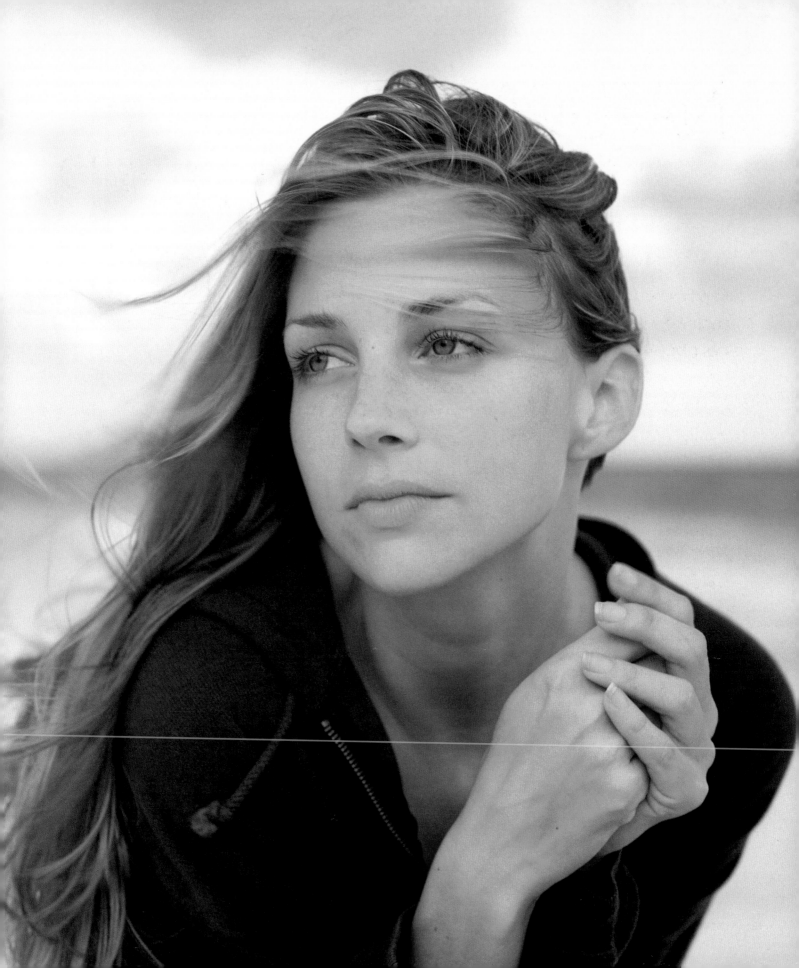

HAIR'S THE FACTS

Your hair really is a barometer of your state of health, both physical and emotional – your tresses won't be glorious if you're stressed out. Here's the lowdown on keeping up your hair – from the inside out

Really it's a wonder that we all look as good as we do when you think of the number of factors that can affect your hair – from eating poorly, sleeping badly, and not drinking enough water (as usual!), to hormonal imbalances and feeling bad about yourself (which, of course, gets worse as the only option seems to be to hide your hair under a paper bag).

By the time you can see it, the strange thing is that your hair is actually dead. Which means it's really important to keep your scalp – where the hair is still living in the follicle – in good nick. So what can we do to keep our hair and scalp in peak condition?

FEED YOUR FOLLICLES

Hair is made of a protein called keratin (the same as nails and skin). Now protein, not surprisingly, needs to be nourished by a protein-rich diet plus plenty of vitamins and minerals. That doesn't mean huge steaks daily – though a little lean red meat, twice a week, is good for your iron\levels, which help hair – but it does mean eating a good helping of protein daily. So aim to eat plenty of these foods below, advises nutritionist Kathryn Marsden – they are brilliant for your general health, too:

● Fresh oily fish (salmon, mackerel, trout, tuna, herrings, sardines, whitebait, anchovies, pilchards, etc); lots of fresh organic vegetables (particularly dark green leaves); salads and fruit (especially figs and dates); pulses (peas, beans and lentils); natural live yoghurt; cold-pressed oils (olive, hemp and walnut); seeds (linseed, sunflower, pumpkin and sesame); wholegrains (brown rice and oats); sea vegetables (kelp, nori, wakame, etc – find them dried in health food stores and sprinkle them over savoury dishes). For lots of good ideas, visit www.whfoods.org

● Drink lots of still pure water – eight large glasses between meals (yes, we know we've said it before…).

● Avoid too much cow's milk or cheese (especially if you have dandruff), also excessive sugar, salt, caffeine, saturated and hydrogenated fats, and processed foods.

● And please don't smoke! (Apart from making you very ill, smoking dries out your hair and makes it smell revolting.)

DESTRESS YOUR TRESSES

Massage your scalp, neck and shoulders. Tightness in these areas can affect blood supply and thus the health of your scalp. Ideally, you want the skin on your scalp to be mobile, like that on your face – try it now, if you're tense or stressed you won't be able to move it at all. Anyone can massage their head (see page 30 for details) and we bet you'll find you love it: we're addicted to it. (And it's the quickest headache-buster and re-energiser ever.) It also loosens dead skin cells and, according to some men, encourages hair growth even on bald/ing areas. (In India, it has been standard practice for millennia; the late John F Kennedy was a devotee and Sarah, when she worked on the men's magazine *Esquire*, interviewed former Labour politician Bryan Gould, who swore that it worked, especially with his head turned upside down – the blood

How to give dandruff the brush-off

For dandruff or other scalp conditions, integrated medicine expert Dr Mosaraf Ali recommends avoiding yeast products and citrus fruits as well as coffee, alcohol, excess salt and sugar. He also suggests using a neem-based shampoo. People with very dry hair and skin should eat plenty of oily fish or consider a fish oil supplement, he says.

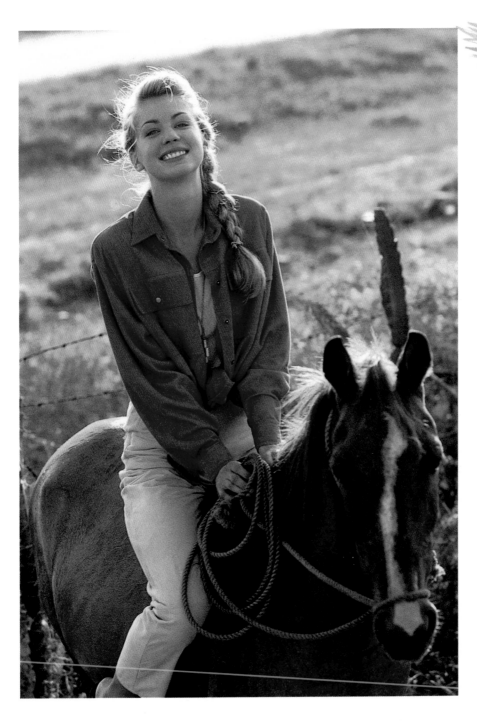

Tip... **For complete protein in a tiny portable package, eat six or so whole almonds daily. Soak them in room temperature water for 24 hours (to help the body absorb the nutrients easily), then peel and nibble through the day.**

to help you fall asleep,' he suggests.

The 4-7-8 Relaxing Breath Exercise (which is on his website www.drweil.com) is utterly simple, takes little time, needs no equipment and can be done anywhere. Although you can do the exercise in any position, it's best to sit with your back straight while learning it.

The only slightly tricky bit is the position of your tongue. You need to put the tip against the ridge of tissue just behind your upper front teeth, and keep it there throughout the entire exercise. You will be exhaling through your mouth around your tongue. This can feel strange at first but it soon comes naturally. Pursing your lips slightly may help.

● Exhale completely through your mouth, making a whoosh sound.
● Close your mouth and inhale quietly through your nose to a mental count of four.
● Hold your breath for a count of seven.
● Exhale completely through your mouth, making a whoosh sound to a count of eight.
● This is one breath. Now inhale again and repeat the cycle three more times for a total of four breaths.

The exact time you spend on each phase of the exercise is not important but the ratio of 4:7:8 is. If you have trouble holding your breath, speed up the exercise but keep to the ratio of 4:7:8 for the three phases. With practice you can slow it all down and get used to inhaling and exhaling more and more deeply.

rushes to it, that way, increasing the effect.) **Manage stress and relax with a regular breathing exercise.** We swear by exercise to calm us down and pep us up – walking, riding and yoga, in particular. The common factor? You breathe well and live in the moment. If you can't get out – and in fact

even if you can, this is worth doing – try this breathing exercise, which integrated health expert Dr Andrew Weil recommends everyone to do twice daily, all your life. 'Use it whenever anything upsetting happens – before you react. Use it whenever you are aware of internal tension. Use it

SCHEHERAZADE GOLDSMITH

We loved Sheherazade's book, *A Slice of Organic Life* (imagine John Seymour's *Self-Sufficiency* – the bible for seventies sustainable living – fused with *Vogue*). And we especially like the realistic approach this beautiful mother of three takes to 'greening' her lifestyle

I came to the organic and green movements as someone who hadn't previously thought about either. I'd grown up on the King's Road and all I cared about was going out and going shopping. I was always a 'why, why, why?' sort of child, and when I met my husband (environmental campaigner Zac Goldsmith) I didn't instantly accept all his green proposals. I wanted to see the evidence – and I still do. It was while I was pregnant that I really started to think about what I was eating – suddenly being responsible for someone else. Now I'm the kind of person who's always asking, 'Why does this supermarket apple look so shiny?', 'Why do we have strawberries in November?'

I never buy things that are 'in fashion'. I choose things I fall in love with, and wear them till they fall apart. If you do that, everything magically goes with everything. Mostly, I'm a jeans girl – usually up to my knees in mud.

I use natural cosmetics where possible but I still mix and match. I'm a huge fan of Jane Iredale's mineral make-up. I discovered it through my dermatologist, Dr Nicholas Lowe, who I went to when I developed adult acne. I was convinced that using the powders would make me look like a New York granny – but they sink in beautifully and don't block the pores, which is important if you have acne. My trick if I'm going out is to apply my make-up, then sit in a steamy bath for 20 minutes.

I use MOP shampoo and conditioner, but I mix and match with less natural stuff like Philip Kingsley hair Elasticizer. Nobody's perfect. You've just got to do what you can, and feel good about it.

My big guilty un-green secret used to be my car: a gas-hungry Golf. Eventually it blew up – but I waited till then to replace it. There's no point replacing a perfectly good car with a more eco-friendly option until you really have to, because so much of a car's carbon footprint is related to the energy used manufacturing it. I desperately wanted to go for the latest turbo fuel-injection Golf, but I thought I'd better get a hybrid, so – rather grumpily – I went to the Toyota garage and bought a Prius [electric hybrid car]. And now I love it: it's roomy, and I feel very smug not having to pay the congestion charge.

I genuinely fear for the future of the planet, and the world we're creating for our children and grandchildren, if we don't make changes to the way we live. My argument is that even if you don't believe in the science – which I do – what do you have to lose by adopting a more eco-friendly lifestyle? I've gained pleasure from everything I've changed about my life – be it eating organically, buying my Prius, shopping at farmers' markets or the satisfaction of swapping a light bulb that's blown for one that's not going to need replacing for years.

'I've gained pleasure from everything I've changed about my life – be it eating organically or buying my Prius'

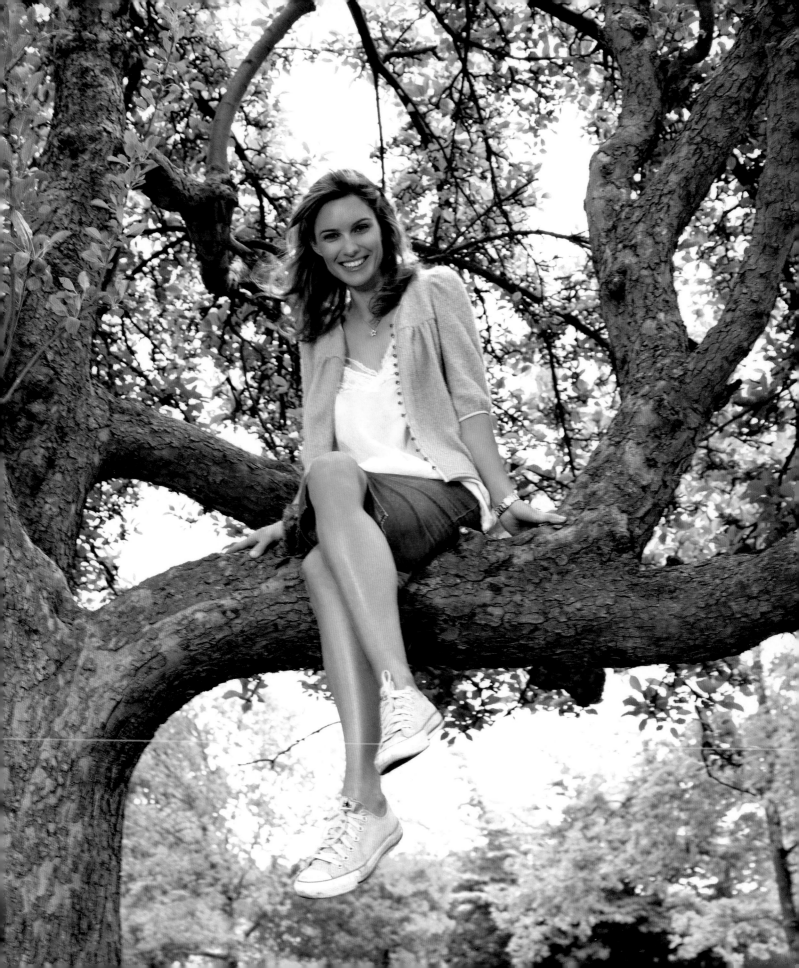

keep it clean

If you look at shampoo advertising, you'd be forgiven for thinking most shampoos come straight from a meadow or a rainforest. But truly natural shampoos are harder to find than hen's teeth…

A lot of shampoo advertising has us foaming at the mouth. A sprig of organic herbs wafted at a shampoo bottle, and brands create an aura of naturalness around their products, meanwhile stuffing them full of harsh detergents (like sodium lauryl sulfate, see below). And don't get us started on the mainstream brand that calls itself 'Organics'…

Daniel Galvin Junior and his sister Louise come from a hairdressing dynasty (their dad, Daniel Senior, used to be the Princess of Wales's colourist). So it created quite a stir in the Galvin household when both Daniel and Louise launched their own ranges – leaving out the foaming agent/detergent called sodium lauryl sulfate (SLS), which is used in so many mainstream haircare lines. 'My family eats organic food and wanted to use organic toiletries,' explains Daniel, 'but I couldn't find any. Many current shampoos contain potentially harmful chemicals such as SLS that not only damage your hair but also your skin and health. Alcohol is bad for hair, too, because it dries it out – yet it's a common ingredient in haircare. And SLS really dries out the scalp.' It's no wonder, believes Daniel, that hairdressers are seeing a plague of 'dry scalp' – and that isn't just a polite word for dandruff, which is a medical condition – but is simply that: dry scalp. (There's some evidence that SLS may cause hair loss, too, by attacking the follicles, and it is likely to irritate skin conditions such as

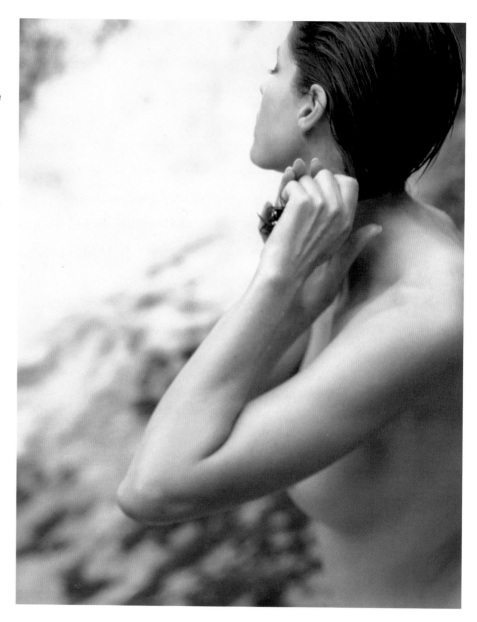

eczema, and may help to trigger asthma attacks too.)

Meanwhile, shampoo commercials – and many hair gurus with a vested interest in selling gallons of shampoo – also have you believe that daily washing is a must. Maybe it's necessary sometimes if you live in an ultra-polluted town – but, to be frank, commercial shampoos seem designed for the purpose of excessive use. Just as using a harsh toner on skin turbocharges oil production, over-washing the hair will strip away the scalp's natural, protective oil barrier – often causing irritation, and a subsequent increase in the production of that oil. So you think you need to wash your hair again… It's a vicious circle.

If you feel you need to wash your hair daily, or very frequently, we would steer all of you away from shampoos based on sodium lauryl sulfate. And the trouble is that sodium laureth sulfate (SLES) – a widely used alternative which has a reputation for being kinder (just) – isn't necessarily the answer, either: 'laureth' ingredients (not just sodium but also ammonium laureth sulfate) can react with nitrogen to produce nitrosamines, which are potential carcinogens.

So what's a chick to do? With the vast numbers of products lining the shelves claiming to be 'natural', it can be daunting to know which ones really are. There are, alas, almost no 100 per cent perfect green and natural solutions. We have done our best here, trialling the gentler, more natural shampoos. But we're optimistic that this area of natural haircare development will grow over the next few years so we will have more choice.

Until recently, choosing whether or not to go with a natural shampoo boiled down to one question: how much do you like suds? But in reality, shampoos don't have to froth

like the cream on a knickerbocker glory to get hair perfectly cleansed. When you try a more natural shampoo (such as the ones listed on page 101), go by what you see in the mirror, and how your hair feels, and get over the idea that mega-foam equals good.

Certainly, we suggest that to maintain a balance and avoid an overreacting scalp, you may want to seek out haircare products that contain gentler washing agents perhaps based on corn or sugar derivatives (such as decyl glucoside,

> *'Many current shampoos contain potentially harmful chemicals such as SLS that not only damage your hair but also your skin and health'* **DANIEL GALVIN**

coco glucoside and lauryl glucoside).

We also suggest trying to cut down the frequency with which you wash your hair, if at all practical. This is beauty heresy – we'll probably be on some shampoo giant's hit list, after this. You may protest that washing less frequently won't work for you; you may even be on the verge of throwing this book across the room, but trust us: the scalp has its own natural balance, and too-frequent washing (then drying – with all the time and energy this gobbles up; also remember that drying is, well, drying) upsets this. With hair washing, you really may discover: less is more.

THE CASE AGAINST HAIR WASHNG

If you're feeling really radical, you could just give up washing your hair completely. Think we're nuts? Periodically, the press discovers the idea of going cold turkey on haircare, and puts someone on a shampoo 'diet' – most recently after UK newsman Andrew Marr said that he hadn't washed his hair for six weeks, yet his hair's condition had improved. The idea is that after a few fairly grim weeks – about six to eight – hair starts to rebalance. The natural fauna, flora and oils in the scalp settle down, so that hair becomes 'self-cleansing', provided you brush it a bit. As one tester reported (after the initial few weeks of hair hell), 'Over the next few weeks, the quality of my hair improved even more – it even started to look shiny. Also, my flaky scalp had completely disappeared.'

To be honest, this isn't really an option for us (though neither of us washes our hair more than a couple of times a week, max). Except when we're on holiday, we like to look a bit more styled and hopefully as chichi as people expect a beauty editor to! But – confession time – Jo's husband Craig hasn't washed his hair since 1967 (he does occasionally use mud treatments), and has a fine head of hair. On Craig's advice, two friends of ours – each with major haircare empires (so you won't get them shouting this from the rooftops) – also gave up washing their hair, and found that baldness began to reverse itself. Now this may be too daring a solution for even the greenest babe, but if the man in your life's losing his hair, what has he got to lose by trying it?

What we'd prefer not to find in our haircare

We essentially agree with John Masters (another of our heroes) as to what – in an ideal world – does not go into a natural haircare/styling product:

● no sodium lauryl sulfate;
● no parabens, DEAs, MEAs or TEAs;
● no GMOs (genetically modified organisms);
● no petrochemicals;
● no animal testing (of course);
● no artificial colours, fragrances or fillers;
● ingredients should be as organic as possible;
● all essential oils should be steam-distilled and not extracted with hexane, which may alter the effect of the oils;
● all ingredients should be as biodegradable as possible;
● Fairtrade ingredients should be used whenever possible;
● packaging should be recycled/recyclable.
We applaud the efforts of those companies striving towards this, but many brands aren't there yet.

HOLIDAY HAIR REPAIR

On the following pages, you'll read our Tried & Testeds for hair products that put back what shampoo takes out, leaving it smooth and shiny. Dr Hauschka – one of the pioneering natural brands – also recommend using their neem hair oil for tresses that are dull, dry, frizzy and weakened by sunshine, swimming and styling. The result, they say, is soft, manageable hair. Sarah also likes to use the Ayurvedic bhringaraj oil – by Pukka Herbs – in exactly the same way.

1 Before applying the oil, stimulate the blood circulation to the scalp: using both hands, fingers apart, start at the temples and move upwards towards the back of the head. Gathering as much hair as possible between the fingers, gently tug the hair upwards, away from the scalp.

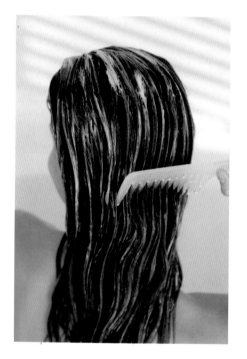

2 Apply oil to the fingers. Massage the oil into the scalp, using small, circular movements, starting at the hairline and working backwards to the base of the head. Cover as much of the scalp as possible. Really dig into the scalp as you massage so that you move the skin itself.

3 Finish by combing your fingers through the hair, from the hairline to the base of the head. Apply more oil to treat the hair, concentrating on the ends.

4 Wrap your hair in a warm towel and leave for 30 minutes or overnight. Wash out with shampoo (it may be necessary to wash and rinse twice), then follow with conditioner.

We love...

Everyone always said it would be impossible to create an organic shampoo that foamed: only chemicals make froth. But the small mother-and-daughter brand Essential Care proved them wrong, and ever since, Jo's been devoted to their Gentle Herb Shampoo, which foams perfectly, leaves hair silky and, a world first, is organically certified by The Soil Association. After trialling Fushi natural shampoos and conditioners for several months, Sarah – who has a thick mane of often strawlike long hair – is very impressed. Her faves are Total Repair Herbal Shampoo and Repair & Soothe Herbal Conditioner.

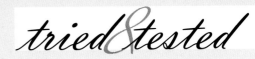

SHAMPOOS

There's a new 'green hair guru' in this category, voted for by testers who've now trialled more than 70 natural and more-natural options. Their verdict? Yes: a natural shampoo really can leave hair clean, shiny and manageable

✿ LOUISE GALVIN NATURAL LOCKS NOURISHING SHAMPOO FOR DRY/DAMAGED HAIR

Score: 8.28/10

Seems the Galvin family is greening the haircare world: talented haircolourist Louise is the sister of Daniel Jr – who already has a shampoo entry in this category. This reasonably priced 'sister' to Louise's (pricey) Sacred Locks range performs brilliantly, according to our testers. In this shampoo targeted at thirsty hair, find Pro-vitamin B5, sweet almond extract and vegetable proteins, plus gentle cleansers. We love the chic black-and-white bottles, and that Louise has off-set all carbon emissions through The Carbon Neutral Company.

Comments: 'Ten out of ten! It transformed hair washing from a misery to a pleasure, as my hair knots so easily' • 'tricky at first, as it's quite runny; once I got the hang of it, it was fine: easy to rinse out, left hair squeaky clean, shiny, bouncy, silky and light' • 'no irritation to my occasionally itchy scalp' • 'great results – though needed conditioner too' • 'smells lovely – reminds me of a chocolate orange...'

✿✿ LOGONA GINGKO REPAIR SHAMPOO

Score: 8.12/10

This German brand was a player in the natural beauty market long before it became a twinkle in the eye of the Estée Lauder and L'Oréal empires; the whole Logona range

is certified natural by the European BDIH scheme (see page 209). Alongside the cleansing agents such as coco glucoside, from coconut, Logona offer a 'phyto-active' complex of calendula, silk protein and wheat bran extract, formulated to restore even dry, damaged hair. The fragrance comes from pure essential oils. Testers loved it.

Comments: 'The best shampoo I have used, giving a lovely shine and cutting down on the frizzies' • 'pleasant smell and did a good job' • 'foams well; made hair smoother, with healthy gloss, and it felt really clean' • 'gave hair body and washed out well' • 'delivered a shine on my not-so-shiny hair!'

★ ✿ DANIEL GALVIN JUNIOR HAIR CLINIC ORGANIC HAIR JUICE

Score: 8.06/10

This winner from Daniel is based on sodium coco sulfate (an ingredient not a million miles from sodium lauryl sulfate, but less refined and less irritating). Accessibly priced, this frequent-use shampoo comes in Honeydew Melon and Ginger & Lime.

Comments: 'I normally dread washing my long hair, but I really enjoyed using this because of the wonderful fragrance; it left my hair beautifully clean and gave it more volume and bounce' • 'very effective; left my hair squeaky clean with no hint of residue, nicely shiny and smooth; easy to put a comb through too' • 'smell and texture great and my hair looked really shiny and healthy'.

✿✿ LABEL.M ORGANIC MOISTURISING LEMONGRASS SHAMPOO

Score: 7.77/10

Toni & Guy go organic! Yeehaw! Creative director Sacha Mascolo-Tarbuck has overseen this project to create a 'green' range, with organic credentials certified by the USDA/NOP. The daily-use shampoo is free of sulfates, and contains organic linseed, blackcurrant seed oil, jojoba, shea butter, rice milk and soya milk powder.

Comments: 'The best-smelling shampoo I've ever used; posh packaging, and left my hair squeaky-clean' • 'liked the delicate lemony fragrance; lathered well, and rinsed out easily; very moisturising' • 'really shiny, glossy hair – several nice comments! The bottle is lasting for ages' • 'my favourite out of the ones I tested; scalp felt very refreshed'.

✿ ORIGINS CLEAR HEAD MINT SHAMPOO

Score: 7.75/10

Our testers loved the wake-up call delivered by this zingy entry, which owes its uplifting fragrance to a trio of essential oils: Brazilian mint, spearmint and *Mentha piperata*. Wheat proteins, which are renowned for their hair-smoothing action, feature in the formula.

Comments: 'My fine, usually lifeless hair had a lovely shine and was even bouncy – a miracle' • 'helped my itchy scalp' • 'loved the minty fragrance' • 'my frizzy hair felt clean and shiny' • 'my hair was revived and manageable – highly recommended'.

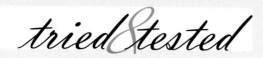

CONDITIONERS

We all dream of silky, lustrous hair, so conditioner is a beauty essential for many women. Happy days: our testers identified several new 'winners' in this category, out of over 50 'greener' conditioners now trialled. NB: this is still a challenging product to formulate in a 100 per cent pure way (look out for Jo's recipes for tress-shiners in *The Ultimate Natural Beauty Book*, for some suggestions...)

GREEN PEOPLE INTENSIVE REPAIR CONDITIONER

Score: 8.95/10

A magnificent score for this conditioner which smooths hair with organic jojoba, quinoa and B vitamins. Our testers trialled it as a slap-on-rinse-out conditioner, but Green People say you can also use it as a hair mask-style 'deep treatment'.

Comments: 'Loved the strong bergamot smell – soothing and refreshing; made my dark, curly hair nice and glossy' • 'my hair was tangle-free after' • 'hair softer, less mad, wiry and frizzy; definitely improved texture'.

NEAL'S YARD REMEDIES NURTURING ROSE CONDITIONER

Score: 8.5/10

The scent of rose helped seduce our testers with this 45 per cent organic concoction, enriched with coconut and olive oils, and antioxidant maple extract. It was 'bliss to use' and shine enhancing. There's a calendula infusion alongside the distilled roses.

Comments: 'Very nice, creamy texture which spread easily; hair felt very soft and bouncy for a couple of days' • 'didn't weigh hair down, was light and soft but not fluffy' • 'love that it's natural – my long hair gets assaulted with London fumes and gunk daily so I don't want to go home and put on more chemicals' • 'lovely rose fragrance and nice gloss, though might be expensive for my long hair' • 'left my hair smooth and shiny'.

ORIGINS CLEAR HEAD MINT CONDITIONING RINSE

Score: 8.18/10

A 'sister' to one of the top-scoring shampoos, this gel conditioner for normal-to-oily hair has a zesty trio of mints (Brazilian, spearmint and *Mentha piperata*), with hydrolysed wheat protein and panthenol to fight flyaways. It does contain silicones, which may build up.

Comments: 'Love the mint fragrance; gave a great shine; good for knots and easier to brush' • 'less static and no product left after rinsing' • 'a hit: wish I'd hidden it from my daughter!' • 'gave me sexy hair!'

FUSHI REPAIR & SOOTHE HERBAL CONDITIONER

Score: 8.1/10

Fushi take an inside-out approach to beauty: at their Harvey Nicks juice bar, they zhoosh up a super-hair-health smoothie. This top-end range uses high levels of active botanicals in products which are made in small batches. This conditioner includes soothing, healing calendula, with invigorating frankincense and neroli, avocado and sandalwood, to repair damage to hair and scalp.

Comments: 'Liked it straight away: ten out of ten for smell; combs through easily; easy to rinse and left hair glossy, shiny and smooth' • 'fab "good-mood" smell, lovely to use, hair feels silky' • 'gives great gloss' • 'practical, elegant packaging'.

★ DANIEL GALVIN JUNIOR HAIR CLINIC HANGOVER HAIR ORGANIC LAVENDER CONDITIONER

Score: 8/10

Daniel Galvin Junior's Hangover Hair – one of our star buys – is designed 'to detox and revitalise' even the most stressed-out tresses. It also comes in Lemongrass & Lime. (NB: the range is not certified organic.)

Comments: 'Good detangler and excellent for the price' • 'hair was more manageable and easier to comb' • 'pleasant fragrance and practical packaging' • 'brought my curly grey hair to fuller, shinier life; my husband commented on how nice it looked'.

AVEDA MOISTURIZING CONDITIONER

Score: 8/10

Aveda already has an entry in the Hair Masks category – see opposite – but this is the slightly lighter conditioning version, in the same (rather pricy!) range. Hair-nurturing ingredients include buruti oil (rich in vitamin A and EFAs), palmarosa, pomegranate – and there's a wonderful fragrance, from vanilla, rose geranium and ylang-ylang essential oils.

Comments: 'Only needed a small amount on my thick coarse hair to give a fantastic gloss, which made my hair dazzle under the lights' • 'made my hair shiny, manageable, hydrated and so glamorous! I wanted to stroke it, it looked so great.' • 'hair smoother and detangled on application; it can be frizzy but this made it silky and easier to blow dry'.

HAIR MASKS

We've never met a hairdresser who hasn't told us that one of the 'top tips for great hair' is to slather on a hair mask once a week. In this category, look for a sensational new number one entry among the rich, intensive, more natural hair masks now available...

❀ LOUISE GALVIN NATURAL LOCKS DEEP CONDITIONING TREATMENT

Score: 8.25/10

No sulfates, no parabens, no silicone, no petrochemicals, no synthetic fragrances or polymers – just lashings of good stuff for hair, including grapeseed oil, vegetable glycerine, jojoba, soy protein – all infused in a zesty way with uplifting citrussy essential oils. This is a second category winner for Louise in this book (her shampoo went straight in at number one in that section, too), and is also certified carbon neutral.

Comments: 'I really liked this conditioner, which is easy to apply; lovely fragrance; made hair shiny and healthy-looking; but do rinse out, comb through, and rinse again – one rinse and it can be a bit unmanageable after' • 'thick, creamy, almost wax-like consistency, really easy to work through; made hair smell fresh and clean' • 'managed frizz, and people commented on the shine and bounce; very effective at enhancing the different tones in my hair' • 'best to ends, not roots, as might be oily; worked best in the gym sauna'.

❀ JOHN MASTERS ORGANICS HONEY & HIBISCUS HAIR RECONSTRUCTOR

Score: 8.10/10

We'd be hard-pressed to find a hairdresser as committed to finding a more eco-friendly route to hair perfection as John Masters. His efforts have paid off with this bestseller (apparently loved by Alicia Silverstone and Sandra Bullock). The once-a-week deep treat is known in New York as 'the saviour of tired hair'. Alongside quality essential oils, it includes soluble sulphur. John also recommends it as a post-colour treatment, and as 'first aid' for dry or split ends. NB: the range is not, as yet, certified organic.

Comments: 'The best thing ever! My hair was transformed into glossy, weighty, swingy stuff – I looked as if I'd just come out of a very expensive salon' • 'I loved this – it smelt amazingly fruity: felt I should be eating it; made my thick, coarse hair feel soft, shiny and silky' • 'good for my frizzy hair' • 'liked the practical biodegradable plastic packaging'.

❀ AVEDA DAMAGE REMEDY INTENSIVE RESTRUCTURING TREATMENT

Score: 8/10

This moisturising formula is powered by certified organic ingredients, including quinoa protein, sandalwood, barley extracts, antioxidant sea buckthorn and alfalfa leaf powder, with a relaxing fragrance blended from essential oils of bergamot, mandarin and ylang-ylang.

Comments: 'Lovely! Dry, frizzy hair became sleek and shiny' • 'excellent to work through my long hair; gave a lovely gloss, more body – and hair stayed in place at long last' • 'I gained an extra day without washing, as it didn't weigh it down' • 'combing it through my fine hair was a dream and the gloss was fantastic' • 'smelt refreshingly of essential oils' • 'a miracle: made my fine, straight hair feel as if it had been professionally blow-dried'.

❀ PHYTOLOGIE PHYTOCITRUS MASK

Score: 8/10

From the French botanical hair specialists Phyto comes this deep tress treat, crammed with natural ingredients, including sweet almond protein, grapefruit extract and shea butter. It's designed to 'revitalise hair left dry by colouring and perming', say Phyto, by eliminating any alkaline residues. They say it works its magic in just two to five minutes.

Comments: 'Made my recently coloured hair feel thicker, glossier and brighter' • 'only needed a tiny dollop' • 'my thick, long hair became smooth and controllable'.

❀ MOP C-SYSTEM RECONSTRUCTING TREATMENT

Score: 8/10

This zesty orange-fragranced creation comes from a brand loved by the stars. It contains a mega-dose of vitamin C from papaya, grapefruit, mandarin, mango, lime and lemon – although overall, it's not quite as natural as those ingredients might suggest. Our testers loved it, though: one even gave it 11 marks out of ten.

Comments: 'My dry, brittle, lacklustre hair felt instantly revived – this is as good as having a professional treatment' • 'an excellent treatment that leaves hair glossy and manageable' • 'this is a life-changing product, truly amazing: it fixed my grey-hair trauma' • 'I will buy shares in the company' • 'I love the cheeky orange packaging'.

the organic HAIRDRESSER

John Masters is the original 'organic hairdresser'. With a salon on Manhattan's Sullivan Street, in SoHo, John very much pioneered the idea of natural – but chic – hairstyling

John's New York salon is a must-visit for wannabe green beauties: beautifully decorated, great sounds – and if you're lucky, you get to pet his rescue dog, Maya (with John, opposite). It's what John calls a 'clean-air' salon, where hairspray and nail polishes are banned. John explained to us that he caught the organic bug at the end of the 1980s: 'Watching friends die of Aids or get healthy too late pushed me to get healthy.' This inspired him to develop his own range of haircare and, later, body- and skincare – all with looks-good-on-the-bathroom-shelf packaging.

We asked him to share his natural styling tips:
● 'If you want to keep energy consumption to a minimum, leave your hair to air dry till it's around 75 per cent dry – then use a blow-dryer.'

● 'Towel-dry hair by patting it, not rubbing it, and hang your head upside down, ruffling hair to add body while it dries.'

● 'I recommend ionic dryers and brushes, which speed up drying time dramatically.'

● 'Hair will wilt if it's still warm when you finish styling. A shot of cool air helps set the style.' (The best dryers have a 'cool' button for that final whoosh.)

● 'A lot of women wash their hair every day because the style doesn't last, not because it's actually dirty. Instead, try spritzing your hair with a water mister, and restyle. You'll save a lot of time that way too.'

Be an ionic woman

A few years ago, Jo stumbled upon an amazing range of ceramic hairbrushes in Harrods' Urban Retreat. It was her first introduction to 'ionic' hairstyling: the ceramic barrels not only reflect hot air more effectively than other brushes but also produce less static and reduced frizz. The result? Shiny hair, with fewer flyaways. As you just read, John Masters recommends ionic technology, to keep drying and styling time to a minimum.

There are now many ranges of ceramic/ionic brushes, including one by John Masters himself, who offers them in three sizes. Aveda also make them, and there's a great range by another US company, Olivia Garden. In addition, several brands now make ionic hair-dryers (available from good suppliers). They all trumpet the word 'ionic' on the label, so that's the magic word to look for.

You kind of need to be a physicist to understand why ionic brushes and dryers are so effective at smoothing hair, but basically they produce a stream of negative (that's good!) ions (or molecules), which neutralise the dulling ions that build up on hair, and attract dust and grime. In addition, says John Masters, 'Negative ions have a positive effect on improving air quality. In my experience, they also provide tranquillity and refreshment. Negative ions are found in nature, specifically by waterfalls and oceans.' At John's salon, the stylists all use Farouk CHI ionic dryers. 'These not only produce negative ions,' explains John, 'but they also have the lowest EMF of all the dryers on the market.' (EMF is the electromagnetic field that is emitted from electrical appliances – not just hair-dryers but wireless networks, illuminated bedside clocks, etc.)

'I recommend ionic dryers and brushes, which speed up drying time dramatically' JOHN MASTERS

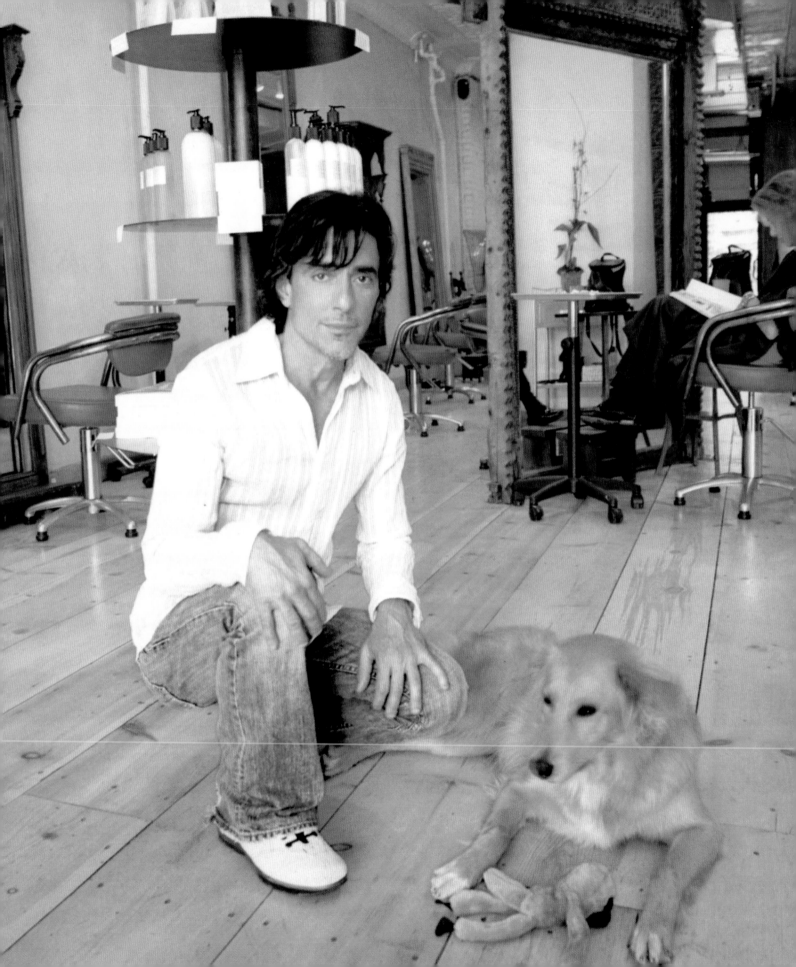

style file

We know that plenty of women resist replacing the anything-but-natural styling products in their bathrooms with 'eco' alternatives – no matter how natural the rest of their life has become – believing that nothing can be as good. But we're here to tell you, it's changing…

Those miraculous gloops and sprays – some of which contain ingredients that aren't a million miles from plastic – ensure one good hair day after another, making them hard to give up. But happily, thanks to innovations from companies such as John Masters, Aveda, Santé and ShiKai (in the States), you now don't have to abandon good hair days in the interests of saving the planet.

Natural styling products use aloe vera gel, for instance, to moisturise and hold hair. Plant waxes and gums aid styling, while a whole variety of plant oils add lustrous sheen and moisture. They may be packed with botanicals such as rosemary to give natural body, or horsetail and nettle to curl and strengthen hair. And instead of a cocktail of synthetic fragrance elements – there are up to a mind-boggling 200 in a single conventional hairstyling product – the essential

oils in natural styling products can positively boost hair and scalp health.

So far, we have to admit there isn't a vast choice if you want to go down the natural styling route. (But sometimes lack of choice can be a real relief, we find.) In fact, if you lined up all the truly botanically based options on the hairstyling fixture of your local drugstore, they'd occupy a tiny corner. That's why we didn't trial styling products for this book: there are not enough out there, right now. But we do list our own favourites.

Although there are relatively few salons using them, the numbers are growing – so keep your eyes peeled: we recently stumbled upon a tiny one in Brighton, called Cuttlefish, when we were walking through the Lanes (on the way to meet our wonderful illustrator David Downton, whose studio is there). Stylists increasingly appreciate them. 'The products aren't as heavy, and I don't get any more complaints from clients about the styling products irritating their skin or making them cough,' says Kathleen Nugent who has switched to vegan, chemical-free products at her Minneapolis salon.

So here's the lowdown on natural styling possibilities – and some tips on how to use the products…

Mousse

Mousse is light in weight and slips easily through hair, yet it holds very well – making it a breeze to apply. Squirt a dollop into your hand and apply with your fingertips to the scalp. As John Masters explains: 'Volume and hold really happen in the first half-inch of hair – that's what supports your style.' We love: Santé Natural Styling Mousse and Aveda Phomollient Styling Foam.

Gel

Heavier than a mousse, delivering longer-lasting hold and/or a more 'piece-y', textured look (in hairdresser-speak). Rub a small amount into your palms and distribute evenly through wet hair. Be sure to run your fingers through hair thoroughly and repeatedly, otherwise gel tends to clump where it's first placed. We love: Santé Natural Styling Gel and Aveda Confixor Liquid Gel.

Hairspray

With styles so natural these days (mercifully), we don't know many women who want their look finished with a solid fixing of spray. NB: although CFCs were banned some years ago, the propellants in hairsprays make them difficult to dispose of and non-recyclable. If you do use spray, the best way is to extend your arm as far as possible and spray from above the head, to distribute evenly. Even with 'nontoxic'

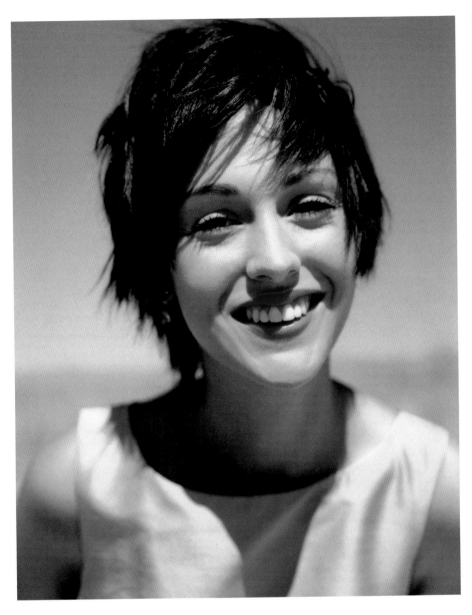

hairsprays, we advise you to hold your breath till the mist settles. We love… actually, we don't. Sorry. But we've heard good reports of MOP (Modern Organic Products) Firm Finish, which is scented with extracts of orange, mango and grapefruit and has (so they promise) 'zero environmental impact', and Aveda Witch Hazel Hair Spray, which says it gives a light-to-medium hold without stickiness or flaking – and of course it contains organically grown witch hazel.

Pomade/wax

This is the perfect product for the funky, chunky look that seems to have become a modern classic – adding control and 'definition' without stickiness. A little goes a long, long way: start with a pea-sized dollop (*un très petits pois* for fine hair), rub thoroughly between your palms and skim through hair, rubbing the ends between your fingers to define them. We love John Masters Organics Bourbon, Vanilla & Tangerine Hair Texturizer – it smells almost good enough to eat.

De-frizzers

We're not really wild about these, but then we don't suffer from the frizzies. Almost all de-frizzers are based on silicones, also known as dimethicone. These are pretty harmless, except that in time, some experts believe, silicones can build up on hair, making it dull – so that you're adding more and more product in an attempt to regain shine. In reality, you just need a teensy amount – the size of a pea, squirted into palms, which you then rub together and work through your hair. There is one stellar entry in the de-frizzing category from our previous books – and we thought the review for Aveda Light Elements Smoothing Fluid was worth repeating here. We love it too.

AVEDA LIGHT ELEMENTS SMOOTHING FLUID
Score: 8.8/10
At the heart of the Light Elements range is certified-organic lavender water, traditionally used in aromatherapy for its antibacterial properties, found here alongside organic jojoba oil, to help moisturise and condition, in a lightweight fluid. Several of our ten testers – not all with dry and/or frizzy hair – gave it full marks.
Comments: 'The best product I've used on my long, highlighted, fluffy hair – totally lives up to its promises' • 'gorgeous smell' • 'light, serum-like consistency is easy to spread on wet or dry hair – the best styling agent ever'.

COLOUR ME RISKY

Fact: most women of a greying age – or with mousy natural hair colour – feel a new surge of self-confidence if they gaze at a gorgeous, subtly-tinted-and-highlighted head of tresses. But is hair dye a case where feeling good might cost more than money?

We have our hair coloured. Have done for years, and probably always will. Jo has wonderful piece-y blond bits in her naturally dark hair and Sarah has a dark rinse plus highlights on her mid-brown hair, which is greying at the temples. We feel great about the results but less secure about some of the chemicals we're slapping on the thin skin of our scalps every six to eight weeks.

There are two main potential problems with hair dyes: they may cause an allergic reaction (which you're warned about on the packet) and they may increase the risk of certain cancers (which you're not). There's no argument that many of the chemicals used – both in the colouring agents (a lot of which come from petrochemicals and some still from coal tar) and other ingredients – are allergenic and may cause severe dermatitis. According to the FDA (the American regulatory body), hair dye reactions include hair loss, burning, redness, irritation and swelling of the face. A recent European Commission report, *Hair Dye Substances and Their Skin Sensitising Properties*, emphasises that 'many currently used hair dye substances are skin sensitisers, and this may be of concern for the health of consumers…often causing dermatitis'. The committee found 27 chemicals which they classified as skin sensitisers.

The problem is that you can be fine with a product for, say, 21 applications, then have an allergic reaction on the twenty-second The safe option is to do a patch test for sensitivity before every application of hair dye, both at home and in salons. (Put a dab of the exact product on your scalp behind the ear or inside your elbow, leave for two days, then look for itching, burning or other reactions.) It is vital when home colouring to follow the manufacturer's instructions to the letter – and the minute.

There have long been questions about the potential carcinogenicity of some chemicals used in hair dyes, particularly one called p-phenylenediamine (PPD) and related compounds. (The 'p' stands for para, but there are several other types of phenylenediamines used in dyes.) PPDs are most commonly found in brown and dark brown semi-permanent and permanent colours. As well as being a 'well-known and potent skin sensitiser', in the words of the EC Scientific Committee on Consumer Products, PPD is linked to an increased risk of various forms of cancer, including bladder cancer, non-Hodgkin's lymphoma, multiple myeloma, leukaemia, ovarian cancer and possibly breast cancer.

However, the evidence of carcinogenicity is confusing. Some large studies have revealed no extra risk but Professor Samuel Epstein, founder of the Cancer Prevention Coalition and one of the world's most knowledgeable scientists on the risks of environmental chemicals, attacks the accuracy of this research. He is clear that 'there is substantial evidence on the carcinogenic hazards of petrochemical hair dyes' with prolonged use. He emphasises that it's not only the colouring agents that are risky: 'There is a whole host of other ingredients – such as detergents and preservatives – which may be toxic or carcinogenic.' His advice? 'Avoid brown and dark brown hair colours, and look at the labels on others to make sure they don't have PPDs in them. There should be an outright ban on PPDs.'

Dr Stephen Antczak, co-author of *Cosmetics Unmasked*, believes that, while there is a risk, other environmental factors are much scarier. We're probably far more at risk of developing a chemically induced cancer through smoking, drinking alcohol or inhaling chemicals from household agents containing synthetic chemicals, paint fumes, aerosol deodorants, etc, he says.

One last thing: progressive hair dyes used to contain lead acetate, but lead and lead acetate have now been banned in hair colours.

If you do choose to reconsider the products you use to colour your hair, the only really natural brand we know of is Logona, which Professor Epstein approves of in terms of ingredients. However, John Masters tells us he's working on a natural colour range to compliment his organic hair care. We will put more details on the website when we have them, www.beautybible.com.

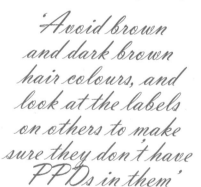

'Avoid brown and dark brown hair colours, and look at the labels on others to make sure they don't have PPDs in them'

PROFESSOR SAMUEL EPSTEIN

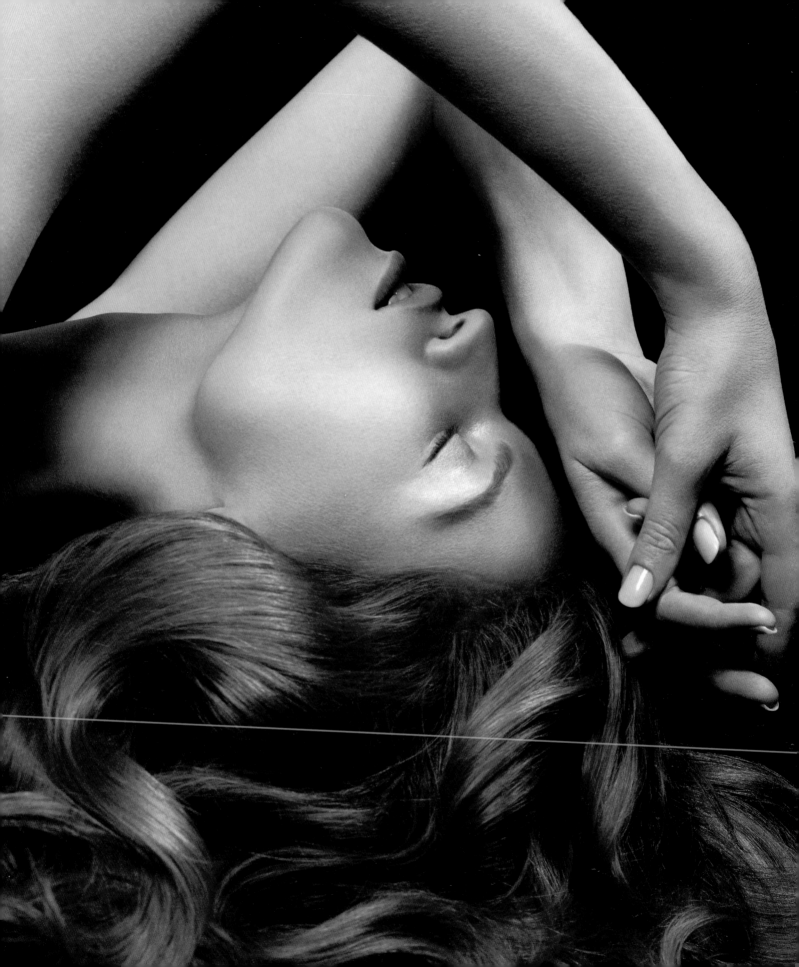

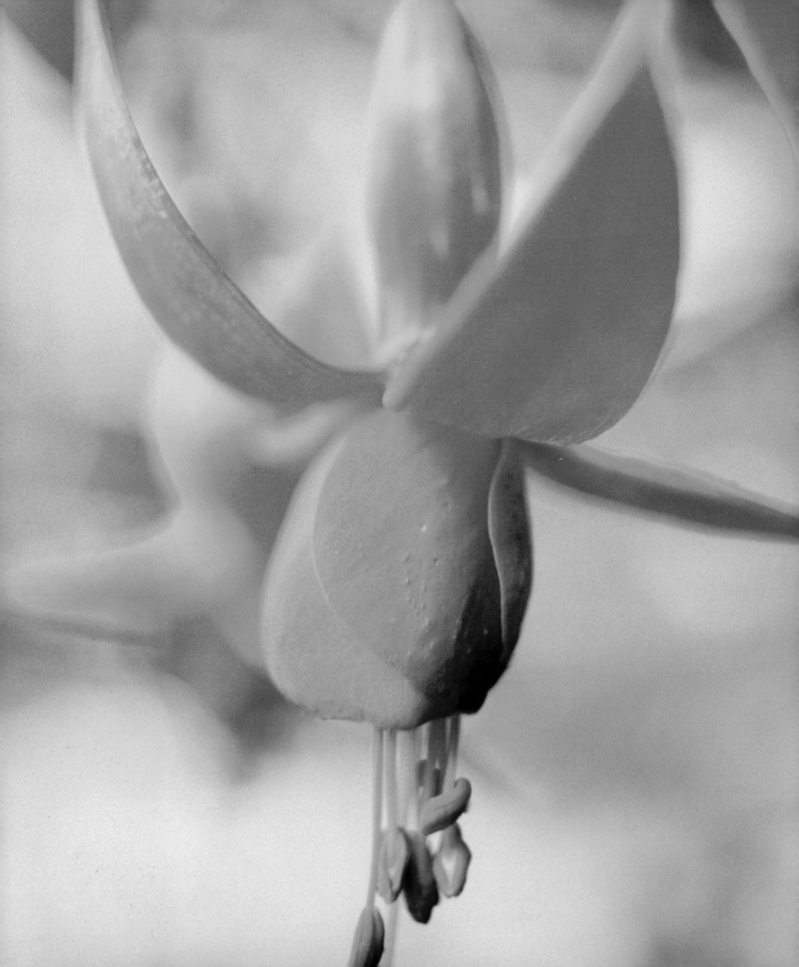

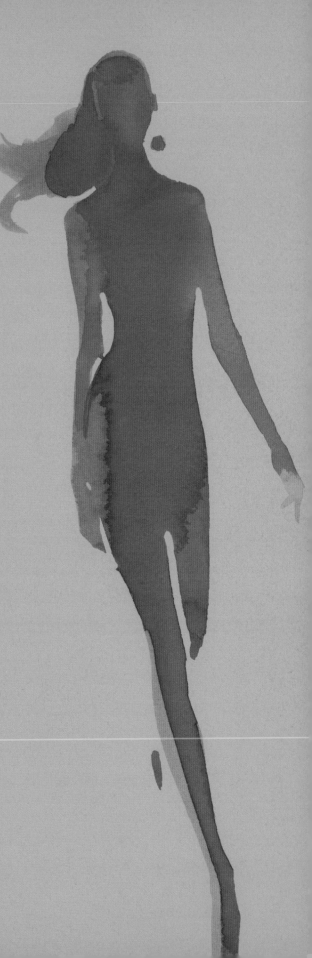

Body

Beautiful bodies are born, yes (especially if your name is Elle, Claudia or Gisele). But we believe all bodies are innately beautiful – think of the amazing job they do – and can become more so with top-to-toe moisturising, blitzing and pampering. And if, like us, you're concerned about the long string of synthetics in so many body preparations, we've found some natural contenders that do the trick terrifically – even making rear views that teensy bit more Gisele-esque!

BE
some body
TO LOVE

A decade or so ago, Jo had a 'light bulb' moment as she put on some body lotion. Watching it sink into her skin, she thought: 'Where's it going?' Trying to live a natural lifestyle, eating organic food, it suddenly didn't make sense to be slathering on a cocktail of anything-but-natural, definitely-not-organic ingredients

Frankly, we have come to be a shade more concerned about what's in the body products we put on our skin because – compared to a few square inches of face – the quantities of lotion, cream, butter and oil slurped up are so much greater. It is absolutely true that the jury is still out about the potential impact on health of many of the thousands of petrochemically derived ingredients in body products. The mainstream cosmetics industry insists that the synthetic ingredients in cosmetics are 100 per cent safe. (Nevertheless, many have still never been tested, and it is a fact that ingredients are quietly removed from the market all the time.)

By contrast, many natural ingredients have been used safely in the 'wise woman' tradition to soften, smooth and shield skin for centuries, millennia in some cases. (Not that all natural products are inherently risk- or irritation-free. Nettles – ouch! – are natural. So is poison ivy.)

But health is not the only issue for us. It's also about sustainability, and how ingredients are produced. We love the idea of Fairtrade body butters, for instance, and we'd rather have the essential oils grown by women's cooperatives in Kenya fragrancing our unguents, thanks, than a molecule invented by a chemist in a Long Island lab.

Today, there's a vast industry out there, aimed at cleaning and softening bodies while ensuring that every nook and cranny smells sweet at all times. We're encouraged to turn our bathrooms into 'at-home spas', havens of pampering, with an armoury of sense-soothing treats within arm's reach. Now we're all for a bit of self-care, and we love a bath as much as the next woman (possibly more…). But we don't like the way that we're encouraged by the beauty industry to be almost Howard Hughes-like in our obsession with cleanliness, and to own an arsenal of products to clean, smooth, deodorise. Certainly – and this is our personal preference – we don't want to slather on layer after layer of chemically preserved gunk when there are other options.

On our own wish list are sustainably produced bath- and body-care products – which means botanically based rather than petrochemically derived. As with the food we eat, we'd rather the ingredients were organically farmed, if poss. And we don't want to be left with a binful of excess packaging tweaking our guilty consciences after we've unwrapped the goodies inside.

We're delighted to say that many of the fantastic products we trialled for this book fit that bill perfectly. So happy slathering…

We don't like the way that we're encouraged to

be almost Howard Hughes-like in our obsession with cleanliness

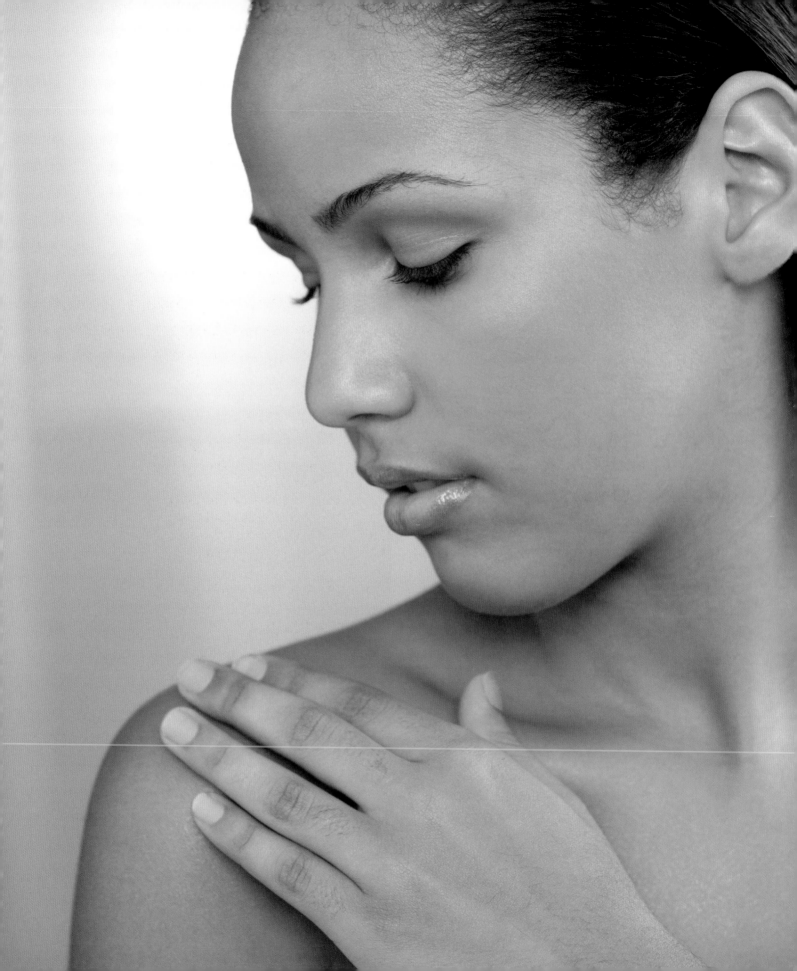

buff stuff

If body-buffing were an Olympic sport, we'd be up there on the podium. Life's too short for many beauty practices in our view – the equivalent of stuffing that proverbial tomato – but scrubbing and brushing pay huge beauty dividends

If you don't do anything else for your body – at all – do body-brush. We won't mince words here: it's the most miraculously transforming action you can take, helping to boost circulation, slough away dead skin cells and – in our experience – is the most effective weapon against cellulite, because it revs up the body's natural detoxing mechanism. (For more on cellulite, see page 131.) And once you've invested in the brush itself, this treatment is virtually free. How to choose the brush? We like either long-handled versions, or those with a strap on top, which slip over the hand – like a horse brush. Bristles shouldn't be too soft or too firm. When brush shopping, use on the back of your hand; if it leaves fine white traces where it's scratched the skin, it's too hard. Sweep in upward strokes towards your heart: from feet to tummy, hands to shoulders (avoiding tender areas such as the breasts), for two minutes each morning. We can't promise you eternal life, but we can promise you a healthier body.

Scrub up nicely

As well as body-brushing, we are huge fans of body scrubs. Scrubs are some of the easiest products to create naturally: salt and sugar can be suspended in oil, then scooped on to skin in the shower or bath, massaged in and rinsed away. At a pinch (literally), you can use a scoop of salt and a slurp of olive oil. In fact, we find that a good oil-based scrub, used at bath time, can all but eliminate the need for body lotion; the oil stays on the skin, leaving it nourished and gleaming, even after you've showered or bathed. (Pat, rather than rub dry, or wander round in a towel for five minutes and let the air do the work.)

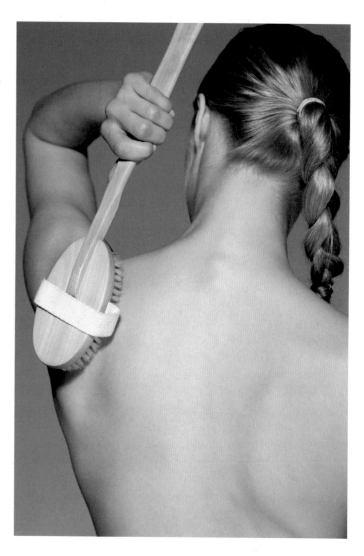

We love...

Neither of us uses a cellulite treatment, because we don't really suffer from this beauty woe. But we do body-brush religiously: Jo with a very fine copper-bristled brush that she found in Germany, and Sarah with the Raffe Body Brush by Origins, a real beauty steal which has the perfect blend of briskness without brutality! The nifty design makes it a breeze to get at most bits of you – though you might need a hand with middle back, if you're not that supple.

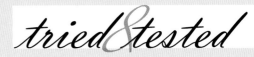

BODY SCRUBS

A good scrub is the fast track to gleaming, glowing body skin – and judging by our testers' comments, happy husbands... We've now sent over 60 natural options to testers, who (in the latest round of testing) found some new fave scrub raves, see below. Prepare for smoother, softer, more vibrant skin...

Salt and sugar scrubs are best used in the bath (where they dissolve, infusing the water with any oils). Those containing pulverised nuts, olive stones or bamboo are best reserved for the shower – or you can find you're sitting on the nutty gritty!

✿ REN MOROCCAN ROSE OTTO SUGAR BODY POLISH

Score: 9.33/10

Very nearly the highest-scoring product we've trialled in 13 years, a new addition to REN's bestselling Rose Otto collection – here, in a soft, sugar-based scrub (with a somewhat luxurious price tag). It also contains stimulating kola nut and Paraguayan tea extracts – and the heavenly scent and buffing action has earned this a tub-side place in Jo's bathroom, too.

Comments: 'My skin looked and felt very dry and scaly; then I used this and it was so much better – I didn't need extra body cream. My partner noticed my skin being very soft – now that's amazing!' • 'my children and partner commented on how nice I smelt, which is a first' • 'I loved everything about it: the smell, texture feel of my skin after, and people round me noticed the subtle scent'.

★ ✿ LIZ EARLE NATURALLY ACTIVE SKINCARE ENERGISING BODY SCRUB

Score: 8.8/10

The buff-you-smooth ingredient in this gel-like scrub is ground olive stones (with smooth jojoba beads), in a lightly foaming blend – perfect to use in the shower. With natural source vitamin E and damask rosewater, it's enhanced by a blend of essential oils with geranium, sweet orange, grapefruit, patchouli and rosemary.

Comments: 'Loved the fresh, clean smell – no need to use perfume after' • 'good texture and lather: hard skin on the backs of my arms has gone, also staved off ingrowing hairs on bikini line after waxing' • 'skin glistened and felt really soft' • 'fabulous!'

✿✿✿ ESSENTIAL CARE ORGANIC COCONUT CANDY BODY SCRUB

Score: 8.33/10

This smells like a tropical island (or a cocktail!), thanks to the super-coconuttiness. It won the 2009 Soil Association Beauty Awards, and – with sugar and cocoa butter – is literally good enough for you (let alone your skin) to eat: at the Natural Products Show, where it was launched, they were serving it on biscuits!

Comments: 'Really liked the coconut smell – fresh and like summer!' • 'skin felt clean, refreshed, relaxed and pampered' • 'I liked the amount of "scrub" in the product: felt as though it was doing what it needed to do' • 'skin felt rejuvenated – helped to remove dry skin' • 'skin pronouncedly less dry' • 'as someone who reacts badly to perfumes, I found the smell of the product perfect' • 'you want to eat it...'

✿✿ PRIMAVERA AROMATHERAPY DETOX SALT SCRUB

Score: 8.3/10

Part of Primavera's 'salt spa therapy' collection, this salt scrub features sea minerals, known for their cleansing and detoxifying powers. An am rather than pm choice, as the juniper, black pepper, ginger, rosemary and basil have a wake-up action.

Comments: 'Skin felt silky-smooth – one of the best scrubs I've ever used' • 'creamy texture, not at all scratchy' • 'soft, gentle texture, like wet sand but not as abrasive; improved my skin greatly' • 'heavenly lemony fragrance' • 'love this – really effective'.

✿ REN GINGER REVIVO-TONIC BODY SCRUB

Score: 8.28/10

Gosh, another winner from REN. Again, this features sugar as the scruffing agent (muscovado and demerara cane), and in this invigorating option you can enjoy the circulation-boosting powers of ginger and ginseng. REN, you scrub up nicely...

Comments: 'Best massaged into damp skin; felt softer and smoother immediately, improved skin tone with regular use' • 'my very dull, lifeless skin with milky white spots was greatly improved, dullness disappeared, white spots completely gone, skin looked full of life' • 'absolutely loved this large tub, which will last me ages; pleasant ginger smell, nice thick texture, skin beautifully smooth'.

come clean

Once upon a time, soap was the only beauty product most people had access to. Now we can choose to bubble our skin clean with body washes and shower gels. But is that such a good idea?

Soap was one of the earliest beauty products (created from wood ash, actually – though quite how anyone got the idea that a pile of cinders would transform into something to get skin clean baffles us). Today, for the non-beauty-minded, soap is still the only 'essential'.

Lately, however, the beauty industry – including the natural beauty industry – has come up with an alternative way to get us clean: the body wash. In general, these are kinder to skin (though the usually plastic packaging is less kind to the planet, if it's not recyclable – so do check on the label). Some do double-duty as shower gels, squirted under running water to create a cleansing foam, and even shampoos.

On the subject of foam, can we have a mini-rant about sodium lauryl sulfate (SLS)? (Yes, another one, just in case you missed it in other sections of this book.) SLS is a foaming agent, as well as the most commonly used surfactant (detergent) and is added to bath products to make them bubbly and foamy. *You* readers send Sarah (who's the magazine's health editor) lots of stories about the benefits of not using products containing SLS. For instance, one asthmatic who routinely had to use two inhalers daily plus other drugs was able to come off them entirely when she stopped lying in a bubble bath for 30 minutes every evening, at the instigation of her daughter who had read something about SLS. Another grandmother endured two years of vaginal itching, being bounced from one doctor to another and prescribed different drugs including HRT and topical products, until a bright young dermatologist seeing her shift uncomfortably in her seat asked if she used bubble bath. She did, she stopped – and so did the itching. For children with eczema, one of the saddest things is that aqueous cream, a routinely prescribed emollient for eczema, itself contains SLS. In one study of 100 children, the aqueous cream caused symptoms including redness, itchiness, burning and stinging in more than half the children using it. 'Aqueous cream, like many other common cleaning agents, contains surfactants, which can thin the skin barrier. If this vital barrier is damaged – particularly in areas such as the face where it's thin anyway – it's easy for irritants and allergens to get in and trigger a flare of eczema,' explains consultant dermatologist Michael Cork from the University of Sheffield Medical School. SLS is the most common surfactant and the most harsh. See why we go on about it?

Keep it short and sweet

We don't shower just to wash ourselves; most of us also use the shower as an opportunity to sing, wake up, warm up and think. (The average American adult, apparently, spends 10.4 minutes in the shower, while teenagers, of course, tend to shower until the hot water has gone.) A short shower is much less water-greedy than a bath, but there's more you can do to keep water consumption down (not to mention the greenhouse emissions from heating it). Ask your plumber about fitting a low-flow shower head. And consider buying a shower timer, which will help you keep water and money from going down the drain: a kitchen timer with a bell is fine (just keep it outside the shower) or look online for the Shorter Shower or Shower Coach. If you want a real challenge, take what's known as a 'navy shower': turn on the water, get wet, turn off the water, soap and scrub, then turn on the water and sluice off. We're told this cuts water (and energy) consumption by a staggering 83 per cent.

We love...

Sarah adores Trilogy Botanical Body Wash: 'This is smooth and silkifying – plus it's packaged in brown glass and lasts for ages.' Jo is a recent convert to body washes and is especially keen on the wonderfully aromatic Balance Me Seven Day Hand & Body Wash, featuring anti-bacterial green myrtle. (It's less messy than soap, but she still suffers eco-guilt at the empty plastic bottle, for which there are still very few recycling facilities.)

Bin the bug-busters

Except in hospital settings, where they may sterilise hands and potentially help prevent the spread of the superbug MRSA, we are not fans of antibacterial hand washes. There is increasing concern about the antibacterial ingredients, which now seem to feature in up to three quarters of liquid soaps, also deodorants, toothpastes, mouthwashes, cleaning supplies, and may be infused into kitchen utensils, toys, bedding, socks and trash bags. Concerns are that they can cause the formation of superbugs, lead to allergies and destroy fragile aquatic ecosystems. The Environment Agency and the World Heath Organisation have called for research into triclosan (aka Microban) following fears about its impact on the environment and wildlife. Instead, use soap or a non-antibacterial hand wash: and wash your hands thoroughly (especially thumbs, which often get overlooked) for at least one minute, before rinsing and drying on a clean, dry towel (damp towels harbour bacteria). As an aside, we are also completely against the addition of antibacterials to chopping boards, food packaging and even the interiors of fridges. If you use good hygiene when preparing food, these are completely superfluous to requirements. If you really want to do something, add a couple of drops of tea tree oil to warm water and wash with a clean cloth.

We don't shower just to wash ourselves; most of us also use the shower as an opportunity to sing, wake up, warm up and think

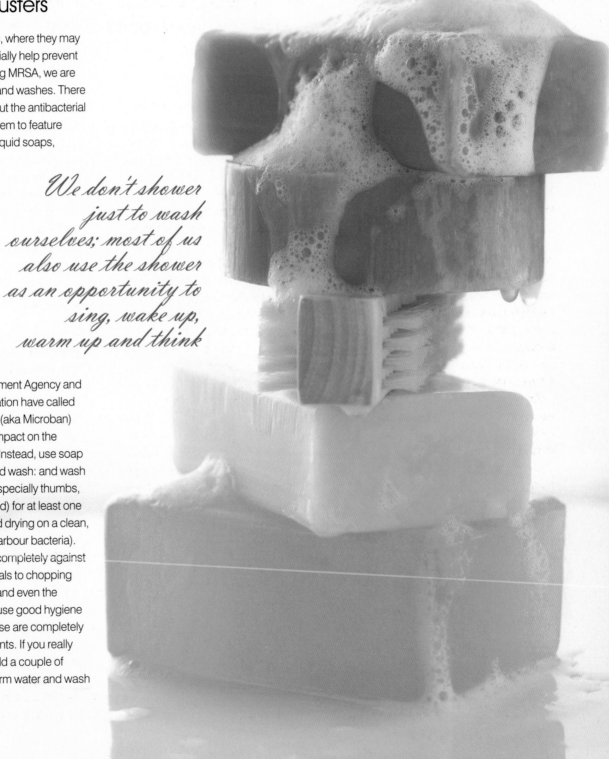

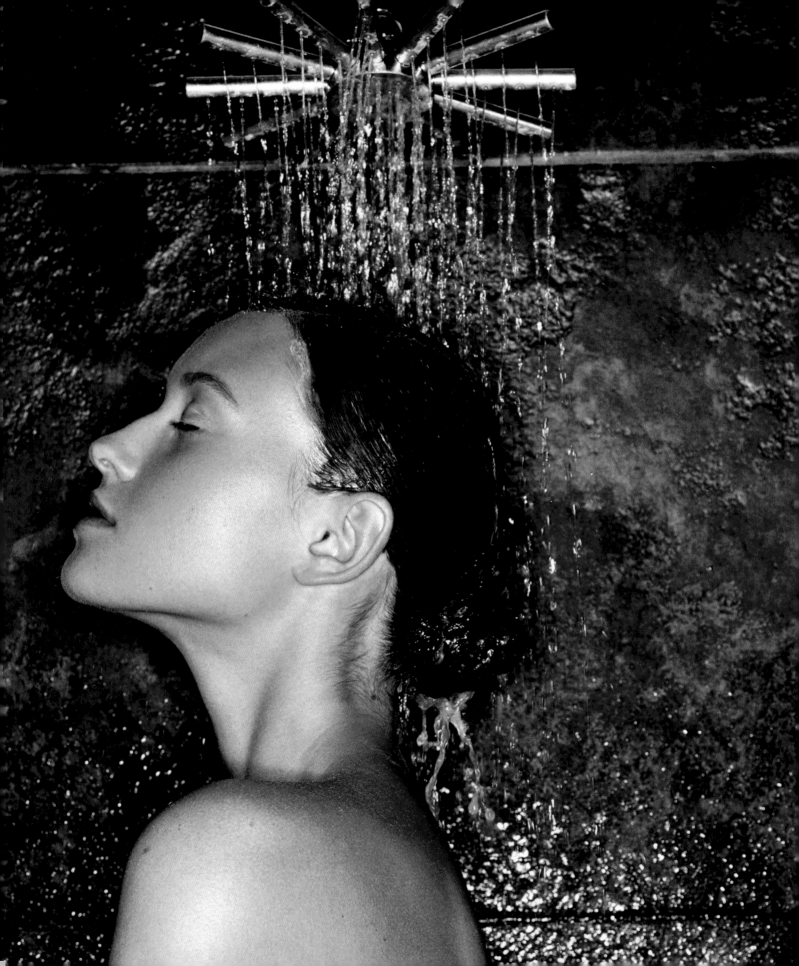

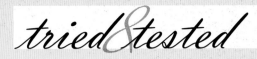

BODY WASHES

This is a booming area: our diligent 'green' testers have now sudsed their way through over 70 body washes (of course every product goes to 10 of them). None of the washes featured here – do look out for one new entry – contain triclosan, or potentially irritating sodium lauryl sulfate (SLS). From a landfill point of view, though, soap still wins – with its minimal, sometimes nonexistent packaging…

✻ TRILOGY BOTANICAL BODY WASH
Score: 9.1/10
An exceptional result for this product from New Zealand natural brand Trilogy. It contains extracts of kawa kawa from the native pepper tree, skin-purifying burdock and a sense-soothing blend of camomile, frankincense and lavender oils. Like all the Trilogy range, the key ingredient at the heart of this wash is certified-organic rosehip oil, known for its cell-regenerating action.
Comments: 'I will definitely buy this again; it has everything you want: gentleness, effectiveness, fresh uplifting scent (even my husband liked it) and it's moisturising – I loved it' • 'more foam than I expected – excellent product' • 'lasts for ages and ages' • 'very user-friendly pump – excellent results'.

✻✻ WELEDA LAVENDER CREAMY BODY WASH
Score: 8.62/10
Weleda offer four options in their Creamy Body Wash range: personally we love the Rose and the Sea Buckthorn, but our testers plumped for Lavender, with its soothing, aromatherapeutically calming effect. All the washes contain organic sesame oil, a natural anti-free-radical antioxidant, vitamin A and vitamin E, and are based on eco-friendly cleansing agents derived from sugar and coconut.
Comments: 'Excellent product – subtle lavender fragrance, not at all old-fashioned, left my skin slightly scented, moisturised, and softer' • 'creamy and rich, left a silky feel, not expensive but feels like a top-quality product – perfect' • 'like the simple packaging and flip top' • 'wonderful and relaxing in the evening; only needed a little bit so lasted for ages'.

✻ REN MOROCCAN ROSE OTTO BODY WASH
Score: 8.6/10
Following on the huge success of their Moroccan Rose Otto Bath Oil (which did so well in our Relaxing Bath Treats Tried & Tested), REN (which means 'clean' in Swedish) created this wash based on mild cleansing agents derived from corn, oats and sugar, which are sulfate-free and therefore gentle on the skin. And then there's that heavenly rose scent…
Comments: 'Lovely, sensible packaging; high-level beauty product with pampering feel – heavenly fragrance' • 'fresh rose scent lingered on my skin' • 'left skin smooth and moisturised' • 'one pump was enough for my whole body' • 'my skin felt gorgeous after – I absolutely love this product'.

★ ✻ NEAL'S YARD REMEDIES GERANIUM & ORANGE SHOWER GEL
Score: 8.43/10
Although not certified organic (unlike many of the Neal's Yard winners in this book), this ultra-natural product does contain organic extracts of calendula, lavender and orange flower, plus organic orange oil, which explains the fabulous uplifting fragrance. (Using their signature glass packaging for a shower product was queried by several testers.)
Comments: 'Lovely refreshing smell; performed really well and you don't need very much; skin feels smooth and clean' • 'little red bumps on my upper arms have reduced – which is great' • 'my skin felt gorgeous after, left a baby oil film – but not greasy' • 'one little drop washed my whole body and left it silky'.

✻✻✻ BALANCE ME SUPER WASH WITH JUNIPER & BERGAMOT
Score: 8.22/10
Since we trialled this product for the hardback edition, Balance Me have reformulated to meet Ecocert organic guidelines, and jazzed up their labels prettily. You'll still enjoy the blend of geranium, juniper, bergamot and lavender, with their stimulating and refresh actions.
Comments: 'Foamed well, smelt great, left me clean, what more could you want?' • 'liked the citrussy aroma very much; good for waking up' • 'foamed brilliantly, you get a generous amount – liked it a lot' • 'kept my skin in good condition' • 'foamed well, skin felt clean and soft, very pleasant and product in smart packaging with flip top'.

BODY LOTIONS

Our many thousands of testers have slathered their way through getting on for 100 natural (or more natural) products in this category alone, to find out which lotions really do ease tight, uncomfy skin, and leave it velvety and enduringly soft. For this Tried & Tested update, we're excited that they've made some new discoveries, see below. As before, all brands mentioned deserve a pat on the (well-moisturised) back

❀ REN WILD YAM OMEGA 7 FIRMING BODY REPAIR CREAM
Score: 9/10

Featuring wild yam (long used in different ways to help menopausal women) to moisturise and help boost skin lipids, this high-scorer also contains sea buckthorn berry oil, a potent source of essential fatty acids. While not totally natural, it is trying hard.
Comments: 'Instantly absorbed, dry areas disappeared and my skin felt as smooth as velvet' • 'my worst areas of dryness – shins and heels – cleared up' • 'light, unobtrusive smell, generous-sized pump dispenser; seems to have banished late-winter scaly skin' • 'my skin was softer – even my husband noticed' • 'I only had one ingrowing hair after waxing while I trialled this – normally I have loads' • 'my new best product for my very sensitive skin'.

★ ❀❀❀ NEAL'S YARD REMEDIES GARDEN MINT & BERGAMOT HAND LOTION
Score: 8.87/10

What's a hand lotion doing in this section? Well, with 1,150 different products to send out, the odd human error crept in and we accidentally sent it out with a body lotion form! It's not really surprising that this Soil Association-certified hand product did well as a body moisturiser: far more products have that versatility than beauty brands will let on. With the clean, green scent of freshly picked garden mint and Sicilian bergamot, in a blend of skin-softening shea butter, jojoba and evening primrose oils, we think it makes a fabulous hand and body lotion.
Comments: 'Attractive minty smell, dispenser gave precisely the right amount, absorbed quickly, makes skin fresh and revitalised, supple and smooth' • 'love the cobalt blue bottle – gorgeous cream' • 'very effective and pleasant to use' • 'my body skin needs a lot of attention but the results of this are worth it' • 'my husband used this too after gardening' • 'wonderful silky texture'.

★ ❀ AVALON ORGANICS LEMON HAND & BODY LOTION
Score: 8.87/10

A good performance for an affordably priced lotion, based on (organic) sunflower, flaxseed and coconut oils, with glycerine and beta glucan, to moisturise and promote cellular turnover. With Organics in the name, you might assume every ingredient is certified organic, which is not quite the case, but it is more natural than many other products.
Comments: 'Zingy, fresh, sharp smell – like home-made lemon curd!' • 'buttery texture which sank in with no tackiness – beats expensive body lotions hands down' • 'my lizard scales were better after two days, and skin as soft and smooth as a baby's bottom after two weeks' • 'I'm a body cream slut but am a convert to this now' • 'instantly softens and moisturises and leaves a fresh lemony scent – really really like this, good gift too'.

❀ KORRES GUAVA BODY BUTTER
Score: 8.77/10

Double oops. Probably because it comes in a pump-action bottle, Jo and the 'beauty elves' dispatched this to be tested as a body lotion, not a butter. Whatever, this is Korres's bestselling creation: rich and moisturising, with shea butter, quince, guava, almond and avocado oil, to boost elasticity. Butter or lotion, it's still a winner.
Comments: 'Thick, luxurious cream, which absorbed quicker than any butter I've tried before – made skin smooth and healthy looking – brilliant stuff!' • 'I really enjoyed rubbing it in, my husband liked the smell, skin instantly softer, and cleared up itchy spots on my shins' • 'divine long-lasting fragrance – leaves slight sheen on skin, was happy with everything about this product'.

❀ BAREFOOT BOTANICALS S.O.S. RESCUE ME FACE & BODY CREAM
Score: 8.87/10

Do you have dry, dry skin? This is Barefoot Botanicals' prescription: a cream packed with essential Omega 3, 6 and 9 fatty acids, which they say can support the skin while it's withdrawing from steroid use. (Useful for babies' cradle cap and eczema, too.) With borage oil, evening primrose oil and shea butter, calendula, burdock, comfrey, chickweed, French lavender, neroli and camomile, it caters for faces and bodies.
Comments: 'Another beautiful natural

clean-smelling product; skin feels like it has a new protective layer, smells wonderful, definitely moisturised' • 'my daughter has nut allergies so this is a must for us; it also calms down her sore eyes when they flare up' • 'a great bonus that one of the principles behind it is to make a cream with sensuality and uplifting aroma' • 'looovely! Light and fluffy, leaving skin really moisturised, with fresh fruity fragrance; used in my office during a flu outbreak, it was the best thing ever for dry, chafed noses, even on my colleague's supersensitive skin'

★ ✿ LIZ EARLE NATURALLY ACTIVE SKINCARE NOURISHING BOTANICAL BODY CREAM
Score: 8.75/10

In response to customer requests for 'skincare for the body', the formulators at Liz Earle came up with this lightweight satin-soft cream, turbocharged with botanicals such as echinacea, betacarotene, vitamin E, shea butter, hops and avocado oil, fragranced with essential oils of orange, lavender, rosewood and geranium, which also have skin-soothing and toning properties.

Comments: 'Ten out of ten! Leaves skin very moisturised – no stickiness – and sweetly scented' • 'my skin was in need of TLC, upper arms dehydrated, tummy crêpey and dry: now they are plump and moist again'

• 'skin feels velvety soft: big difference on knees, heels, elbows' • 'love the smell of summer fields' • 'Ten out of ten – I have bought it several times'.

★ ✿ YES TO CARROTS C IS SMOOTH BODY MOISTURIZING LOTION
Score: 8.7/10

One of several winners from this US brand (they also have ranges called Yes to Tomatoes and Yes to Cucumbers). The 'signature' ingredients in the carrot range are organic carrot juice, pumpkin, sweet potato and melon, here formulated into a rich lotion. (To our noses, the fragrance is baby powder-ish – and rather comforting.) The generous Yes to Carrots bottles and tubs are very economical, and worthy Beauty Steals.

Comments: 'Ten out of ten, for light creamy texture, immediately absorbed, good packaging, skin immediately moisturised and comfy; with regular use skin felt more healthy and supple' • 'slightly disappointed that it doesn't smell of carrots! But like the light fresh fragrance and silky lotion; excellent packaging, gave softer skin and areas of dryness improved' • 'quickly absorbed and very effective'.

✿ ✿ GREEN PEOPLE BODY BLISS LOTION
Score: 8.57/10

Rose, green tea and shea butter are the 'star' ingredients in this divinely-scented body lotion, which is certified by the Organic Food Federation. Green People were pioneers in the natural beauty field,

but unlike some early brands whose formulations are 'stuck in a rut', the GP team is constantly working to improve textures – and this lush lotion lives up to its name.

Comments: 'Top marks for this lovely light rose-smelling cream which sank in instantly; my skin felt immediately smoother' • 'really nice product with a feel of luxury – no greasiness after use' • 'Ten plus! Adored this soft smooth and deliciously scented cream; my legs are prone to dry scaly patches and there was a definite improvement after a week; at last I have smooth shiny skin.'

✿ INDIA HICKS ISLAND LIVING SPIDER LILY BODY CREAM
Score: 8.44/10

Clever Crabtree & Evelyn asked the beautiful India Hicks (one of our 'green goddesses', see page 146) to help create a bodycare and home fragrance range inspired by her enviable Bahamas lifestyle. The range is free of parabens, mineral oil, sodium lauryl sulfate and propylene glycol, and this particular fresh-scented cream is rich in antioxidant olive and grapeseed oils, with lashings of mango, shea and avocado butter.

Comments: 'A joy to smooth in – seemed to melt, left skin soft with a lovely subtle smell' • 'also used this on my face and that felt great too – very blissful indeed' • 'utterly moreish, very pampering – the sort of thing they would apply to you in a spa' • 'the wide-necked glass jar would suit the poshest of bathrooms' • 'a real treat to be told that I smell nice after using this!'.

We love...

Well, we just love body moisturisers – practically any – to slather on from top to toe. Sarah goes for a combi of oils in the bath followed by Miracle Lotion by Seven Wonders, stuffed full of herbs and oils for instant visible hydration – works on fingernails too. Jo prefers the richness of body butters (see overleaf), and has several tubs stacked precariously on her bedside including Dr. Organic Aloe Vera Body Butter (from a new-ish range at Holland & Barrett), and the luscious Aromatherapy Associates Enrich Body Butter, which contains murumuru butter and babassu oil, and delivers a serious patchouli punch.

better butter

Body butters are nature's skin-cocooning bounty: pressed from seeds and nuts, they can instantly restore suppleness and smooth even the driest skins. And now body butters sometimes come with an extra 'feel-good' factor: Fairtrade ingredients

Although they're a relatively new concept in the West, butters have been used around the world for body-care for centuries: they are especially skin-compatible, with nutrients and healing properties that sink in easily. With the exception of shea butter (which can be used straight from the tub), most are incorporated into a blend of carrier ingredients, which softens the butter and makes it easier to apply; we tested many of these blends (see opposite), and our testers loved them. Butters are now increasingly available as Fairtrade products, with ingredients sourced directly from Third World cooperatives – a trend we wholeheartedly support. Here's what the best-known beauty butters can do for your skin…

Cocoa butter

Pressed from the seed kernels of the cacao tree, *Theobroma cacao*, cocoa butter is rich, sumptuous, smells of chocolate and melts into skin at body temperature, boosting suppleness, soothing skin and acting as a barrier. It's also high in antioxidants. It is commonly used for sunburn, scars, stretch marks, wrinkles and for softening rough, dry skin.

Mango butter

This is a great source of essential fatty acids and naturally contains antioxidants. It is one of the most universal butters, because of its incredible moisturising powers and versatility. Pressed from the seed kernels of the mango tree, *Mangifera indica*, it's often used to prevent stretch marks, restore skin elasticity and in sun protection.

Shea butter

Derived from the vegetable fat of the African karite tree, *Butyrospermum parkii*, shea butter is rich in vitamins A, E and F among others. An intense moisturiser, it's a boon for all sorts of skin conditions, from itchiness, rashes and eczema to dermatitis, dry skin and nappy rash. It's said to enhance skin renewal, increase circulation and even promote wound healing.

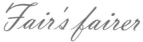

Fair's fairer

The Body Shop, to their credit, pioneered the idea of 'community trade ingredients' in their beauty products, setting up projects to purchase specific ingredients such as shea butter and cocoa butter from disadvantaged Third World communities. They now source 25 natural ingredients from community trade projects, from Caribbean bananas to Namibian marula oil.

The idea is that community trade (now widely called Fairtrade) provides growers with a secure market for their ingredients. Jo has first-hand experience of this: Green & Black's Organic Chocolate, which she started with her husband Craig Sams, was the first product to carry the UK's Fairtrade mark, certifying a fair price and a rolling five-year contract for the Belizean farmers who grow cacao for top-selling Maya Gold. Before Green & Black's came along, the farmers had received plenty of aid, which encouraged them to grow rice and annatto (a yellow colouring), but there was no secure market for either, which meant that when the aid projects timed out, the farmers were back to square one.

So Fairtrade really is the most positive way forward for these communities. We would encourage you to support products that contain Fairtrade ingredients whenever possible. Like we say, beauty with an extra feel-good factor.

BODY BUTTERS

Nature, as we said on page 122, has created some amazing natural butters that melt into skin, leaving it velvety. Here are our testers' top choices – including some new options, to answer even the thirstiest body's SOS

★✿ YES TO CARROTS C THROUGH THE DRY SPELL DELICIOUSLY RICH BODY BUTTER
Score: 9.29/10

This somewhat ludicrously named budget brand from the US got an exceptional score for this shea-butter-rich treatment for ultra-dry skin, which also features antioxidant ingredients derived from (yes) organic carrot juice, sweet potato, melon and pumpkin, as well as jojoba and avocado oil. We certainly applaud their 'Seed Fund', which ploughs some profits into a charity offering seeds, equipment, irrigation and know-how to poor communities. (We find the fragrance rather powdery and uncarrot-y, but testers loved it.)
Comments: 'Love the fresh natural smell, and soft, easy-to-apply texture, almost like lovely thick yoghurt; skin is instantly smooth, soft and feels quenched. And the price is incredible!' • 'Was absorbed quicker than roadrunner, bliss to use – smelt of a cross between your mother's make-up bag when you were little and Play-Doh;' • 'skin looked fresh and happy' • 'smelt heavenly'.

✿ NEAL'S YARD REMEDIES ROSE BODY CREAM
Score: 8.85/10

A truly impressive score from this product, one of Jo's own faves (she slathers it on to feet every night). With a pretty rose scent (and the regenerating powers of rose oil), this ultra-moisturising blend owes its skin-cocooning qualities to organic shea nut butter; there's hazelnut, avocado oil and calendula, too. In a hefty glass jar that's definitely for the boudoir rather than the sponge bag, it lasts for aeons.
Comments: 'Made skin look healthier and smoother' • 'rose is one of my favourite essential oils; worked a treat on my scaly feet and bumpy arms' • 'pleasing to use: really great for dry elbows and feet' • 'my last pedicure was weeks ago and my feet still look good' • 'texture like ice cream'.

✿ KORRES GUAVA BODY BUTTER
Score: 8.62/10

Korres's luxurious, pump-action body butters are easy to use (and look pretty smart). The Guava option (this Greek brand offers a choice of five) harnesses this fruit's healing, nourishing properties; it's rich in vitamin C and B-complex vits. To restore elasticity and smoothness, there's shea butter, sunflower oil, avocado oil and quince extract, too.
Comments: 'Liked the rich texture, sank in quite quickly; skin felt smooth and nourished' • 'skin instantly hydrated' • 'might have preferred a lighter perfume but the fruity, slightly sweet smell was pleasant' • 'loved this – my skin felt nourished, instantly looked and felt better' • 'brilliant, this product really works; loved the no-mess dispenser and my skin looks younger than for a long time'.

✿✿✿ CIRCAROMA SOFTENING BODY BUTTER
Score: 8.6/10

Circaroma are very, very good at body-nurturing. This deeply moisturising, creamy butter is certified organic by the Soil Association, and features shea butter, vitamin E and almond oil to replenish and rehydrate, together with geranium flower and lemon zest, which, they promise, has a 'detoxing' effect. Their tip? Soften the butter in your hands first, for ease of application.
Comments: 'Made skin instantly softer; you can also use it as a hair conditioner' • 'natural lemon/geranium smell and rich wax-like consistency' • 'definite improvement in skin on knees and elbows' • 'hydrated better than a good body oil; skin looked "alive" and felt smoother and softer' • 'particularly good for dry patches on legs'.

✿ KORRES YOGHURT BODY BUTTER
Score: 8.5/10

Ah! Another impressive Korres winner, which ranked just a fraction behind the Guava Body Butter, above. Why yoghurt? It's a natural, anti-inflammatory source of lactose, proteins, minerals and vitamins, delivering comfort to dry skin in combo with almond, sunflower, avocado oil, shea butter and glycerine.
Comments: 'Great product with a lovely fragrance, really nourishing, and calms down irritated dry skin; quite costly so perhaps a present?' • 'my boyfriend said I smelt like a newborn baby and had skin like one!' • 'lovely thick, buttery texture, didn't feel greasy or tacky and I could put on my pj's immediately' • 'smoother skin and fewer bumps on my post-pregnancy tummy; loved the fab pump; much more economical'.

glisten up

There's nothing bodies love more than being nourished with soothing and smoothing oil. Listen hard and you can almost hear your skin slurping up that goodness…

Body oils can be a 100 per cent natural way to nourish skin and leave it supple. (Bugs can't breed in oils, so they don't need preservatives.) But not all body oils are created equal: many (including baby versions) are made from mineral oil (paraffinum liquidum, on the label), which can block pores. By contrast, natural oils – such as sweet almond, grapeseed and olive – are highly skin-compatible. Around the world, oils are revered for their anti-ageing powers: Berber women, for instance, keep skin velvety-soft with the oil from the argan tree; and show us a smooth-skinned, bikini-worthy Frenchwoman of uncertain age, and we'll show you a body oil devotee. In fact, we'd say body oils are the ultimate body-care choice for the wannabe natural beauty…

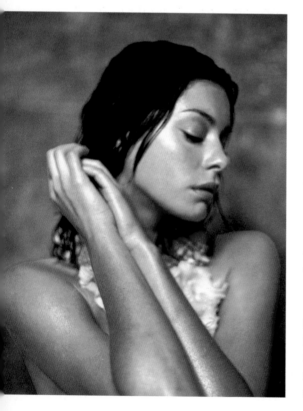

BODY BOOSTER

Our friend Kathy Phillips is one of our beauty heroes: former *Vogue* beauty director, author of *The Spirit of Yoga* and *Vogue Beauty*, and now overseeing beauty coverage in the magazine's Far Eastern editions, she also created This Works, a heavenly range of aromatherapy-based beauty treats – including some of our favourite bath and body oils. A living advertisement for her own range, she's got super-supple skin (not to mention a super-supple body, due to daily yoga). So we asked Kathy for some self-massage tips that will restore – especially feet and legs – after a weary day.

Says Kathy: 'Cranial osteopath Michael Skipwith told me recently that the body is under more strain from sitting at a computer all day (subtly using one side of the body too much and jutting the neck out too far) than it would be after jogging

evenly for several miles. Have you noticed how tiring it is to stand all day when you seem to be doing nothing? How legs feel heavy, tight and puffy? Whichever way you acquire muscle tension and tightness, regular stretching and relaxing are needed. And simple, regular massage with essential oils – every day, if you can – will make a noticeable difference. Jean Valnet, the "high priestess" of aromatherapy, lists both clove and ginger for their analgesic and anti-rheumatic effects, and lavender for almost everything, from regulating the nervous system, to burns, acne and even alopecia. I created my own blend, Muscle Therapy (with warming, stimulating clove, black pepper and ginger), which I rub hard into calves, lower back, neck and shoulders – even hips, if they are sore. After a warm bath is ideal.

'To soothe tired legs, de-puff ankles and relax tight calves, massage body oil in flowing, upward movements from ankle to knee and thigh, using the whole hand to cup and roll the flesh. It's important not to forget a good pummel with your thumbs at the feet too – and flex your feet back and forward to get at those reflex points. This way, you are massaging in the oil to boost circulation, as well as to nourish and moisturise. "Putting your feet up" is such a brilliant expression, in addition, and one of the first yoga exercises I do after a long day is to lie on my back and just put my legs in the air – so simple and so therapeutic.'

BODY OILS

Beauty Bible has now trialled more than 50 different botanically-based oils, each over a period of some weeks. As usual, we wanted our testers to tell us: do they sink in fast or leave skin like an oil slick? Are they good for massage? Do they smell gorgeous? Post-anointment, here's the verdict…

❀❀ AROMATHERAPY ASSOCIATES ENRICH MASSAGE & BODY OIL

Score: 8.95/10

We love this, so we're not really surprised it did so incredibly well. (We're especially keen on the wonderful essential oil fragrance – think geranium, tuberose, ylang-ylang, vanilla…) The body-nurturing blend features macadamia, evening primrose, coconut and olive oils, and we find the pump-action bottle less messy to use than some oils.

Comments: 'Ten out of ten! I have fallen in love! A great massage and body oil which leaves skin beautifully, subtly scented, and nourished, no oily residue' • 'excellent pump delivery, very attractive smell, oil absorbed quickly' • 'seductive fragrance, and skin immediately softer and had a sexy sheen' • 'fantastic! Does exactly what it promises – instant and ongoing improvements'.

❀❀ ESPA DETOXIFYING BODY OIL

Score: 8.66/10

Espa promise this oil, tangy with grapefruit, cypress, juniper berry, lemon and eucalyptus, can 'combat the effects of toxins, relieve water retention and assist the fight against cellulite' and several of our testers supported this claim vociferously.

Comments: 'Loved this! My dry skin feels shiny and moisturised; saggy upper arms better toned' • 'décolletage less dry and crêpey, eczema patches cleared up a treat' • 'my cellulite has improved vastly; limbs feel firmer, with the sponginess gone' • 'skin super soft and much more even toned'.

❀❀ JO WOOD USIKU ORGANIC BODY OIL

Score: 8.65/10

We're thrilled for our fabulous friend Jo Wood (see overleaf) that our testers voted for her body oil. Echinacea and St John's wort work to reduce irritation or redness, while the rich blend – in its stylishly Biba-esque glass bottle – includes Arctic bilberry, which contains high levels of antioxidant vitamin E and fatty acids.

Comments: 'Really gorgeous smell; left skin feeling luxuriously smooth – it's on my birthday list!' • 'skin immediately softer and smoother and plumper, good on heels; found it difficult to control the amount that came out of the glass bottle' • 'very easy to apply on damp skin; only need a little' • 'my favourite of the products I tested – I loved the way it made me and my skin feel calm and happy'.

★ ❀ THE BODY SHOP SPA WISDOM MONOI MIRACLE OIL

Score: 8.5/10

This multi-tasker (for skin, bath or hair) is one of the most natural products on The Body Shop's shelves, with just three oils: coconut, monoi de Tahiti and babassu. Monoi, from Tahitian gardenia flowers, gives the exotic fragrance, while babassu comes from The Body Shop's community trade project, giving 12 rural Brazilian communities of women the chance of regular work.

Comments: 'Smells like heaven and a treat to use' • 'gave a dewy shimmer and softness to skin' • 'worked magic on dry skin' • 'amazing as a hair oil, left overnight' • 'made skin glow'.

❀❀ CLARINS RELAX BODY TREATMENT OIL

Score: 8.31/10

Clarins recommend this 100 per cent natural formulation – based on wheatgerm and hazelnut oils with a calming blend of bitter orange, camomile and geranium – to combat fatigue and tension after physical activity.

Comments: 'Gave a lovely sense of wellbeing and soothed a sore knee and tense neck' • 'gave me a smooth bottom' • 'left nice sheen and made me feel irresistibly sexy' • 'luxurious smell' • 'I only ever use this product'.

We love…

We're major aficionados of body oils. Jo favours REN Moroccan Rose Otto Ultra Nourishing Body Oil and we both slurp on This Works Skin Deep Dry Leg Oil, the best thing for flaky shins. NB: don't forget neat sweet almond oil, or that beauty staple – olive oil.

JO WOOD

Jo Wood is the ultimate rock chick: gorgeous, glamorous, young-at-heart, looks amazing in a miniskirt – even in her fifties. We have plenty of reasons to admire her: she not only came through a messy break-up from Rolling Stone Ronnie with great dignity (and a new lease of life), but Jo Wood Organics – her range of award-winning, certified organic fragrances, bath & bodycare products, which reflects her own passion for organic living – goes from strength to strength. We love it – and we love Jo…

'When I began to put good things into my body

I started making my own organic skin and body oils to give to my girlfriends after my brother gave me a book called *The Fragrant Pharmacy*. Ronnie said: 'You'll never get that together,' when I told him I wanted to launch my own organic bath and body range. So I thought, 'I'll show him'. And I'm so glad that I did and proved to myself and everyone else what I could achieve.

I became health-conscious when I was mis-diagnosed with Crohn's disease. They put me on steroids and said that I would be on them for the rest of my life. I thought, 'I can't be doing with this.' I met a herbalist who asked me what I ate, and I told him: 'Kentucky Fried Chicken – I love convenience foods.' He told me that I had to clean out my system.

When I changed my diet, quit smoking and drinking and began to put good things into my body and on to my face, I suddenly felt and looked ten years younger. I'm now happier with myself than I've ever been, and that reflects in my face.

First thing in the morning, I brush my teeth – and my tongue. Then I brush my body with a body mitten – taking it slowly, working up from the soles of my feet, using circular movements towards the heart. It helps the lymphatic system remove toxins, makes you tingle all over, and it's great for keeping cellulite at bay.

If you really care about your health, it's not enough to just eat organic. You also need to make sure that you don't overload your skin with synthetic products.

I found that yoga fitted in perfectly with my new, clean life. It's all about being calm, about living well and in harmony with the universe, about respecting your body and the planet. I wish I had more time on the road to do yoga – that's when I could really do with it!

I'd like people to be as happy and energetic as me. If you have a good organic diet, it not only affects your health, it affects your mind, too. It makes sense that if you're not polluting your body with chemicals, you feel so much better in yourself. My family says, 'The trouble with you is you've got so much energy.' But my mission in life is to get everyone feeling as good as I do.

I was born patient. I'm a Pisces and a good listener. I sacrificed my career to raise a family. I couldn't be as famous as my husband and I didn't want to compete. So I looked after him, raised the children, was supportive. I was a grounding influence. Now that chapter in my life is closed, but I find that I have so much to look forward to. For the first time in my life, I'm really taking care of *me*, spending tons of time with my growing troupe of grandchildren and enjoying doing the things that *I* want to do. And about time!

and on to my face, I suddenly felt and looked ten years younger'

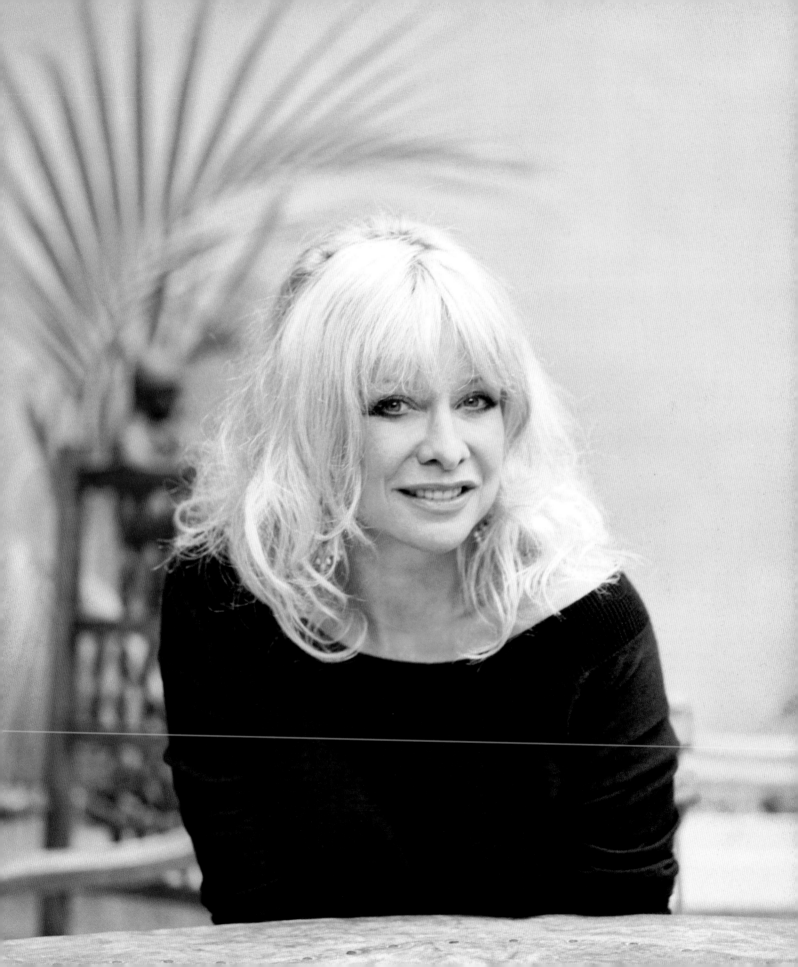

TO SWEAT
or not to sweat

Horses sweat, men perspire, women 'glow'. That's news to us girls! As we hurtle through modern life, most women we know work up more than a little 'glow'. But with the ongoing controversy about the impact of deodorants and antiperspirants on health, we keep being asked: what's safe to use?

We've probably had more anxious e-mails to our website, www.beautybible.com, about deodorants than any other subject. It's a beauty hot potato. And a health one too. The National Cancer Institute (NCI) in America is cautious, saying 'researchers are not aware of any conclusive evidence linking the use of underarm antiperspirants or deodorants and the subsequent development of breast cancer.' But, of course, absence of conclusive evidence is not conclusive evidence of absence.

The doubts started with a highly publicised study by Dr Philippa Darbre in 2004 which highlighted a possible link between deodorants and breast cancer, after parabens were found in breast tumours. The parabens, it was mooted, could act as oestrogen mimics and promote the growth of breast cancer cells (see below). A later US study also suggested a link when using deos was combined with underarm shaving in young girls, giving an average earlier diagnosis of 9.6 years. The thinking: tiny nicks caused by shaving could allow chemicals from deodorants and antiperspirants easy access to the body.

Now, these studies are small and the protocols incomplete. There was no definitive evidence in the Darbre research that the parabens in the tumours, for instance, actually came from deodorants rather than any other beauty products such as body lotion (or even food).

But the NCI says aluminium-based compounds (which are used to block sweat glands) might also pose a problem. 'Some research suggests that aluminium-based compounds, which are applied frequently and left on the skin near the breast, may be absorbed by the skin and cause oestrogen-like (hormonal) effects [the same mechanism as parabens]. Because oestrogen has the ability to promote the growth of breast cancer cells, some scientists have suggested that the aluminium-based compounds in antiperspirants may contribute to the development of breast cancer.' They conclude that 'because studies of antiperspirants and deodorants and breast cancer have provided conflicting results, additional research is needed.'

Some cancer physicians suggest that, meanwhile, it's worth avoiding these compounds. And we know from scrutinising the labels that although the deodorant industry has poured scorn on these studies, many manufacturers have quietly removed parabens from their products.

But, of course, none of us wants to be a Sweaty Betty. One paraben-free option is a deodorant 'crystal': damp it and swipe – and you're meant to stay fairly sweat-free. These are based on natural mineral salts, and, just to make life confusing – when you're trying to avoid antiperspirants with aluminium in – this mineral salt is generally called alum (or ammonium alum). But this alum is not the same as the questionable aluminium ingredients found in antiperspirants, and works effectively to prevent body odour by forming an invisible topical surface film, which inhibits and kills odour-eating bacteria. Overleaf see our testers' recommendations for other natural products.

NO SWEAT

These lifestyle shifts are worth considering to minimse 'glow'!
- Try to limit your consumption of caffeine, alcohol and spicy foods, which all increase sweating and body odour.
- If you eat meat, avoid red meat, which changes body odour. (Vegetarians rarely pong, in our experience.)
- Wear loose-fitting clothing to keep skin cool, and always choose natural fibres.
- Follow de-stressing techniques in this book (see pages 94–95); a lot of body odour is triggered by flight-or-fight stress hormones, rather than heat.
- We find that washing armpits with hot water rather than soap can make a difference (the bacteria seem to 'recolonise' faster after removal with soap than with plain water).

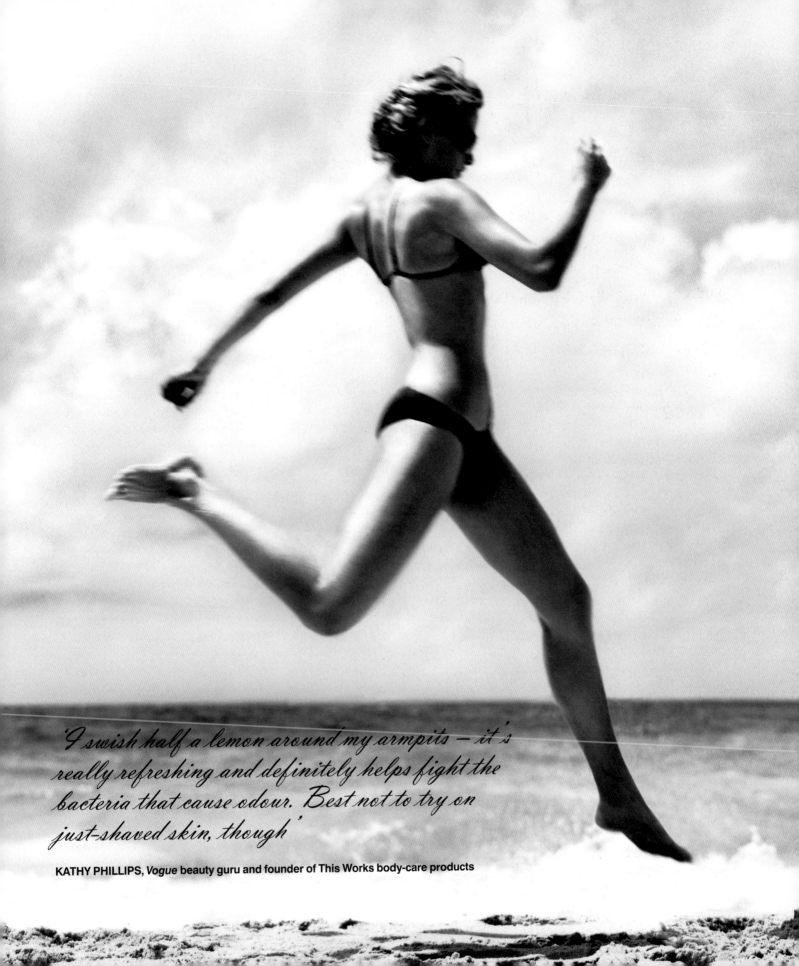

'I swish half a lemon around my armpits — it's really refreshing and definitely helps fight the bacteria that cause odour. Best not to try on just-shaved skin, though'

KATHY PHILLIPS, *Vogue* beauty guru and founder of This Works body-care products

NATURAL DEODORANTS

There are now many natural paraben- and aluminium-free deodorants based on bacteria-beating (it's the bugs that cause the whiff) ingredients such as witch hazel, coriander and thyme – and natural minerals that have an extraordinary effect. We tried many more for this edition but none scored higher than the products below. But do remember that everyone has different 'glow' patterns, so you may need to try more than one

❀❀ DR HAUSCHKA DEODORANT FRESH
Score: 8/10

This roll-on in glass packaging is formulated in two versions: a herb-scented Fresh version (which our testers trialled), with sage and witch hazel to purify and invigorate (they say) and Floral, scented with jasmine and lilac essential oils and relying on neem leaf and sage extracts to soothe and purify. Odours are absorbed, we're told, without clogging the pores.

Comments: 'By far the best natural deo I have found' • 'I ride a motorbike and go to the gym, but this kept me dry, with no hint of smell' • 'no white powder or stickiness, and very pleasant smell; felt fresh and dry all day and evening' • 'didn't sting after shaving' • 'keeps you dry in all conditions' • 'I used this straight after waxing and felt no pain'.

★❀❀ URTEKRAM LIQUID DEO CRYSTAL
Score: 7.21/10

Urtekram is a small Danish brand – the name translates as 'good things'. This glide-on deodorant contains the natural ammonium salts that prevent bacterial growth in a user-friendly format. It comes in three versions: Flower, Green and White (the one we trialled), which has a neutral scent.

Comments: 'This kept me fresh all day and evening – even at an aerobics class' • 'a good functional product' • 'roller-ball was very controllable, nice size for travelling; I felt

clean and fresh, with no hint of a whiff after nights out' • 'felt confident that I was fresh and dry' • 'compared well with my normal deodorant' • 'felt fresh all night, despite being crammed in a busy pub'.

★❀ GREEN PEOPLE ALOE VERA GENTLE CONTROL ROLL-ON DEODORANT
Score: 7.05/10

This alcohol-free (therefore no stinging) product, which also avoids aluminium, is based on naturally occurring ammonium salt to fight germs, which has been combined with zinc ricinoleate (from castor oil) to deodorise, along with olive leaf extract, antiseptic essential oils and floral waters.

Comments: 'Ten out of ten – it kept me fresh and dry through a night out' • 'I stayed fresh all day and didn't feel that this was going to have any adverse health effects' • 'I sweated on a long walk but didn't feel sticky or smelly' • 'I was sceptical, but am now a convert'.

★❀ THE BODY SHOP ALOE ANTI-PERSPIRANT DEODORANT
Score: 6.88/10

From what is one of The Body Shop's most natural ranges, this product has been recently formulated for ultra-sensitive skins. (We love The Body Shop's pioneering stance on everything from sex trafficking to ending animal testing, but we wish they'd walk their talk a bit more on natural ingredients.) It contains community trade aloe vera gel,

which is very gentle on skin, and provides vital income for farmers – so three cheers to The Body Shop for that, at least.

Comments: 'Spot-on compact packaging with good size roller-ball; kept me dry and odour-free; more effective than my usual deo – I will buy this now' • 'kept me fresh during my showjumping lesson' • 'worked just as well as any other deodorant I have used; liked the herby smell' • 'left my skin soft and worked very well; will continue to use this'.

★❀❀ CRYSTAL BODY DEODORANT STICK
Score: 6.88/10

US businessman Jerry Rosenblatt created this line in 1985, after a visit to France, where he discovered that many French people swear by mineral salt deodorants. A traditional 'rock' deodorant, it is handily packaged in a swivel-up stick that makes it simple to use (although you have to damp it before using, which a couple of testers found tedious). Fragrance-free and non-sticky, it promises not to affect clothing, even silk.

Comments: 'Easy to use – just wet and apply; dried very quickly and kept me fresh all day and evening' • 'didn't sweat at all and felt really fresh – nice alternative; natural and effective' • 'no residue from this rock crystal; I felt a bit tacky but not sweaty and definitely no smell' • 'I was, surprisingly, very happy using this: no white marks, one application is enough and the crystal will last you for ever!'

thigh society

We don't usually approve of the tabloid press being snide-y about celebrities' figures, but the fact they pick on dimply derrières and untidy thighs just proves the point that cellulite is no respecter of figure, age, diet – or income. About nine in ten of the girl gang have the same problem. So what's to do?

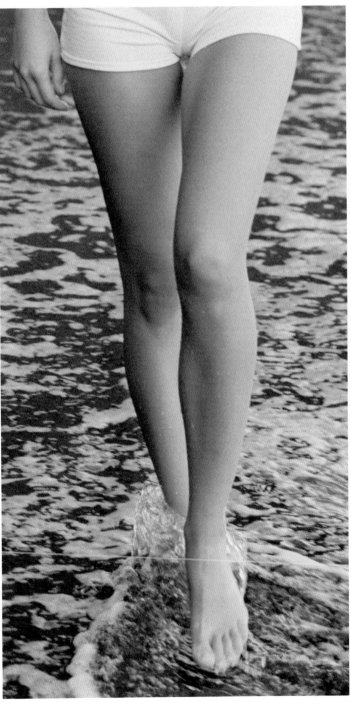

We would love to say there's a magic solution to cellulite but we'd be fibbing. As we explained before, we're lucky in that we only have the titchiest bit of mattressing: we put that down mainly to eating organic food (some experts think that the body encases toxins such as pesticides, preservatives and colourings with fat to make them safe). And neither of us take the contraceptive pill or HRT, both of which have long been linked to cellulite. Plus we have been pretty good about following this five-point, ditch-the-dimples plan for a very long time.

- Eat fresh organic food (see overleaf).
- Take well-chosen supplements (see overleaf).
- Have a vigorous daily walk, plus do plenty of stretching exercise, eg yoga, swimming and dancing. Walk up and down hills and stairs as much as possible.
- Invest in a pair of leg-sleeking FitFlops, the sandals with the built-in gym, also now as fur-lined boots for colder weather.
- Use firming moisturisers (see our Tried & Tested results, page 133).

EAT AWAY THE DIMPLES

Getting rid of cellulite is not about eating less, but eating enough of the right things. In his book *The Cellulite Solution*, dermatologist Dr Howard Murad of the University of California, Los Angeles, explains that button-back chair look is caused when the skin cells get dehydrated and weakened; this lets fat cells push into the middle layer of the skin (dermis) and show through the surface. But the cheering thing is that by repairing, rehydrating and strengthening your skin through what you eat and drink, you can help push these cells back below the surface.

Food friends

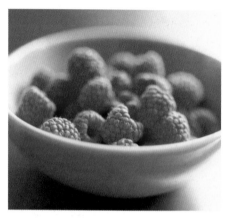

- Fine protein, such as oily fish, shellfish, eggs, poultry, game and tofu.
- Vegetables and salads, especially green leaves, onions and garlic.
- Fruit, especially blue, purple, red and pink types such as blueberries, blackberries, cherries, red grapes, raspberries and strawberries.
- Water – drink a glass of hot water with a squeeze of lemon first thing, then sip-sip-sip your way through the day, aiming for eight large glasses in all.
- Fresh juices – blend cucumber and watermelon and toss in a handful of torn fresh mint leaves for a divine detox drink.
- Olive oil and herbs – the best things to dress salads and cook with.
- Whole grains, such as brown rice, oatmeal, sprouted grains and sugar-free muesli (see recipe, right).
- Brazil nuts and almonds – full of essential nutrients: aim for three brazil nuts daily and six almonds.

Food foes

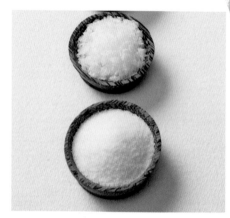

- Sugar.
- Salt.
- Fried, processed, canned and preserved foods.
- Foods containing yeast.
- Fungal foods (blue cheese, vinegar and mushrooms).
- Gluten in bread, pasta, cakes and biscuits.
- Animal fats (red meat) and dairy produce (except for yoghurt – choose sheep's or goat's if possible).
- Caffeine and alcohol.

Figure-friendly habits

- Always eat a protein-rich breakfast: muesli with live natural yoghurt, eggs and bacon (organic please), or a fruit/soy smoothie.
- Don't let yourself get hungry during the day: eat every two to three hours.
- Carry a small bag of mixed nuts and seeds – or crunchy crudités – with you to avert the candy bar munchies.

Recipes

Smoothie: whiz together a cupful of mixed berries (frozen is fine), 40g (1½ oz) chunks organic tofu and 2 tablespoons live natural yoghurt, with a little apple juice if you like.
Muesli: for one portion, mix 1 tablespoon porridge oats, 1 teaspoon runny honey, 1 teaspoon milk and 2–3 small apples or 2 small pears, grated.

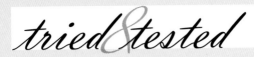

CELLULITE TREATMENTS

Can any product really tackle unsightly lumps and bumps? Surprisingly, perhaps, our testers say 'yes' – in tandem with lifestyle shifts. They found a new, effective – and budget-priced – derrière-blitzer among the supposedly firming natural lotions, potions and oils (more than 25 different options, in all) which they have now trialled for both the hardback and paperback editions of this book…

Our challenge to the panellists: use two assigned products, each on one thigh/hip/buttock only, for comparison, over a period of months. While not exactly morphing anyone into Elle Macpherson, some products did appear to make a difference. If treating your cellulite will make you feel happier in a swimsuit, then give these a try. But be prepared to use them religiously. And if not, remember: that's why Elizabeth Hurley re-created the kaftan…

★✿✿ WELEDA BIRCH CELLULITE OIL
Score: 8.28/10

We have searched for a long time to find a cellulite treatment which our testers have found to be truly effective. There were some early products in this category –we're talking 15 years ago – which our first panellists found incredibly impressive. Later, the European Cosmetics Directive required complete ingredient disclosure, and those products had to be reformulated. But the great news is that this 100 per cent natural oil from Weleda – packed with the circulation-boosting elements from young organic birch leaves, rosemary and ruscus, in a wheatgerm-and-jojoba base – really does deliver impressive results in this challenging category.

Comments: 'Following the clear instructions for this attractive smelling oil, my skin feels much better, smoother and more refined; texture is better and cellulite looks much improved: it encourages me to work on skin brushing, diet and exercise' • 'sank in quickly, improved skin texture, making it softer, smoother and less bumpy' • 'good value in an overpriced market' • 'I'm really sceptical about cellulite products but this one is worth continuing with alongside regular exercise, etc'.

★✿ LIZ EARLE NATURALLY ACTIVE SKINCARE ENERGISING HIP & THIGH GEL
Score: 7.37/10

The gel-like texture of this product makes it a breeze to apply, then get dressed straight after – by which time, this 'energising tonic for the micro-circulation' has sunk in perfectly. Stimulating botanicals include butcher's-broom, ivy, horse chestnut, plus a ten-oil blend incorporating grapefruit, sweet orange, eucalyptus and peppermint. As with most cellulite products that we trial, some testers were underwhelmed – but others were impressed, and all liked using it.

Comments: 'Skin felt moisturised and soft, and appeared smoother, less lumpy and more pliable; thigh 5mm slimmer after six weeks – I would buy it' • 'uplifting smell; lovely non-sticky gel that sank in quickly, leaving skin cool, tingly and very smooth' • 'cellulite still there but not so noticeable' • 'I lost an inch off the top of the treated thigh, but I don't think it affected my cellulite' • 'skin felt tauter and less like cellulite – my husband noticed and he didn't know I had been trying this product; I lost 1cm off my thigh. I would buy it before a special occasion' • 'cellulite less noticeable; skin firmer and tighter'.

✿✿ ELEMIS CELLUTOX ACTIVE BODY CONCENTRATE
Score: 7.3/10

This is essentially a massage oil for problem zones, combining almond and vitamin E oils with active botanicals including juniper, lemon and sea fennel. Note that it is more appropriate for use at night-time as it's an unctuous oily blend that could mark clothes.

Comments: 'Very impressed; firmer skin and less orange peel' • 'skin smoother and less rough' • 'cellulite looked less dimply' • 'leg slightly less lumpy' • 'after six weeks a dramatic difference, with smoother, more toned thighs and soft skin; also improved stretch marks' • 'I look and feel firmer'.

✿✿ DECLÉOR AROMESSENCE CONTOUR
Score: 6.95/10

Get this! After four years of research, Decléor claim that it's possible to reduce your cellulite by breathing in the blend of essential oils – basil, black pepper, hyssop, grapefruit, clary sage – in this 100 per cent natural oil. Apparently, inhaling it kick-starts the body hormonally to work on excess fat reserves.

Comments: 'Easy-to-follow instructions; texture of skin soft and smooth; after six weeks, possibly firmer' • 'a fragrant product with results my boyfriend noticed: smoother skin, less dimpled, 2cm reduction in thigh size' • 'medicinal smell, so you think it must be doing you good' • 'lost an inch, though cellulite wasn't reduced' • 'more toned'.

RAINBOW HEALING

Colour affects us profoundly: whenever you choose what to wear, or a paint colour, you're instinctively using its ability to influence your state of mind. But colour is also employed in physical healing, from the medical use of coloured light to the more esoteric chakra therapy

Look around you. Can you see anything that isn't coloured? Think of your sense of wonder when you see a rainbow, or, on a smaller scale, the enchanting dappled light when sunlight shines through a window pane on to a white wall. There's a huge range of invisible colours, too: the sun emits short-wave ultraviolet light, for instance, and white light is a mix of every hue.

Doctors use coloured light for skin conditions, including psoriasis, and also areas of pain: a recent study shows its effectiveness in hand, knee and ankle pain. Many practitioners of traditional and alternative medicine systems (most originating in the East) incorporate chakra therapy into their work. Chakras are centres of energy, ascending from the base of your spine to the top of your head. Each of the seven major chakras is linked to one of the colours of the rainbow, going from the red base chakra up to violet at your crown. Chakras – the word means circle or wheel – were first identified by yogis in Ancient India, more than 4,000 years ago. They may sound 'new age' but, like the meridians (the energy

lines used in acupuncture), they are now beginning to be validated by modern science.

Leading neuroscientist Dr Candace Pert dazzled the scientific world with her discovery of the opiate receptor in the brain in 1972, which allowed her to map the pathways between our minds and bodies. (For more about this, read her compelling book *Molecules of Emotion*.) Her research also led her to investigate the chakras. In physical terms, she says, the chakras correspond with sites of 'very important peptides' or VIPs (in fact, they're vaso-intestinal peptides), chemical messengers that are crucial in connecting the brain and the immune system. Dr Pert describes the chakras as 'mini brains' – key points of electrical and chemical activity where information is received, processed and distributed from and to the 'body mind'.

A little story to explain why Sarah takes chakras seriously. After a terrible riding accident in 2002, she was given morphine for several months for the pain. The combination of the psychological trauma and the opiate drug catapulted her into black holes of suicidal depression and appalling panic

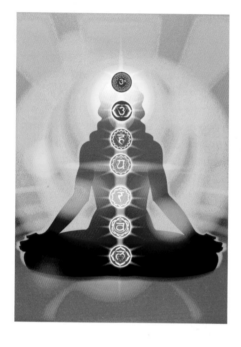

attacks. She tried everything. Nothing made a difference. One day, she saw an alternative therapist who worked on her chakras. Driving home later, she felt a glimmering of her old self – and hope – returning. The therapist (Gillian Hamer, who is also a health sciences lecturer, nutritionist and reflexologist) told Sarah that her base chakra – which is associated with a sense of self, physical survival and stability – was totally depleted and others partially so. Gillian used various techniques to replenish the energy of the chakras. For Sarah, it was a turning point, which led over several months to a full recovery.

So you might want to take care of your chakras, we think.

Colour tricks

Colour light therapist Colette Prideaux-Brune suggests choosing green if you're feeling jangly and unbalanced: 'Wear any shade or take a walk in a park.' If you're feeling mentally tired and have a lot of brain work to do, sit in a yellow room or put a bunch of daffs on your desk. On a dark, joyless day, go for orange: a bowl of fruit, a candle or a silk scarf will do the trick.

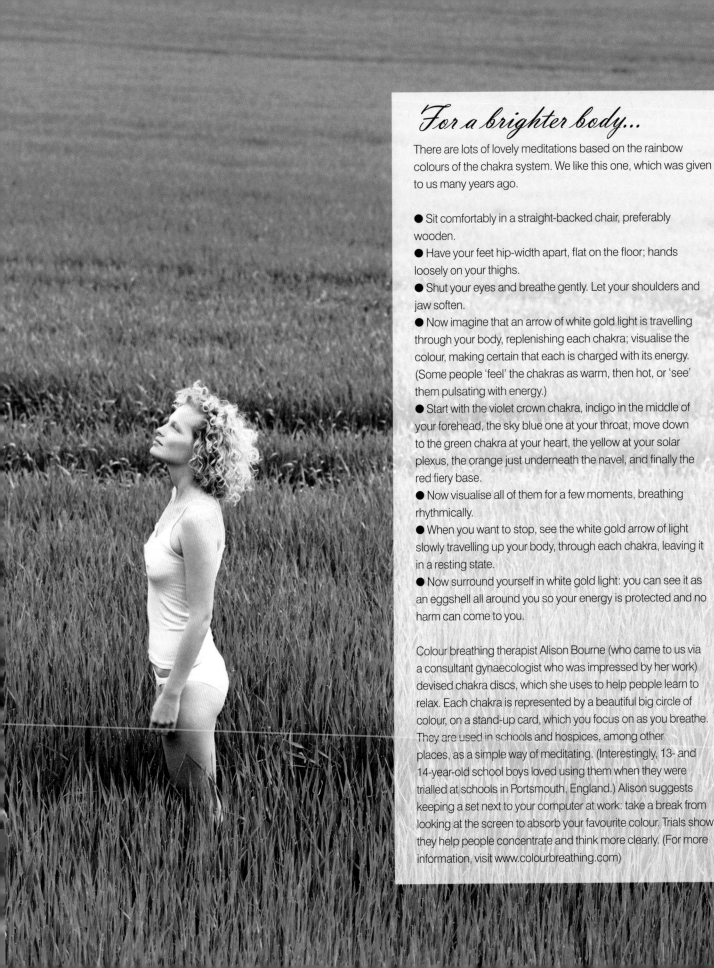

'For a brighter body...

There are lots of lovely meditations based on the rainbow colours of the chakra system. We like this one, which was given to us many years ago.

● Sit comfortably in a straight-backed chair, preferably wooden.
● Have your feet hip-width apart, flat on the floor; hands loosely on your thighs.
● Shut your eyes and breathe gently. Let your shoulders and jaw soften.
● Now imagine that an arrow of white gold light is travelling through your body, replenishing each chakra; visualise the colour, making certain that each is charged with its energy. (Some people 'feel' the chakras as warm, then hot, or 'see' them pulsating with energy.)
● Start with the violet crown chakra, indigo in the middle of your forehead, the sky blue one at your throat, move down to the green chakra at your heart, the yellow at your solar plexus, the orange just underneath the navel, and finally the red fiery base.
● Now visualise all of them for a few moments, breathing rhythmically.
● When you want to stop, see the white gold arrow of light slowly travelling up your body, through each chakra, leaving it in a resting state.
● Now surround yourself in white gold light: you can see it as an eggshell all around you so your energy is protected and no harm can come to you.

Colour breathing therapist Alison Bourne (who came to us via a consultant gynaecologist who was impressed by her work) devised chakra discs, which she uses to help people learn to relax. Each chakra is represented by a beautiful big circle of colour, on a stand-up card, which you focus on as you breathe. They are used in schools and hospices, among other places, as a simple way of meditating. (Interestingly, 13- and 14-year-old school boys loved using them when they were trialled at schools in Portsmouth, England.) Alison suggests keeping a set next to your computer at work: take a break from looking at the screen to absorb your favourite colour. Trials show they help people concentrate and think more clearly. (For more information, visit www.colourbreathing.com)

JUST SAY *(natural)* S-P-A-A-A-H...

You choose natural and organic products at home. But what about when you book into a spa or a beauty salon? At last, the spa world is getting in on the natural act

We can think of several big name spa brands whose treatments certainly have a natural aura about them, but which – actually – are almost entirely based on petrochemicals. You have to be pretty vigilant to distinguish between the marketing hype of so-called 'natural' spa products and the real thing. There are very few lines that are genuinely pure and chemical-free – and what makes life harder is that in a spa setting, you probably don't get to see the packaging for what's being slathered on your skin.

We have both lain, seething, as ill-informed beauticians told us that what they were about to massage into our bodies was 'entirely natural', when we knew that it contained literally dozens of chemicals. If you ask most spa therapists whether their products are 'natural', they will tell you they are. This is because most spas only train their therapists in the effectiveness of the essential oils used, completely ignoring the chemical carriers that make up the bulk of the products. In most cases, you can only find out exactly what's in the bottle, jar or tube by scrutinising the ingredients list on the retail products that the salon usually offers for sale.

At last, however, some natural and organic brands are devising beauty treatments to teach to therapists. In the USA, this is obviously seen as a potential boom, with the launch of a trade publication called *Organic Spa Magazine*. In the UK, Circaroma, The Organic Pharmacy, and The Spa at Pennyhill Park Hotel all offer truly organic spa treatments, and Dr Hauschka's treatments are about as natural as it gets. Espa's products and treatments are becoming increasingly natural, and their oils are entirely so.

Most aromatherapy treatments are a good natural bet: they are based simply on carrier oils and essential oils – and we can't recommend Aromatherapy Associates' massages too highly, if you're lucky enough to find a spa/salon that offers them. Jo's own Wellington Square Natural Health Centre in Hastings, Sussex, offers natural beauty therapies using Lavera products, among other pure brands (though it might be a bit of a schlep just for a facial or a massage).

If a spa/salon claims to offer 'organic beauty treatments', do ask which organic body certifies the products used (or indeed the treatments themselves in some cases). This will put the salon on the spot – and if they're hyping the treatments, might encourage a more honest stance in future. What we really want to see is honesty, so that beauty-seekers can make an informed judgment. We don't like 'greenwashing' in any form, simple as that.

There are other eco-issues to think about when considering spa treatments. Nowadays, of course, no self-respecting hotel is built without a spa, but this addition considerably increases the power and water demands of the building. Consider one of the most popular trends: the monsoon shower; huge amounts of water can be used momentarily in the name

Bathtime is an opportunity for self-healing. Focus on self-awareness from

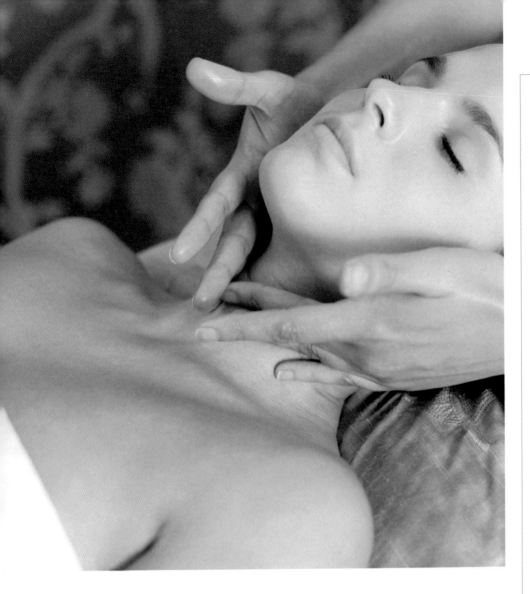

You don't have to move out of your own lovely home if you don't wish to. You can re-create some of the pampering spa rituals in your own bathroom. So pile up the organic cotton towels, put a Do Not Disturb sign on the door, light the scented candles, turn on some relaxing music and chill out…

Treats to make at home

● Try this (slightly messy) body treat from The Oriental Spa Bangkok (where Jo went on her honeymoon): the enzymes will help soften skin, while fruit acids will gently exfoliate. Blend 2 ripe papayas in a food processor till smooth, then add 2 drops of mandarin and 2 drops of vetiver essential oils. Wrap yourself in clingfilm or a (reused) length of bubble wrap, winding it tight. Lie on a towel for 20 minutes, then shower off.

● Noella Gabriel, director of treatments and product development for Elemis, suggests the following: 'Blend 7 drops of your chosen essential oils with 1 tablespoon of ordinary milk before adding it to the bath. This helps the water and oil to mix, allowing the oils to be more easily absorbed into the body.'

● Soften and smooth your body all at once: mix a small carton of plain yoghurt (which is hydrating and has skin-toning lactic acid) with a cupful of oatmeal flakes, which exfoliate gently. Apply to the body in circular motions, then rinse.

of your wellness (typically, these emit 50 or so litres of water a minute, or more than three times the rate of a normal shower). And the water in the spas' sundry steam rooms, showers and pools needs to be treated in the same way as a regular swimming pool – usually with chlorine, which remains the cheapest (and potentially most environmentally harmful) way to disinfect communal water.

Heating spas also gobbles up plenty of energy. Spas that rely on natural thermal springs, such as the world-famous Bath Spa, or those in Europe's spa towns, clearly need far less energy for heating water than those powered by fossil fuels, and you might want to consider that when you're booking a spa break. Encouragingly, there's innovation on this front: the spa at Titanic Mill – a former textile factory in the North of England that's been converted into apartments, a hotel and conference venue with spa – is being powered by a photovoltaic solar installation. Three green cheers for them. (By the way, we're adding a Green Spa section to www.beautybible.com, which will update you on any organic treatments on spa menus or all-organic spas.)

head to toe, and on relaxing every organ in your body, one by one'

HORST RECHELBACHER, founder of Aveda

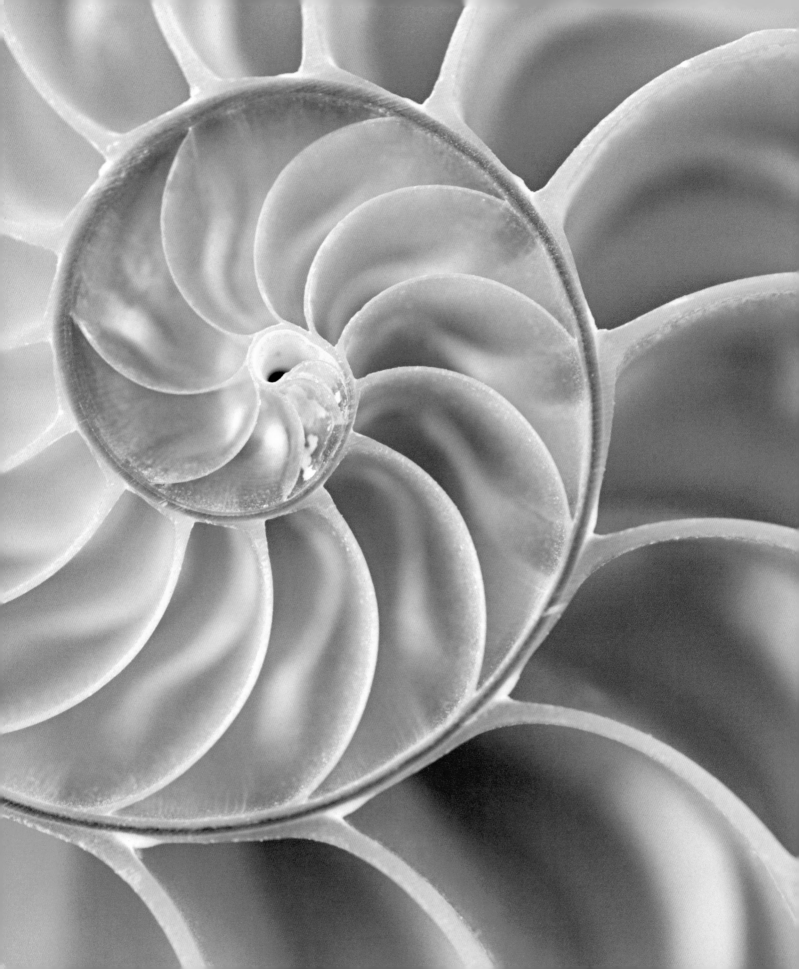

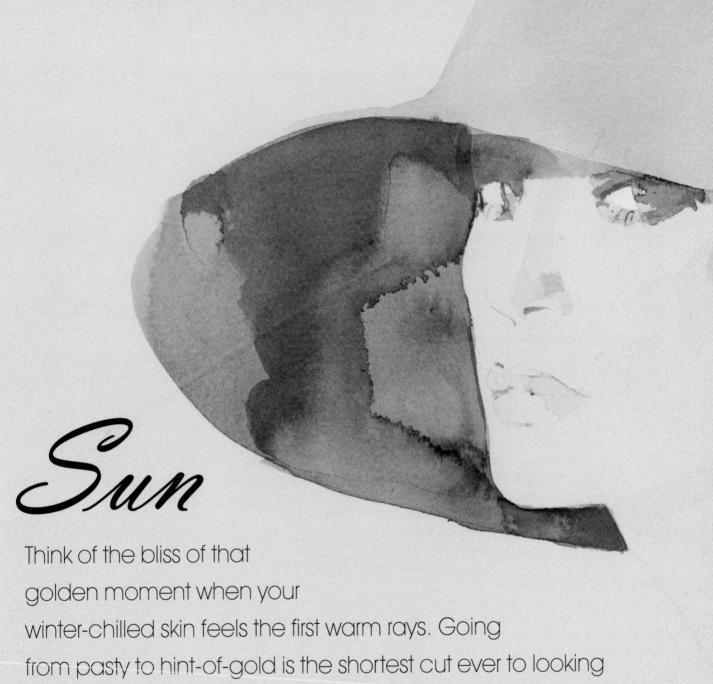

Sun

Think of the bliss of that golden moment when your winter-chilled skin feels the first warm rays. Going from pasty to hint-of-gold is the shortest cut ever to looking glam. It's undoubtedly mood-enhancing, and now, thank goodness, it seems a dose of sun really is good for us. But there's still debate over the risks and benefits of sun preps. Here we give you the best advice on safe-sunning.

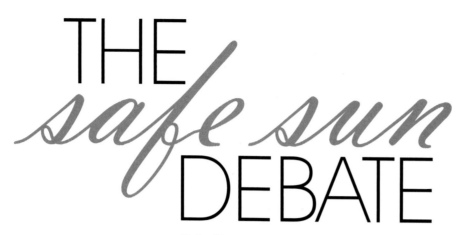

THE *safe sun* DEBATE

It's in. It's out. It's good, it's bad… In one breath we're warned that exposure to UV light increases our risk of cancer; in the next that we need the sun to help our bodies make beneficial vitamin D. And then there's the argument that sun preps themselves could be risky… So what's the truth?

For centuries, right up until the 1960s, it was the fashion to be lily-white – it meant you were 'genteel' enough not to work in the fields, so any beauty worth her parasol covered up from head to toe. Then, as holidays abroad became a status symbol, copper became the 'It' shade for skin. But with the hole in the ozone layer came the threat of skin cancer from ultraviolet sunlight. Doctors wagged their heads and said we should stay in the shade, or slather ourselves with sun preps. Recently, however, we've been told that we need sunlight to help our bodies make vitamin D and also that some sun preps could be harmful in themselves. Here, we weigh up the sun-exposure pros and cons.

The good

Fact: the sun is good for you. As well as making you feel, well, sunny, it allows your body to make vitamin D, a hormone and micro-nutrient that helps protect you against various types of cancer (including colon and prostate cancers and, ironically, melanoma), as well as osteoporosis, multiple sclerosis, diabetes and other chronic diseases.

But you don't need to sunbathe for hours to produce good vitamin D synthesis in the skin: just ten to 15 minutes daily of bright sunlight (not noon-day heat) on unprotected skin. If you're outside a lot, you'll get plenty of sunlight even wearing a sunscreen, because no product blocks 100 per cent of UV light. If you have fair skin, do wear a sunscreen,

says consultant dermatologist Dr Nicholas Lowe; people with dark olive or black skin may like to expose their skin without sunscreen for 15 minutes daily.

The bad

Fact: ultraviolet (UV) light from the sun causes skin damage. In a nutshell, UVA causes ageing and UVB burning. The longer-wave UVA, which can pass through clouds and glass, penetrates deeper into the skin, damaging collagen and elastin, and speeding dryness, wrinkling, brown spots and croc-type skin; it can also affect the immune system, damage DNA and may increase the risk of malignant melanoma. UVB rays are stronger, have an immediate impact and are primarily responsible for sunburn and skin cancers, but they're blocked by glass.

The sun prep issue

There's continued scientific argument over the safety and effectiveness of the different types of sun-protection products. The two main choices are:

● Chemical sunscreens or filters, which absorb the UV radiation and turn it into supposedly harmless thermal energy.
● Physical barriers or blocks, usually based

on the minerals titanium dioxide and zinc oxide, which in their natural state reflect UV light away from the skin.

Chemical sunscreens Some experts maintain that commonly used chemicals in sunscreens can penetrate deep below the surface of the skin where they act as 'endocrine disrupters', which may be linked to breast and other hormone-related cancers. Industry experts respond that, although molecules from chemical sunscreens have been found in the body some days after use, they are at such low levels that they're unlikely to cause any harm. However, according to leading American skin-cancer specialist Dr Sheldon Pinnell, these screens allow solar radiation into the bloodstream where they may create harmful free radicals, which could damage our DNA. There is also an accepted risk – albeit less serious – that chemical screens may aggravate allergies such as asthma or eczema, or other skin sensitivity problems.

Physical barriers The debate here centres on whether they remain on the skin surface. No one doubts that the bigger-sized (coarse

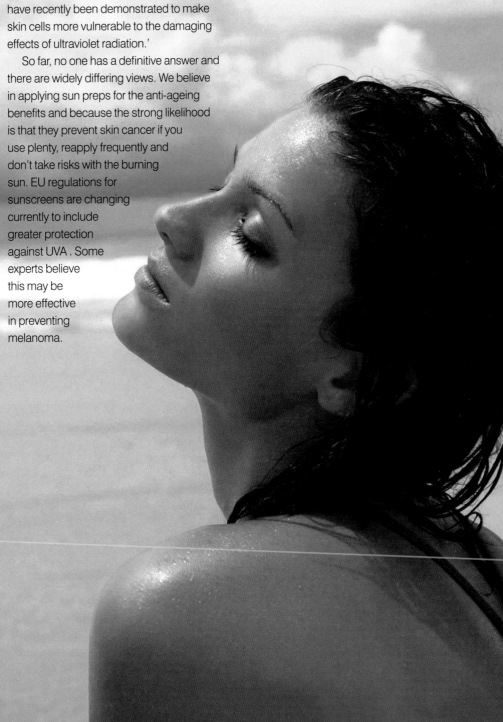

grade) particles do, but they leave a white veil, which takes some time to disappear and may not go completely until you bathe. So scientists came up with 'micronised' – finely powdered – versions of the minerals and, recently, ultra-fine ones, also known as nano-particles, which are some 500 times thinner than the width of a single hair.

In order to keep these on the surface and provide an efficient barrier that doesn't 'drop off', the particles are coated in other chemicals such as silicates and aluminium hydroxide. Despite research showing they probably stay on the skin, some experts fear that the finer grades of these particles (particularly nano) may penetrate in the same way as the chemicals, posing risks to the lungs and other organs. Professor Samuel Epstein of the University of Illinois School of Public Health, chairman of the Cancer Prevention Coalition, is particularly concerned about the penetration of nano-particles, which he regards as a significant potential danger to health. They may absorb UV light in the same way as chemical sunscreens, rather than bouncing it away from the skin, which would raise the risk that they too could transport solar radiation into our bodies.

So do sun preps really work?
While experts agree that sun preps, liberally and frequently applied, can certainly prevent skin ageing, there is a question mark over how effective they are in protecting you against all skin cancer. So far, there is only evidence that they protect against squamous cell cancer, not against basal cell cancer or malignant melanoma; although the presumption is that by preventing sunburn and damage to the immune system and DNA, they should do. Although the use of sunscreens is going up, so is the rate of malignant melanoma; but this may be due to the fact that people wearing sunscreen don't apply sufficient amounts frequently enough – and then

stay out in the sun for dangerously longer periods. It may also be due to use of paraben preservatives, particularly for men, according to dermatologist Dr Nina Wines: 'New research suggests that men may be genetically pre-programmed to develop more skin tumours than women. Parabens have recently been demonstrated to make skin cells more vulnerable to the damaging effects of ultraviolet radiation.'

So far, no one has a definitive answer and there are widely differing views. We believe in applying sun preps for the anti-ageing benefits and because the strong likelihood is that they prevent skin cancer if you use plenty, reapply frequently and don't take risks with the burning sun. EU regulations for sunscreens are changing currently to include greater protection against UVA . Some experts believe this may be more effective in preventing melanoma.

the tan COMMANDMENTS

The BIG thing to remember is this: human skin is not designed to be roasted in the sun. (If you develop moles or sun spots, please do get them checked out.) And fair-skinned lovelies should aim for a honey colour, which will last, rather than deep copper, where you run the risk of ending up like a crocodile in the Sahara...

● Tan gradually: you don't want to look like a perambulating lobster, let alone have your holiday spoilt by the pain of peeling, sunburnt flesh – so no exposing lily-white limbs to the sun for hours.

● Slop on the sun preps: it's worth it for the definite protection against sunburn and skin ageing and the probable protection against skin cancer. And using sun preps means a much better chance of a gorgeous, long-lasting tan. Do use an after-sun, too, see page 149 for Tried & Tested after-sun products.

● Remember: sun preps should be applied liberally on all exposed areas – including the backs of your legs, nape of your neck, ears and bosom – from spring to autumn, every two hours if you're in the sun. Apply 20–30 minutes before going out so that you don't spend time unprotected. Use a generous amount (lab tests use about two to four times more than we usually do) and stroke over the skin rather than rubbing in, which reduces protection.

● Given the uncertainties about the formulations, we suggest that you opt for your favourite type of broad-spectrum sunscreen with four- or five-star UVA protection plus UVB (which is measured as an SPF). Use SPF15 on your face and body if you have dark skin, which tans easily; stay with SPF30 if you are fair-skinned, out on the water or have a family history of skin cancer – and, crucially, for children. (Products above SPF30 don't give much additional protection, according to Cancer Research UK.)

● Look for water-resistant or waterproof formulas so they're not washed away if you 'glow' – but do reapply after swimming.

● Choose formulas with skin-cherishing antioxidants, such as vitamins C and E, pomegranate, green tea, raspberry, Pycnogenol and coenzyme Q10, to help repair any skin damage from the rays that got through.

● Recent research shows that you can really up your sun protection and anti-ageing by applying a dedicated antioxidant serum to your skin just before a sun prep. Pharmacist Shabir Daya recommends

There's nothing more life-enhancing and confidence-boosting than post-holiday sun-kissed skin. But it takes time and vigilance to achieve. Here's our lowdown on how to get glowing – slowly and safely

Vitamin C Anti-Ageing Face Serum by John Masters, which also contains vitamins A and E to neutralise damage; the vitamin C enhances collagen production and helps protect against environmental ageing. We're also trying Jurlique Herbal Recovery Gel, which is rich in extracts of green tea, grape seed, turmeric, rose hip oil plus vitamins C and E.

● Take an antioxidant supplement to support the skin's defences: we're opting for Imedeen Tan Optimizer, which does double duty minimising sun-induced ageing, and should also help you develop a golden tan more quickly.

● Stay in the shade from 11am to 3pm (10am to 4pm in very hot countries), when the sun is high and the radiation most intense. If you're not indoors, apply sunscreen to any exposed areas.

● Invest in big-brimmed (at least 6cm) hats, in fine straw or fabric (think Rene Russo in The Thomas Crown Affair); avoid baseball caps, which expose the vulnerable ear tips.

● Wear sun-protective clothing such as high-necked kaftans in super-sun-protective unbleached cotton or other closely woven fabrics in dark shades, such as deep sea green, indigo and blue/black. If you can see through fabric when it's held up to the light, the sun's rays can penetrate through it to your skin. Remember, too, that if the fabric is stretched tight, or gets wet, it can lose much of its sun-protective capacity.

Eye essentials

UV rays enter your eyes too and may increase the risk of eye disease, particularly cataracts. Make sure contact lenses and reading glasses have a built-in UV filter: check this with your optometrist. Sunglasses are an excellent way of protecting your eyes from UV light: go for big 'Jackie O' frames, with wide arms for maximum protection and look on the label for the CE mark, which shows they conform to European standards, also the British Standard BS EN 1836:1997.

SUNCARE

The suncare industry's in a state of flux, as new guidelines force manufacturers to reformulate so that products offer a better balance of UVA/UVB protection. Some brands are disappearing – but our testers trialled new options, identifying a second Neal's Yard favourite (see below). These products avoid the chemical ingredients that trigger photo-reactivity; they are also formulated without the petrochemical derivatives and preservatives that give most sunscreens their long-as-your-arm ingredients list (and which can often trigger sensitivity)

★ ✿ NEAL'S YARD REMEDIES LEMONGRASS SUN SPRAY SPF10
Score: 7.92/10

Organic soya, sesame and wheatgerm oils have been blended with skin-nourishing horse chestnut in this spritz-on sun protector, which has a low SPF10. The spray format is handy – but we're not convinced the blue glass packaging is that practical for the beach (or the excess baggage quota). It contains a chemical sun screen (octyl methoxycinnamate). Several testers used it on their faces and were quite happy with it (Neal's Yard Remedies confirm it is gentle enough for the face). Reactions to the lemongrass smell varied, so we suggest smelling it in a store before investing.

Comments: 'This worked surprisingly well initially, but wore off faster than my usual brand, what with sweat and travelling, so I had to reapply often' • 'the fragrance, as with most Neal's Yard products, was very pleasant and fresh; sunscreen was absorbed quickly and felt nice on my skin' • 'light liquid which sank in quickly; my face looked freshly moisturised, but no noticeable oiliness; my skin didn't react at all to the sun; I would use this on a daily basis because of the easy application and moisturisation it gave' • 'I liked the sheen it left on my skin' • 'I've not used this range before but, based on this product, I would like to'.

✿ GREEN PEOPLE EDELWEISS SUN LOTION SPF15 WITH TAN ACCELERATOR
Score: 7.92/10

With a water-resistant formula, Green People promise three actions for this cream: sun protection (against UVA and UVB rays), based on titanium dioxide, natural cinnamic acid and edelweiss extract; antioxidants (from green tea, olive leaf and that edelweiss extract again, plus vitamins A, C and E), and a 'natural sun tan accelerator'. They say it's suitable for medium complexions – and a percentage from sales goes to the Penny Brohn Cancer Care centre (which we're great supporters of). It is not certified organic, but does contain 84 per cent organic ingredients.

Comments: 'I love this product: on the one sunny day, my fair skin became slightly browner – usually it just goes a bit pink' • 'as a dark-skinned tester, I noticed a little bit of a white cast on the skin, but that went away when it had sunk in' • 'after using this on holiday, my skin was more moisturised than it would usually have been' • 'nice simple packaging; easy to use' • 'heavenly – very natural fragrance, completely unlike a sun lotion' • 'effective sun prep and left skin very soft – I would buy this product' • 'left a "film" on the skin which wasn't obvious to onlookers, but I felt protected' • 'my legs can get very dry, but they felt smoother and better moisturised for several days after using this' • 'I was dubious about a natural sunscreen but was pleasantly surprised – my skin seemed to like it a lot better than my normal one' • 'very effective and a lot less greasy than my usual product'.

✿ LIZ EARLE NATURALLY ACTIVE SKINCARE SUN SHADE BODY PROTECTOR SPF15
Score: 7.55/10

This product from a very popular brand with an excellent mail order service worldwide (as well as stores in London, New York and Tokyo) is formulated without chemical sunscreens – such as benzophenones, benzene derivatives or cinnamates – which can trigger allergic reactions in the sensitive-skinned. It includes potent antioxidants from natural-source vitamin E, pomegranate and green tea, and has a physical UVA/UVB barrier in the form of ultra-fine titanium dioxide and zinc oxide. Jo is one of the fans of this mineral-derived sunblock. Testers were also very happy using it on their faces.

Comments: 'Skin felt wonderfully silky; perfect for using on the face too' • 'really loved this product – it was extremely moisturising and I didn't burn at all' • 'gorgeous luxury product – at a reasonable price for the quality – which was very good to my skin' • 'I like a physical sunscreen such

GREEN SCREENS

None of these natural brands uses nano-particles. (Other natural/organic brands do, because they are convinced they offer superior sun protection.)

ECOLANI UVA/UVB FULL SPECTRUM SPF15 SUNSCREEN: water resistant with titanium dioxide, plus organic walnut oil, rosehip oil, squalane, green tea extract and evening primrose oil.

KIMBERLEY SAYER ULTRA LIGHT ORGANIC FACIAL MOISTURIZER SPF25: light, non-pore-clogging protection for normal, oily and acne-prone skin, with titanium dioxide and zinc oxide plus sea algae.

SANTÉ SUN SPRAY SPF15 (see below)

TREVARNO DAY CREAM WITH SPF15: this organic product contains fine-grade particles of titanium dioxide, plus moisturising essential oils and soothing herbs. (Their Rose and Jojoba Moisturiser with SPF15 is particularly suitable for dry and more mature skin.)

WELEDA SUN LOTION SPF15: waterproof, with zinc oxide and titanium dioxide, plus extract of edelweiss and other botanicals.

---

as the one in this product – I feel it's much better than overloading my skin with lots of chemicals' • 'this protected my fair skin all day, leaving it soft and moisturised'.

✿ NEAL'S YARD LAVENDER SUN SCREEN SPF22
Score: 6.88/10
Sensibly, Neal's Yard package this in a lightweight, smallish-sized tube rather than their signature blue glass. It's 44 per cent organic – and as we've said, we like the way that Neal's Yard are completely straight about their organic percentages. Offering higher protection for skins that may burn easily, its rich blend incorporates shea nut butter, sesame and sunflower oils combined with soothing herbs, lavender essential oil - and a sunscreen blend based on zinc and a

cinnamon-derived sunscreen agent.
Comments: 'I loved the freshness; had a cooling effect, and the side I used it on was slightly paler – ie, more protected – than the other' • 'delicious lavender fragrance, not overpowering and not "old lady"! No white marks ' • 'left a subtle sheen which lasted several hours; liked the user-friendly tube and will go on using it on face and chest'.

✿✿ SANTÉ SUN SPRAY SPF15
Score: 6.45/10
Not exactly a stellar score this, but several testers did rate it so we felt we should add it to the list. In a spray canister format, it's a very mild, non-irritating formulation ideal for sun-sensitive and generally touchy skins, and, so Sante tell us, for children, thanks to its gentleness. The formula features

herbal extracts, organic aloe, sesame and sunflower seed oils, and a sun-protective blend of zinc oxide and titanium dioxide – the particles are not nano/ultra-fine in size, so it can leave a slight white veil.
Comments: 'Used it walking at 15,000 feet in windy mountains and it was really moisturising, but I needed to reapply it frequently for sufficient protection' • 'reassured by the subtle white sheen because it meant there really was a barrier against the sun' • 'easy to use pump spray – I would much rather use natural mineral protection than synthetic chemical screens' • 'used this on holiday in Portugal – it sank in quickly with no stickiness; pleasant fragrance that left an almondy smell on skin; preferred it to my mainstream brand, even though I had to reapply it more frequently'.

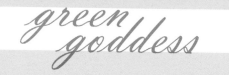

INDIA HICKS

We love (and envy) how India Hicks manages to look so gorgeous without a scrap of make-up. We love her sense of humour, and her down-to-earth attitude to looking good. She's our ultimate 'desert island' beauty: a devoted mother of three, an international supermodel – and now creator of her own natural beauty line…

'Regular going-to-bed and waking times help our bodies

Living on an island makes you very aware of the planet's resources – because everything here has to be shipped in. It makes you very conscious of how much you consume – from fresh water (which is in scarce supply) to electricity. When the weather's bad – something I worry will become a more common occurrence with the chaos of climate change – the power goes down. I remember one year, when I was breast-feeding, we were plunged into darkness. I'd just pumped a whole load of breast milk and frozen it, and the freezer was melting. All I could think was: 'Oh no, weeks of work wasted!'

I try to buy organic food for my family when I can, but unfortunately it's very hard to get here. We did have a go at growing our own tomatoes, but they need so much water and TLC it didn't prove practical. The only thing we've had any success with is corn – by accident; our parrot throws his food around and somehow the maize germinated!

Since moving to the Bahamas, I've become aware of using fruits, flowers, leaves and stems for beauty – and for health. I was thrilled to be asked to create my own range – India Hicks Island Living – for Crabtree & Evelyn, which fitted with this more natural approach to beauty. It was definitely important to me that the products shouldn't have ingredients such as sodium lauryl sulfate and parabens – but just as importantly, I wanted the packaging to have a life after the product had been used up. So the woven box for the candle can be used for cotton wool; the glass tub of bath salts makes a perfect vase. It's a way of thinking that I've become used to.

You know what? The more the houses on this island become massively interior decorated, the more I relish the fact my curtains don't quite fit any more, or that the puppy's chewed the rug.

I've never been a high-maintenance beauty. I don't go to the gym: to work out, I run on the beach every day for miles, and I carry my sons. Although when they're teenagers, I may have to find another way to firm my upper arms!

I hate to admit it, but I never even wore sun protection until a few years ago. Now I'm more cautious, and I also wear hats more often and have great respect for the sun. Although here we have a natural remedy for sunburn: the bark of the gamalamee tree, also known as 'the tourist tree', as tourists burn and peel like the red bark of the tree!

Make-up? I wear it when I'm being photographed, but the rest of the time I don't bother.

We shouldn't underestimate the importance of sleep. When we sleep our bodies heal and grow. We're meant to sleep for between six and a half and eight hours a night – undisturbed. Exercise aids sleep enormously, and regular going-to-bed and waking times help our bodies recognise when to rest. A good mattress and a clear conscience also help…

Nothing makes a person more beautiful than happiness. I gain great happiness and true contentment from my partner and my children, unconditionally loving them and being loved in return; my family are the roots from which I grow. What else makes me happy? My friends with their support and loyalty, and my home life and surroundings.

In all honesty, I really don't give much thought to how I look. Living in the Bahamas, I've realised that beauty can't be stereotyped. Every skin colour, every ethnicity, every hair and body type and every age are accepted here – and to me, beauty has never looked so good…

recognise when to rest. A good mattress and a clear conscience also help'

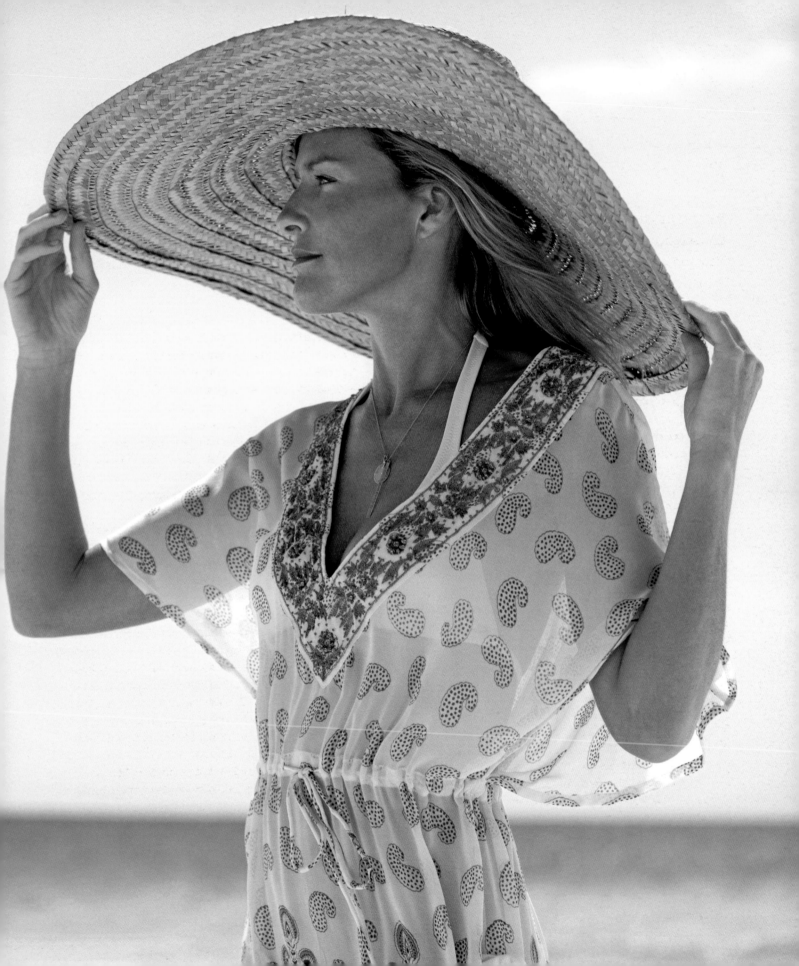

tips for trips

Over the years, we've done quite a bit of travelling. Nowadays, Jo reduces her carbon footprint by only ever travelling by train (except for the rare transatlantic crossing, when boats might just be too slow) and Sarah usually only goes as far as a horse, car or train can take her. But we know lots of you go further, so here are our favourite tips on travelling happily – by whatever means – to help you arrive gorgeously!

● Build up your oomph to catch that early plane or train – and help fight off other people's germs – with Pukka Organic Chywanaprash, a totally delicious Ayurvedic blend of fruits, honey, herbs and spices. Take a teaspoon or two daily, from a week before departure (and whenever you're stressed).

● To reduce jet lag, Kathy Phillips, founder of This Works aromatherapy company and beauty director of Condé Nast Asia, who is a frequent long-haul flier, recommends Enada by FSC: this form of vitamin B3 is proven to reduce jet-lag-induced brain fog and sleepiness. She takes it 30 minutes before the end of a flight on an empty stomach – that should be enough but, if necessary, you can take one a day until your body clock is regulated.

● Always travel in loose, non-crush clothes (cashmere is perfect) and comfy shoes. Above all, avoid tight waistbands and pointy shoes.

● Pack needfuls, such as good books/music/change of shoes in a rucksack (you can get chic ones now), so that you don't end up having to carry heavy bags at the other end.

● Don't wear make-up; if you're flying, slather moisturiser on face and hands continually. Slick on tinted moisturiser, mascara and lippie/gloss just before you arrive. Remember to check in-flight regulations on liquids, creams, etc, before travelling.

● Eye masks are the biz on planes and trains if you want to catch up on sleep or repel chatty space-invaders.

● If you're prone to travel sickness, try acupressure Sea-Bands.

● Flight socks (aka compression stockings, which are available from your local pharmacy) help prevent swelling and reduce the risk of DVT (deep vein thrombosis).

● Dr Scurr's Zinopin Long Haul is a scientifically proven natural remedy with ginger and pycnogenol to prevent DVT, travel sickness, swollen ankles, calf cramp and sluggish circulation.

● Sip lots of still water – cabin air in planes is drier than the Sahara – and avoid alcohol on planes (apart from maybe one glass of holiday-spirit champagne) and, of course, if you're driving.

● Take fruit and crudités to snack on; on planes, pre-order a veggie meal and/or fruit platter.

tried & tested

AFTER-SUN

Despite trialling several new 'green' after-suns for this paperback, our fave sunscreen is still the aloe vera plant: 100 per cent natural and effective, and deserving of a place on every kitchen windowsill. However, the following products – including one new winning entry – made a good impression on our testers…

For weather reasons, some of these after-suns had to be tested more like body lotions than post-sun skin-soothers. Testers still got a pretty good idea of the products' cooling and nourishing powers, if not their tan-prolongability.

✿ YIN YANG PH-AMINO GOLD DEFENCE LOTION
Score: 8.27/10

Yin Yang say this offers 'natural protection from the sun', but it doesn't have a measured SPF, so we supplied it to our testers as an after-sun. This daily face and body cream is packed with antioxidant vitamin E, plus apple cider vinegar to balance the skin's pH level, along with coconut oil and wheatgerm oil (rich in amino acids) to help skin maintain a youthful, healthy appearance.
Comments: 'My skin felt soft and smooth after application – this lasts for hours, too; it also smells delicious' • 'I burned my shoulders and it relieved the redness' • 'absorbed amazingly quickly' • 'I like that it can be used on face and body' • 'would be good for hot children as it's absorbed quickly and doesn't leave a sticky residue'.

★ ✿✿✿ GREEN PEOPLE COOL AFTER-SUN
Score: 8.2/10

The skin-cooling, instant soothing power of this after-sun is down to aloe vera and oil from the herb corn mint, blended with lavender, rosemary and marigold to give a lovely fragrance. This is Jo's favourite after-sun, which she also gave to Angela, a pale-skinned visitor who'd been seduced by the seaside sunshine; Angela went to bed red and woke up lightly golden-toasted. The formula is alcohol-free and is organically certified by the Organic Food Federation.
Comments: 'Lovely product with fresh minty fragrance, which gave an immediate cooling sensation; like a body lotion, which softened as well as soothed and cooled; excellent packaging in soft tube that releases the lotion in the amount you require – ten out of ten' • 'easy to apply, absorbed quickly and relieved redness' • 'light and cooling; immediate relief' • 'easy to carry and use'.

✿ LIZ EARLE NATURALLY ACTIVE SKINCARE SUN SHADE BOTANICAL AFTERSUN GEL
Score: 7.87/10

This light, cooling gel is packed with antioxidant green tea, pomegranate and natural-source vitamin E, to fight free radical damage. Like all of the Liz Earle suncare range, it is subtly fragranced with lavender.
Comments: 'Soothed tight, hot skin immediately; incredibly hydrating – skin felt moisturised but not sticky; gorgeous smell' • 'fabulous: instant relief' • 'absorbed quickly; I liked the transparent panel, so you could see how much product was left'.

★ ✿✿✿ NEAL'S YARD REMEDIES ALOE VERA COOLING SPRAY
Score: 7.21/10

This Soil Association-certified after-sun is spritz-on. The plastic bottle makes it ideal for travelling. Cooling aloe vera gel is blended with nettle extract and helichrysum to take the sting out of sun-stressed skin, and there's a lemon-and-lavender whisper of scent. Testers didn't think it was as moisturising as a cream would be.
Comments: 'Easy to apply, absorbed easily, very cooling, and soothed and moisturised red skin instantly' • 'my skin felt soothed and regenerated after one application' • 'it's always good to spray, rather than rub, when you have sunburn' • 'attractive bottle and light, pleasant fragrance' • 'I used it while working in India and it was great on hot days: I would definitely use this again' • 'it really helped a nasty rash and swelling on my arm, a reaction to a euphorbia in my garden'.

We love…
If we can't get our mitts on an aloe plant, our favourite after-suns are aromatherapy base oils such as sweet almond, peach kernel or jojoba. Any favourite bath or massage oil is good. Jo also sloshes on olive oil with gay abandon.

easy glowing

Brilliant faking is a cinch today, with modern formulas streaks (or no streaks) ahead of the early self-tanners. They also leave skin sun-kissed gold rather than ten-carat carrot. But a little bit of prep is worth it every time…

Time spent prepping means the difference between a patchy, uneven finish and a can't-tell-it-from-real, Riviera tan. Fact: at a recent swimwear fashion show we were speaking at, the real-women-size models all had orange-peel skin and mega-curves, but they sloshed on some instant tan, strutted down the catwalk like princesses – and looked fantastic.

A word of warning, though: some fake tans boast an SPF, but that will only last for the first two hours after you apply it. Remember: a fake tan does not protect you from the sun's rays.

Here's our advice:

● Do a patch test the night before to make sure you like the colour, and that your skin is not sensitive to the product (allergic reactions are rare but have been reported).

● De-fuzz your legs 24 hours before to ensure smooth, even results. (NB: don't expose just-waxed or shaved skin to the sun, or to sunscreens; or you risk a rash.)

● Remove dry skin with a body scrub (see page 115 for T&T winners) and/or loofah, concentrating particularly on dry patches

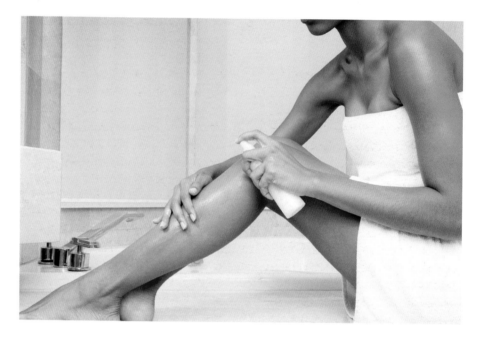

such as elbows, knees and heels. Or make your own – the simplest and one of the most effective is a 'sludge' of olive oil and salt.

● Polish your face with a wet muslin square or wash cloth, or a very gentle facial exfoliant (see page 39 for T&T winners).

● Moisturise lavishly from top to toe,

particularly the bony bits like your knees, ankles and elbows.

● Apply the self-tanner thinly and evenly; you can always add more if you want a deeper colour, but you can't go backwards.

● Wash your hands well after applying any type of tinted cream or fake tan and use a damp cotton wool pad or cotton balls to wipe off areas that don't normally tan, such as the armpits, soles of feet, nipples and fingers. Also wipe off the area around your eyebrows, hairline and jawline.

● Always leave time to dry off completely – if you have to leap out quickly, or you're opting for a salon tan, wear dark undies and loose clothes.

We love…

We're both outside a lot, so we tan slowly and naturally. To tidy up white patches, or jump-start our legs into summer, we mix a self-tanner with our favourite face and body moisturisers to create our own hint-of-a-tan product. (We'd been doing this for years before the beauty industry caught on.) We also make our own tinted make-up with the clever, all-natural Santé Bronzing Fluid.

SELF-TANNERS

Natural brands are trying hard to come up with self-tanners – but in truth, they can't get around the fact it's a chemical called DHA (dihydroxyacetone) which turns skin biscuity brown (and with some products, decidedly biscuity-scented); although DHA does originate from plant sources – sugar beet or cane, or sunflower seeds – it goes through a number of lab processes. So: there's still no totally natural way to fake a tan – but our panellists have added one new 'discovery' to this list, from Lavera. Do remember to exfoliate and moisturise first!

❀ ORIGINS THE GREAT PRETENDER
Score: *7.88/10*
The great thing about this shimmery tinted body gel is that you can see exactly where you've put it, so you can tell which bits you still need to do. It contains a significant proportion of natural ingredients, including sugar-derived DHA and vegetable glycerine, infused with summery-scented essential oils of peppermint, orange and rosemary. The colour develops, darkens and dries quickly, promise Origins. Blend, blend, blend is their mantra for application.
Comments: 'After using this I was pleasantly surprised by the nice golden-brown result' • 'lovely shimmery particles which were great for evenings out – and didn't last after the initial application' • 'the tan stays even over days' • 'this product was absorbed into the skin very quickly' • 'very nice pepperminty smell'.

❀ GREEN PEOPLE SELF TAN LOTION
Score: *7.42/10*
Green People recommend buffing your skin first with their Organic Sugar Scrub to create the smoothest possible surface. This non-greasy formula has been formulated with organic aloe vera and rosehip oils to soothe and nourish, softly scented with rose geranium, sandalwood and vetivert – a blend that Green People

say is suitable for both men and women.
Comments: 'The only self-tanner I have used that did not smell like one – hooray! Nice, fresh smell from the tube and when drying' • 'I used it before going to bed and my skin had a gentle sun-kissed glow in the morning; it was a very realistic colour – not at all orangey – which needed topping up after two to three days' • 'this was very easy to use and smooth on to skin; dried within a few minutes of application with no tacky film on the skin; it also gave a nice, subtle glow; I didn't notice any problems with it rubbing off on to my clothes, and it left no blotches or marks as it wore off' • 'I love the natural formula, the no animal testing policy, and that it supports the Penny Brohn Cancer Care centre'.

❀ LAVERA SELF-TANNING LOTION
Score: *7.09/10*
Suitable for use both on body and face (though we always suggest going 50/50 with moisturiser, the first time you try this), this German product – in no-nonsense packaging – features aloe vera, vitamin E and green tea for extra skin nourishment, and is subtly scented with rosewater, lavender flower water and essential oils.
Comments: 'Having had breast cancer I am wary of using fake tan on my upper body but would happily use this: sinks in

quickly and gives a lovely, natural, very light golden colour – needs daily top-ups, though' • 'very pleasant to use, flowery smell when applied and then nothing; sinks in quickly, leaving a smooth silky finish and pale honey colour' • 'absolutely realistic light gold; I would have given it ten out of ten if they'd included gloves'.

★ ❀ LIZ EARLE NATURALLY ACTIVE SKINCARE SUN SHADE BOTANICAL SELF-TAN SPRAY
Score: *6.65/10*
High levels of organic aloe vera and natural source vitamin E help make this spritz-on self-tanner extremely smooth to apply, while the blend of pure essential oils – sweet orange, rosemary and geranium – give it a delicious initial smell. The DHA in this does come originally from sunflower seeds, to give the golden glow.
Comments: 'Gave a delicate tan that took about two hours [some testers said longer] to develop and lasted about three days' • 'absorbed fast and smelled pretty on application, but don't wear white underwear until it dries properly!' • 'lasted for about a week' • 'I had to do a few goes over a number of days to notice a good colour; after that, it was lovely and natural and easy to maintain that desirable glow by just topping up every other day'.

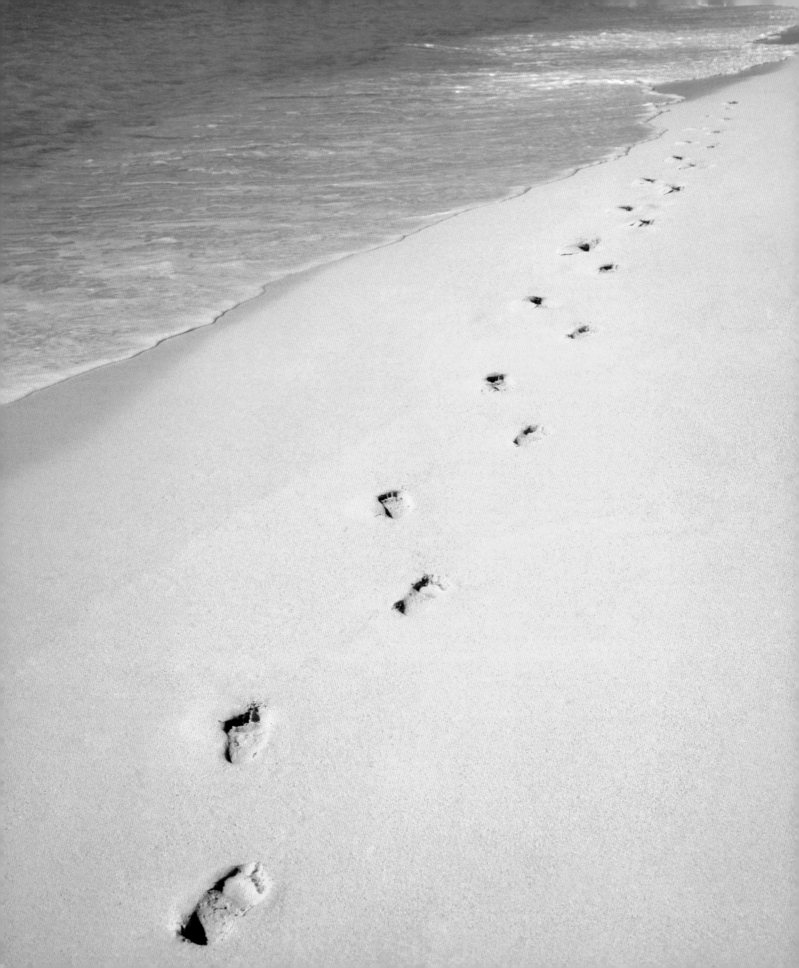

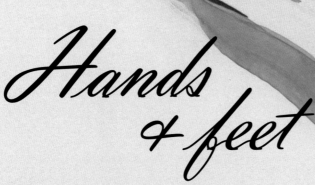

Hands & feet

Feet ground us to the earth and, according to some ancient cultures, are the foundation of good health. We agree. With our hands, we perform a gazillion useful tasks each day – and express ourselves to others. Over the next few pages, you'll find more natural ways to take care of – and pretty up – your hard-working extremities, giving them the TLC they richly deserve to make them touch-me soft, super-smooth and (most importantly) strong.

going to extremities

We like our hands (and feet) to look as pretty as the next woman's. But in the grand scheme of things, it's far more important to keep them supple, strong and dexterous than as perfect as a hand model's. So is it possible to have gorgeous-but-'green' hands and feet? Absolutely. In this chapter, the world's leading 'natural nail' gurus share their secrets

As any wannabe-green goddess understands, it can be tough to be an environmentalist and a femme fatale at the same time, especially if you like to paint your nails (which most females of our acquaintance do, ever since childhood). Let's face it: nail polish comes pretty far down the list of life essentials – but, more than that, it ranks as among the most toxic cosmetics you're likely to find on a typical dressing table. What's more, the chemical solvents in conventional nail polish can, over time, weaken nails and make them brittle.

The 'big three' questionable ingredients in nail polish are:
- toluene,
- formaldehyde,
- di-n-butyl phthalate (aka DBP, or phthalates).

Toluene is a neurotoxin, which affects the nervous system, potentially causing symptoms such as tiredness, confusion, weakness, drunken-type actions, memory loss, nausea, loss of appetite, and hearing and colour vision loss. Yet, extraordinarily, it is permitted to make up to 50 per cent of a nail polish.

Formaldehyde, banned in cosmetics in Japan and Sweden, is a respiratory irritant and has caused cancer in animal studies; it is considered a likely human carcinogen. When DBP (also used in hair spray) is absorbed by the body it accumulates in fat cells: research has shown that it's an oestrogenic chemical, linked to reduced sperm count in men and possibly menstrual disorders, miscarriages and premature births in women. The US Cosmetic, Toiletry and Fragrance Association maintains that DBP presents no health risk. But Kevin Donegan, director of communications for the San Francisco-based Breast Cancer Fund (which focuses, unlike so many cancer charities, on the environmental causes of disease) says: 'If there is evidence that an ingredient causes or is suspected of causing cancer or birth defects, cosmetic companies should not be using it in their products. Phthalates have clearly been demonstrated to cause harm.' High exposure can occur temporarily in your home simply from using nail polish, according to the US Agency for Toxic Substances and Disease Registry.

Good news for those who live in the EU: phthalates are now banned under an amendment to the European Cosmetics Directive. And in the US, Max Factor and Cover Girl, Clinique, Sally Hansen, OPI, Orly and MAC polishes have stopped using this ingredient. Many others proclaim their toluene- and/or formaldehyde-free status. Brands that are free from the big 3 include Zoya and Butter London, L'Oreal Quick Dry, Nars, OPI, Elizabeth Arden, Avon, Cover Girl and Revlon Quick Dry/Top Coats.

However, here's a hallelujah moment! There is a new nail polish technology to gladden the heart (and brighten the fingertips) of green goddesses. While there's no such thing as a completely 'eco' nail paint, the new generation of nontoxic, water-based polishes do avoid the solvents and plasticisers typical of conventional products. Water-based brands include Suncoat, Acquarella and Honeybee Gardens, while Santé, Priti and Adorée are leading the way in the more-natural fingertip field; with the current boom in 'back-to-nature' beauty, expect more to hit the shelves soon.

We have to admit, though, there is a slight downside: in our experience, they may not 'set' as fast (although a drop of almost any kind of oil on to each nail, five minutes after you've painted them, speeds things up), and the finish, while good, isn't quite as 'glassy'. The upside is that some of them peel off so you don't need to use polish remover, and they allow nails to 'breathe' better.

Tip... **Use products containing toluene and other chemicals in well-ventilated areas, advises the US Agency for Toxic Substances and Disease Registry. So always apply nail polish in a large room, with the windows open (weather permitting). Put the tops tightly on to bottles afterwards so the chemicals don't evaporate into the air.**

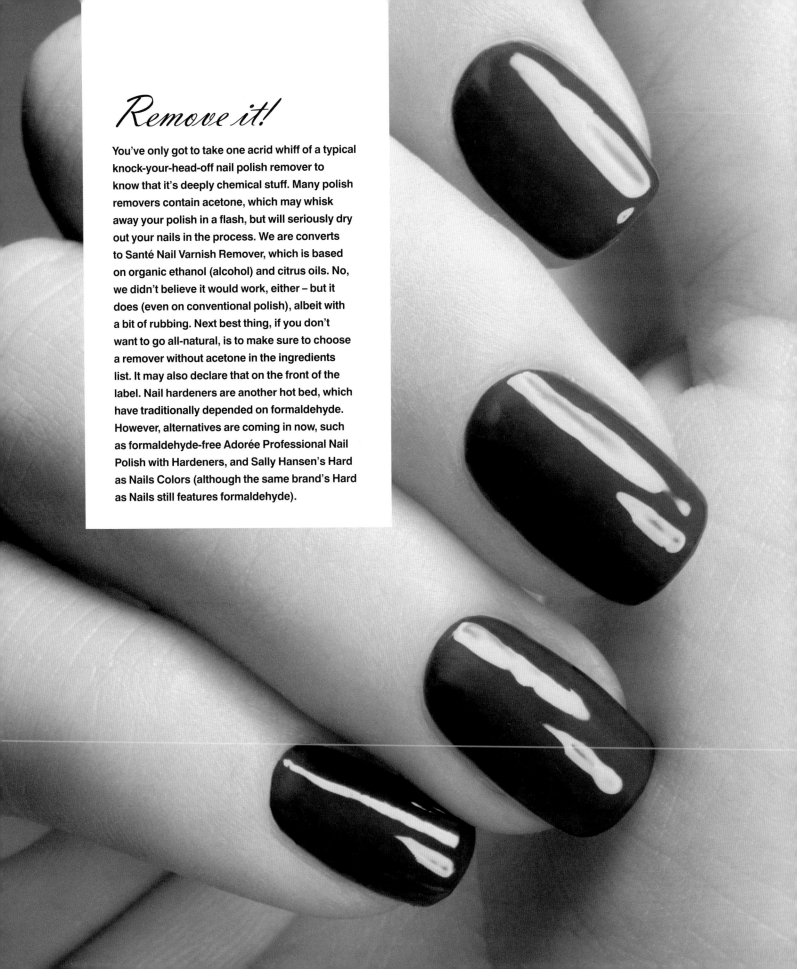

Remove it!

You've only got to take one acrid whiff of a typical knock-your-head-off nail polish remover to know that it's deeply chemical stuff. Many polish removers contain acetone, which may whisk away your polish in a flash, but will seriously dry out your nails in the process. We are converts to Santé Nail Varnish Remover, which is based on organic ethanol (alcohol) and citrus oils. No, we didn't believe it would work, either – but it does (even on conventional polish), albeit with a bit of rubbing. Next best thing, if you don't want to go all-natural, is to make sure to choose a remover without acetone in the ingredients list. It may also declare that on the front of the label. Nail hardeners are another hot bed, which have traditionally depended on formaldehyde. However, alternatives are coming in now, such as formaldehyde-free Adorée Professional Nail Polish with Hardeners, and Sally Hansen's Hard as Nails Colors (although the same brand's Hard as Nails still features formaldehyde).

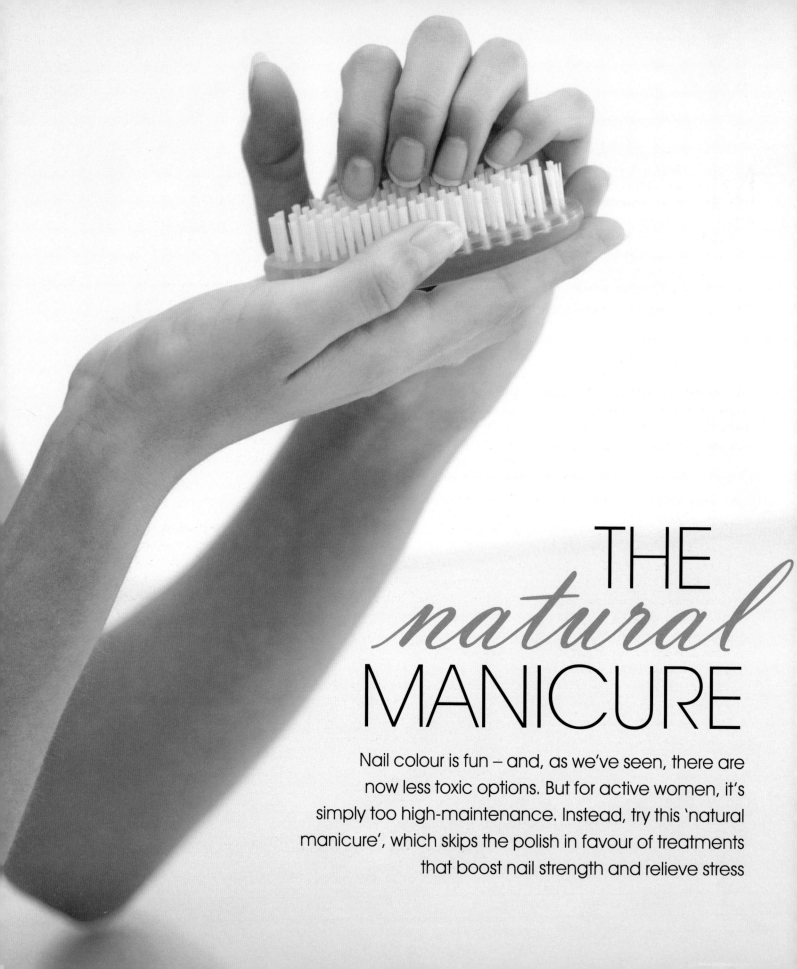

THE *natural* MANICURE

Nail colour is fun – and, as we've seen, there are now less toxic options. But for active women, it's simply too high-maintenance. Instead, try this 'natural manicure', which skips the polish in favour of treatments that boost nail strength and relieve stress

Many women – including Jo – hold their stress in their hands; when she's angsty, she'll discover that she's made two tight fists without even realising it. Releasing that pent-up stress relaxes the whole body, so the following truly natural manicure can work to relieve all-over tension.

Kim d'Amato founded New York's first 'organic' nail salon, Priti (just north of Nolita in Manhattan). Though she sells her own range of (more) natural nail polishes, some clients prefer to have their nails buffed till they gleam – which, says Kim, 'also helps boost nail growth, by stimulating blood flow to the nail bed'. Follow these steps to naturally gorgeous hands…

1 **Trim hangnails.** Use nail nippers – very, very carefully – to clean up any ragged skin around the nail. Do not cut cuticles – the delicate skin where the skin meets the nail – as these help protect the skin from infection.

Tip… **The biggest favour you can do your hands is actually to keep them agile by playing the piano, embroidering, doing needlepoint – even typing. Take up yoga, which will give you amazingly strong wrists (think cobra pose and downward dog). If your hands start to become stiff as you get older, you could try cutting out nightshades from your diet (potatoes, tomatoes, aubergines), which are linked with arthritis.**

2 **Soften rough skin.** Soak your hands in a basin of warm organic full-fat milk for several minutes. The lactic acid in milk helps dissolve dead cells and softens cuticles; the natural fats in milk are also good for dry skin. If hands are grubby, use a scrub on them too. Make your own by mixing roughly equal amounts of organic brown sugar, olive oil and organic honey. For grimy nails with dug-in dirt, try rubbing with a lemon quarter.

3 **Push back cuticles.** Using an angle-tipped nail stick lightly wrapped in a whisper of cotton wool, gently push back the cuticles towards the base of the nail, clearing the nail surface for buffing.

4 **Shape nails.** Using a nail file (see Fab Idea, above right), shape nails into squares with rounded corners, which makes them more resilient to cracks and snaps. File in one direction only – no sawing back and forth.

Fab idea…

The best nail file? Naomi Andersson of Green Hands (a natural-as-poss nail-care company, based in the UK in Herefordshire) has this tip: 'If you don't own a glass file as yet, hurry up and get one. Every nick, catch, dent – file it. Each broken nail, file to the length of the shortest.' It's 'a-stitch-in-time' thinking: if you file a nail that has started to split, you'll prevent it from turning into a much worse break.

5 **Buff nails till they gleam.** Use a smooth-surfaced buffer to buff the entire surface of nails, using a side-to-side motion. Do this gently but swiftly, and don't allow heat to build up. (If your nails are weak, don't do this too often as it can make them more fragile.)

6 **Moisturise and massage.** As a final step, rub hands with warm almond oil, avocado oil or light olive oil – working into cuticles especially, to help stimulate nail growth. Or we suggest applying one of the winning hand creams from our Tried & Tested (see page 162).

'Buffing helps boost nail growth by stimulating blood flow to the nail bed'

KIM D'AMATO, founder of New York's first 'organic' nail salon

nail tips

It's a mystery to us that our hair and skin can be strong and lustrous while our fingernails, which are made of the same protein (keratin), are weak, flaky and dry. We've just managed to find a (multi-pronged) solution, so here's our advice…

Here's a thought: we've come to the conclusion that much of the problem must be to do with the tough life our hands endure because invariably – despite our raggedy fingernails – our toenails are quite well, thank you. Just reflect on a day in the life of your fingernails: continually abused in one way or another, exposed to water and paper (one wetting so it makes your nails swell, the other drying so they shrink, a cycle that repeated often enough makes them brittle and fragile) and pollutants of all kinds (including harsh chemicals in nail polish and remover), seldom covered up or protected – no wonder they show the strain.

So apart from a total life shift where you lie on a sofa 24/7, languidly raising a perfectly manicured hand to summon what or who you need, what can you do?

In no particular order, here's what works for us. Remember it takes up to three months for a new nail to grow in, so don't expect instant results, although you should start to see improvements within two to four weeks.

● Use lots of hand cream, very often – as often as you drink a glass of water (so that's eight times a day, isn't it?) and certainly every time you've had your hands in water.

● Massage in a good nail oil at night, and during the day if possible. The best we know is Dr Hauschka Neem Nail Oil (you only need a drop, literally, so it's not that costly). Naomi Andersson of Green Hands also recommends using cuticle or olive oil 'or even old lip balms in pots, massage all over the nail and around the cuticle area every night'.

● Wear gloves to protect your nails whenever you can – for washing up and any other wet/dirty jobs. And if you can bring yourself to pull on thin gloves while you're

Eat lots of good omega-3 fats, in oily fish, walnuts and freshly ground flax seeds

opening mail or handling paper for any reason, your nails will reward you! (We think it would look very chic to wear stretchy velvet or silk gloves at your desks…)

● If you rashly disregard the advice above, dig your nails into a bar of soap before you do any dirty work – such as grooming horses (Sarah) or pricking out seedlings (Jo).

● Never abuse your nails by treating them as screwdrivers, grout-cleaners or for digging up flints in your field (as Sarah does!).

● Eat lots of good omega-3 fats, in oily fish, walnuts and freshly ground flax seeds.

● Make sure you get enough protein, see the recommendations for feeding your hair on page 94. Iron deficiency is a common cause of brittle nails, as it is of thinning hair, so if you suspect a problem, have your iron levels measured. If they're low, consider a gentle supplement such as Floradix or Spatone (the iron tablets often recommended by family doctors may cause digestive side effects, according to Dr Ivor Cavill of the University of Wales College of Medicine, an expert in anaemia).

● Consider supplements. In Sarah's case, a daily supplement of the trace mineral silica, which is often deficient in our diet, plus omega-3 oils and a chlorella supplement such as Sun Chlorella A, have revolutionised her fingertips.

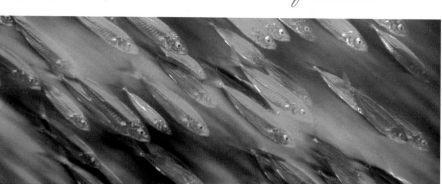

NAIL STRENGTHENERS

Chemical nail hardeners can work short-term miracles, but use them for longer than necessary, and your nails will become brittle and prone to snapping. Massaging a couple of drops of natural nail treatment into your nails and cuticles each night takes much longer to deliver results, but at the end of the testing period, our panellists found these winning products delivered the equivalent of the nail Holy Grail

✿✿ GREEN HANDS CUTICLE OIL AND NAIL STRENGTHENER

Score: 8.61/10

This intensive combination of cold-pressed jojoba and sweet almond oils is enhanced with neroli and frankincense, which gives a warm, lightly spiced fragrance. Green Hands (a British brand that is happy to ship worldwide) say this product is ideal for peeling and brittle nails, and should deliver results within four weeks. They are hoping to achieve Soil Association organic status for it (check www.beautybible.com for a status report on that). Testers were impressed, although it took some a while to figure out exactly how to use the dispenser.

Comments: 'Pleasant smell: my splitting nails are stronger, more flexible and less brittle – I would buy this again' • 'nails stronger and did not split or flake once, more flexible and seemed much longer than usual; cuticles softer – I was surprised by how much difference this made' • 'I am a nurse and the cleaning products we use are so strong my nails suffer terribly; they now look better, are stronger and a lot smoother, and don't break so easily – I would recommend this product to everyone' • 'improved condition of my nails, particularly cuticles' • 'my yellow nails are now white, with less ridging; it's also cleared up the red, itchy skin at the base of each nail; nails now look lovely with no polish – it looks as though I have a French manicure'.

✿✿ THE ORGANIC PHARMACY LEMON & NEEM NAIL OIL

Score: 7.51/10

Neem is well-known for its antifungal and nail-strengthening abilities (so it's good for toenails too). In this nail-booster, neem is blended with jojoba and wheatgerm oils, plus lemon essential oil. The Organic Pharmacy also suggest applying it overnight beneath a rich hand cream before slipping on cotton gloves. Several testers liked the product but marked it down because of problems with the pipette dispenser.

Comments: 'Nails stronger, straighter, whiter, with fewer bumps; they broke less and there were fewer sore, dry bits on cuticles; a bit messy to use but the improvement made it worthwhile' • 'fantastic smell and nails looked better and healthier' • 'my rubbish nails were transformed – stopped peeling and cuticles are almost bearable!' • 'made a huge difference to my cuticles' • 'made an obvious improvement to the condition of my nails' • 'nails stronger and cuticles softer'.

✿ ✿ DR HAUSCHKA NEEM NAIL OIL

Score: 7.45/10

In a pump-action bottle, this nail treatment also contains neem leaf extract, this time blended with peanut oil, apricot kernel oil and camomile, to encourage nail growth and soften cuticles. Just a drop or two massaged into the base of each nail at bedtime is all you need – but remember to do it religiously. Personally, we also like the Dr Hauschka Neem Nail Oil Pen, which dispenses a tiny amount of oil through a slanted foam tip for pushing back cuticles, but our panellists trialled the bottle version. Several testers who usually used this product but trialled others for us said they preferred this one.

Comments: 'Nails stronger and more flexible; the thumb nail no longer splits – evidence it must have really strengthened that one' • 'improved very dry cuticles, nails looked much better too; I really liked this product once I found you only needed a couple of drops for both hands' • 'nails less broken and ragged, looked shiny and were easier to push back – I used it on my toenails too' • 'liked the fresh smell, and parched cuticles looked better almost immediately'.

✿✿ DECLÉOR AROMESSENCE ONGLES

Score: 7.33/10

This aromatic treatment oil from a company with a long reputation of such products features essential oils of myrrh, lemon and parsley, in a base of castor, hazelnut and avocado oil. It should be massaged into the base of nails nightly.

Comments: 'Nails tougher – flexible not brittle – and skin around them conditioned' • 'nails pinker, perhaps from the frequent massage' • 'easy to use; left nails with a slight sheen; good for stopping flaking'.

HEAVENLY HANDS

Top of our list of desert island beauty essentials would be hand cream. Our job description means we work constantly with paper, which strips hands of all their natural oils. On our desks, by our taps and beside our beds, you'll find hand-restoring treats – preferably pure and natural

Because all the women we know are on a constant beauty quest for great hand creams, we've devoted lots of space to the results of the Tried & Tested hand creams that we sent out. (And there were plenty of them.) You might like to know, though, that you can cut down on your hand cream use by using a handmade soap that hasn't had the glycerine removed. (Ironically, the glycerine is often removed and sold to hand cream manufacturers – and if that isn't evidence of collusion to make us buy more beauty products than we really need, we'd like to know what is.) For ultra-pampering, you might also occasionally like to give hands a 'mask

treatment'. Slather on the same mask you're using on your face, keep your hands still for 10–15 minutes, then rinse. The bath is ideal for this; just keep your hands above the water-line.

Personally, we prefer natural hand creams. Our reasoning? We apply a lot of the stuff. Scoops and scoops of it: for sheer volume, probably more than any other product we use. We try to eat organically, even live organically, so it makes sense to pamper our hands as naturally as possible too. (Not least because hands touch food – and food goes into our mouths; and if you haven't washed your hands religiously so do the chemicals.)

We love...

Sarah's hands need TLC as flowers need water, what with riding, gardening and the rest of country life. As well as automatically putting any face/body creams or balms she's using on her hands too (also any sunpreps), she slathers on Seven Wonders Miracle Lotion, oozing with natural oils and herbs, which treats hands and nails – as it says – miraculously. Jo keeps a jar of high-scoring Circaroma Replenishing Hand Cream on her desk and enjoys each application: 'It's like being whisked to the May rose harvest in Grasse.' Balance Me's velvety-rich hand cream is another favourite – also sinks-in-fast Jurlique Purely Age-Defying Hand Treatment.

Citrus scrub

Fact: hand creams will penetrate better and work their plumping magic for longer if you exfoliate hands first. This low-tech, zestily scented hand scrub makes at least ten treatments; keep it in a jar or plastic tub by your bath, and work it into skin from hands to elbows a couple of times a week – especially if you're a gardener.

3 tablespoons freshly ground sunflower seeds (use a herb grinder or blender)
3 tablespoons oatmeal
3 tablespoons flaked sea salt, such as Maldon
3 tablespoons finely grated orange peel
3 drops grapefruit essential oil
3 drops orange essential oil
a small bottle of sweet almond oil

Mix thoroughly all the ingredients except the almond oil in a bowl, and store in a sealed glass jar. When you're in the bath or shower, take a scoop of the mixture, add a few drops of sweet almond oil from the bottle to make a paste and rub all over your hands, paying particular attention to areas of hard, dry skin.

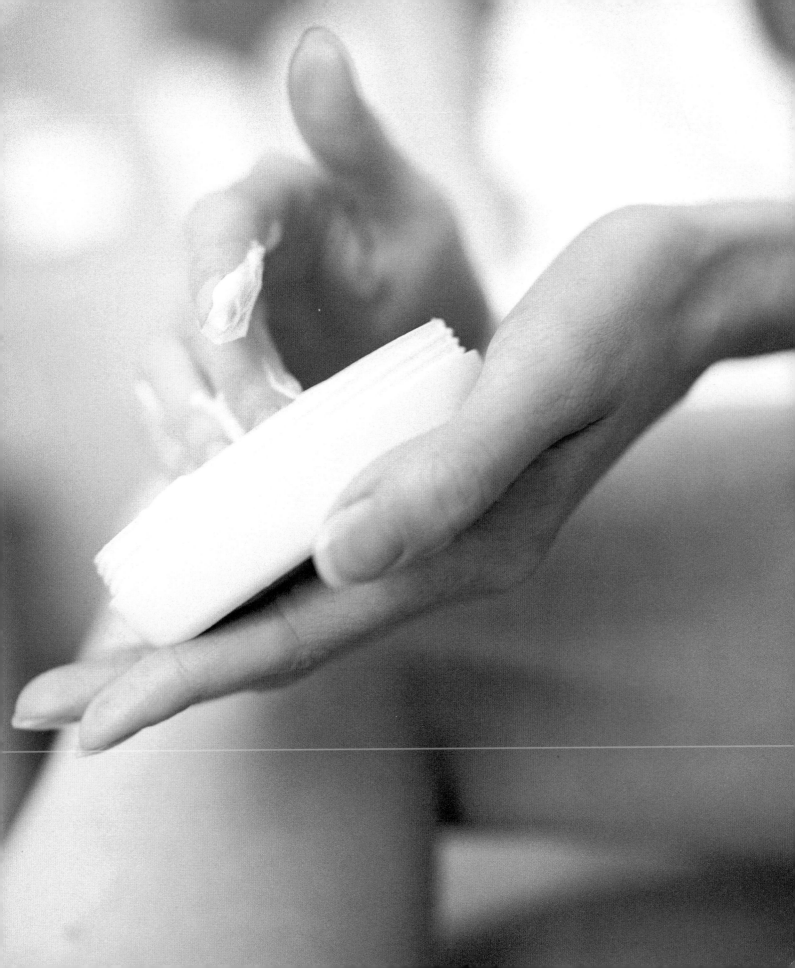

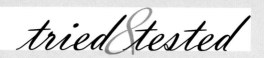

HAND CREAMS

Hand cream is the product that most of us use more often than any other – and the perfect one, we believe, sinks in fast but leaves skin like velvet. It doesn't make our hands sticky. And it should smell like heaven. A tall order for a natural product? Not according to our testers, who've been trialling some new natural entries (now over 70 eco-options tested, to date) – and identified some more crèmes de les crèmes…

❀❀❀ CIRCAROMA REPLENISHING HAND CREAM WITH ROSE FLOWER

Score: 9.10/10

A truly outstanding result for this natural cream from a tiny British aromatherapy brand (which will ship worldwide). All the products are virtually handmade, in small batches. This is based on organic rose water, rose attar, geranium and ultra-moisturising shea butter.

Comments: 'Smells fantastic – real rose scent, not synthetic' • 'very good for dryness, nails and cuticles, and seemed to have a whitening effect' • 'silky feel, sank in right away – a real treat' • 'my hands look younger and brighter – the best hand cream I've ever used' • 'a scar on the back of my hand is less noticeable – my hands are soft as cashmere and blissed out'.

❀❀❀ NATURETIS NOURISHING DRY HAND OIL

Score: 9/10

This is a wild card, because it isn't exactly a hand cream, but a once-a-week hand treatment that our testers loved for its silkifying effect, based on sesame, sunflower, apricot kernel, macadamia nut and jojoba oils. (Actually, Naturetis recommend it's used after the 'matching' exfoliator, which this group of testers didn't even get to try.) Entirely preservative-free, it's organically certified by Ecocert in France (Naturetis is a young French brand, now available in 150 countries). According to our testers – and, gosh, how they loved it – this 'dry oil' (more of a serum according to some testers) really does sink in fast – but still one for beside the bed rather than the kitchen taps, we feel.

Comments: 'An instantaneous winner! I was in need of a miracle worker for dried-out hands and the first application gave immediate relief' • 'a total must-have item: I used it every day as I loved the effects so much: the results of prolonged use were fantastic' • 'a luxurious product, which is well-packaged and has a pump-action dispenser, feels lovely to use and smells beautiful' • 'a little went a long way and absorbed quickly; a real pampering therapeutic treat to use' • 'my nails looked noticeably better after the first application, very healthy and smooth instead of my usual dry cuticles and hang nails; after a few weeks my nails were less brittle and didn't flake and break off as usual' • 'improved the condition of my hands, skin looked almost glowing and supple, and the tone seemed more even' • 'lovely and glossy to use, like a satin veil' • 'divine smell, like a burst of wild blooms'.

❀ JURLIQUE ROSE HAND CREAM

Score: 8.81/10

Jurlique offer a trio of similar creams – and this rich version just pipped the existing entry – Lavender Hand Cream, see below – to the post. (We tested for the first time, for this book, even though it's been around for ages.) Jurlique tell us it's 'rich in the living energy of rose, calendula and violet, to deeply moisturise and restore smoothness' – but you tell us: whatever, it's just a great cream. (NB: you lot do seem to love rose fragrances…!)

Comments: 'Lovely packaging, small enough for handbag, thick but spreadable cream with wonderful delicate rose smell; very moisturising for nails and nail beds too' • 'ten out of ten; amazing! This smelt heavenly, sank in quickly, kept skin moisturised – staying on my hands even after washing, didn't need to reapply all day, big improvement in nail area too' • 'perfect! No residue just a lovely silky feeling. I would definitely buy it'.

❀ JURLIQUE LAVENDER HAND CREAM

Score: 8.77/10

Alongside soothing lavender, this rich but non-greasy cream features rose, calendula, camomile, honey, soya lecithin, macadamia nut oil and aloe among its ingredients. Jurlique recently had a 'brand makeover' (and, we couldn't help noticing, quite a price hike), so the outside is now as lovely as what's in the jar/tube.

Comments: 'Very hydrating – and I have the driest hands in the world' • 'can't stop looking at my hands – they look ten years younger' • 'divine fragrance' • 'my daughter – who is a nursery nurse and prone to dry, sore hands – liked this as well' • 'it also made my elbows soft'.

★ ✾ DR. ORGANIC BIOACTIVE SKINCARE 100% MANUKA HONEY HAND & NAIL CREAM

Score: 8.62/10

This very reasonably-priced range from Holland & Barrett features some really delectable products, even if they aren't quite as 'organic' as the labels suggest. (Only the 'bioactive' ingredients, in some cases, are actually certified.) Our testers really loved this, in its hefty tube, at an un-hefty price: a luxuriously-textured yet sinks-in-fast cream that is an absolute must for honey-lovers, because of the straight-from-the-honey-jar smell.

Comments: 'Very good on dry skin especially "gardeners fingertips", gave a good sheen to nails; excellent overnight treatment under cotton gloves for my son's eczema, after three nights the patches had gone' • 'lovely, good-enough-to-eat honey smell; hands felt very soft and smooth, a fantastic handcream and great value – also worked well on dry knees'.

★ ✾ LIZ EARLE NATURALLY ACTIVE HAND REPAIR

Score: 8.43/10

The tube-sized version of this silky hand treat was so popular that Liz Earle and her team launched a handy, chunky pump-action bottle (which you'll find on our own desks). That probably tells you all you need to know about this sinks-in-fast cream, which contains skin-strengthening echinacea and hops, moisturising panthenol (vitamin B5), antioxidant vitamin E and betacarotene, and is subtly aromatic with bergamot, camomile, neroli and lavender.

Comments: 'Excellent packaging, perfect consistency – rather like a Mr Whippy ice cream – silky to apply, hands felt incredibly smooth and nails benefited from regular use' • 'not oily so I don't have problems opening a door after I've put it on' • 'works a treat, hands felt soft and silky' • 'skin felt in better condition and looked smoother,

---

> *Mentioned in dispatches:*
> though this section is all about creams, our testers really raved about **YES TO CARROTS PAMPERING HAND & NAIL SPA:** an oil-based salt scrub which brightens, nourishes and leaves hands baby-soft, they tell us.

---

nails seemed to shine' • 'heavenly fragrance' • 'my hands look and feel great: my husband asked if I had been for a manicure'.

✾ ORIGINS MAKE A DIFFERENCE REJUVENATING HAND TREATMENT

Score: 8.31/10

This product includes rose of Jericho (a desert plant), plus trehalose (from corn sugar), sea algae, skullcap and meadowfoam seed oil. Almost every tester rhapsodised about its softening qualities and the improvement to nails and cuticles: three saw a difference in age spots.

Comments: 'Startlingly effective; you only need a five pence-sized dollop and within seconds it's like you've pulled on silk gloves; also it's stopped my eczema, which is a miracle' • 'lovely smell; improved smoothness/softness in seconds – slight reduction in age spots over three weeks' • 'immediately softened and enriched skin' • 'my dry hands looked soft and cared-for straight away' • 'perfect consistency, not runny, greasy or sticky' • 'nails shinier and cuticles more groomed' • 'it's very pampering – a little goes a long way so, although it seems expensive, it's worth it' • 'a brilliant hand cream'.

★ ✾ A'KIN UNSCENTED INTENSIVE HAND, NAIL & CUTICLE TREATMENT

Score: 8.25/10

If you don't like the scent of your hand cream to clash with your perfume, this is your best bet. In fact, this nourishing treatment has been specifically created for those with sensitivities, allergies and fragile skin, and is suitable, say A'kin, for anyone with eczema or dermatitis. This Aussie brand uses GMO-free ingredients and some organic ingredients (though the products themselves aren't certified).

Comments: 'Very good for tackling dryness, my hands were cracked and it sorted them out immediately; also fixed my ragged cuticles and helped smooth out hangnails' • 'works well as an overnight treatment: I applied it thickly and in the morning had lovely soft skin' • 'made my hands soft straight away' • 'really easy squeezy tube' • 'just the right size to go in my bag and the packaging is simple and elegant' • 'a good cream for when you need something light and unscented'.

how to have GREEN FEET

Naomi Andersson of Green Hands salon (which includes feet, too) gave us her secrets...

This simple at-home pedicure proves it's possible to reduce your carbon footprint while still having glamorous toes

1 **Set the scene.** Make sure you've gathered everything around you; we don't want you doing back-flips with slippery feet while heading for the bathroom cabinet to fetch something that you forgot. (Get the phone and remote handy too.) You will need: a bowl to soak your feet in, some scrub, a nail brush, a foot file if you have one, a nail file, massage oil, cuticle oil, nail polish remover, nail polish, foot cream (or a product like shea butter).

2 **Soak.** Remove any old polish, then file the nails straight across, filing in one direction only. (Don't saw backwards and forwards; the heat you build up can damage your nails.)

3 **Scrub.** Naomi uses a so-simple mixture of organic brown sugar, organic olive oil and organic honey in her scrubs. (You can add a few drops of your favourite essential oils to this mix if you like.) Take each foot in turn and work between the toes, all around the heel and especially on any dry skin you have, but be gentle across the upper arch of your foot: the skin is thinner

and more vulnerable here. If you have dry and cracked heels, overzealous removal will leave your feet sore; instead, get into the habit of moisturising heels before bed. Don't abrade rough skin continuously, it will make it worse; instead, gently run an emery board over the area daily if necessary, and use a foot file once a week (see Bastien Gonzalez's tip below). One of the best ideas for cracked heels is to apply your old natural lip or face balm directly to the heel at bedtime, and massage in to improve blood flow. PS If the balm comes in a stick, you'll want to keep it for feet only, in future!

4 **Rinse.** Pop your feet in the bowl and rinse off, pat dry with a lovely fluffy towel (Naomi uses organic towels from www.greenfibres.com). Wrap one foot in the towel while you pamper the other.

5 **Cuticle care.** Gently push back your cuticles and wipe away any accumulated dead skin from around the corners of your toenails. (You can use the

rounded end of a glass nail file for this.) Naomi recommends massaging in a small blob of Santé Nail Fluid on each cuticle. (We suggest you could also try one of the top-scoring nail treatments in our Tried & Tested Nail Strengtheners on page 159.)

6 **Massage and moisturise.** Gently massage in your chosen oil, with your fingers and palms, from below the knee. Work in sweeping movements, with one hand following the other alternately. (When massaging, as with body-brushing, make sure you direct all firm pressure massage in an upward motion to encourage blood flow towards the heart.) After you've done the sweeping movements, use pincer movements over the fleshy parts of your lower leg. Repeat this around your upper and lower foot. Then work over the toes with circular movements of your fingertips. Finish by rotating each toe in turn. Repeat on the other leg.

7 **Sweep nails clean.** Use a damp corner of your towel to wipe over each toenail so you have an oil-free surface for polish to stick to. If your nails are exceptionally oily, wipe them with a damp towel or the smallest dab of acetone-free nail polish, then dry the nail area with a towel or tissue.

Tip.... **Our friend, medical pedicurist Bastien Gonzalez, advises that if you buff feet, 'Little and often is best. Just use a foot buffer very lightly. Applying too much pressure compacts the layers and actually makes for harder skin.'**

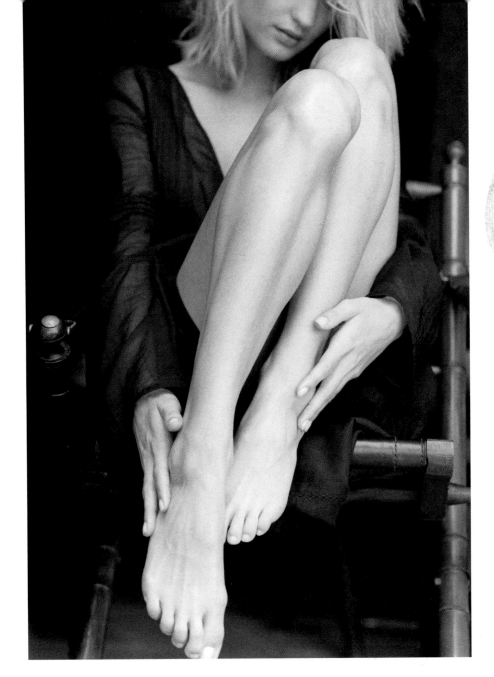

We have tried every foot buffer going, but are now converts to an amazing foot file by Alida. A bit like a giant Microplane cheese grater, this is a metal tool which – with the lightest skim over feet – whisks away rough, hard skin to leave feet baby-soft. It's designed to be used on wet feet, but Jo prefers to use it before bathing or washing her feet at night (her mustn't-miss last-thing-at-night ritual). As for creams? Jo is big on foot nourishment and slathers on ultra-rich Saaf Organic Foot Softening Balm. Sarah really really tries to cream her feet every night cos it makes such a big difference. One of her eternal favourites is all-natural Gilden Tree Nourishing Foot Cream, with an aloe vera (rather than water) base. There's also a great Exfoliating Foot Scrub in the same range.

8 **Polish.** Use a clear base coat to protect nails from staining. Allow the base coat to dry thoroughly before applying colour. This is not the time to rush; if you're running out of time, just do the base and wait until another time to add colour.

9 **Top coat – and put-your-feet-up time.** Wait around ten minutes for all your coats to have dried properly. Naomi uses the Suncoat range, with Suncoat Crystal Clear as a finishing touch, adding:

'This is mysteriously cloudy until dry, but will protect your colour polish and give it a super-shiny appearance.'

10 **Admire and do nothing.** Leave any slight smudges until your nail polish is completely dry; these will come off easily using a cotton bud dipped in polish remover (the skin around your toenails will be so well-moisturised that any polish will rub off very easily, so don't risk spoiling your paint job by fiddling with it now).

PUTTING A
spring in your step

We walk. A lot. In fact, when we both lived in Notting Hill in London, we would schedule meetings the other side of Hyde Park so we could have a good yomp, swapping ideas/news en route. But if you want to walk a lot, your feet have to be healthy. The bonus is that happy feet equal a happier you

Our feet are two of our most exquisitely constructed body parts, each consisting of 26 bones, 30 joints and 115 ligaments. But if this delicate machinery breaks down, the knock-on effect can be pain in our knees, hips and back, as well as the feet themselves. So – apart from ditching those toe-crunching stilettos – how can you make sure your feet are functioning at their best? As well as the crucial importance of massaging in a good cream daily, we've learnt that if you have a foot problem of any kind, the best thing is to consult the professionals.

● Have a pedicure (by a qualified podiatrist who also has an eye for beauty – or you can exit feeling rather hacked about and dismal) every six months. If you have hard skin build-up, go every three months.

● If you have a corn, get it removed as soon as possible by a chiropodist/podiatrist. Do not delay, it will get worse and be more difficult to remove – and you will be in agony. NB: most experts do not advise using a corn plaster (or paint) because they damage surrounding healthy skin.

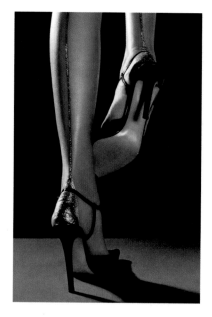

● Our feet absorb three to four times our body weight (and up to ten times when we're playing sport). According to the experts at Footwise, a groundbreaking shoe-shop-cum-foot-clinic in London, up to 80 per cent of people suffer from 'over-pronation' – where the arches have flattened and the feet roll inwards, potentially causing the legs and hips to shift inwards too. Less common is over-supination, where a high arch causes the foot to roll outwards so the feet have less effective 'shock-absorption', leading to pain in the hips and knees. To arrive at a diagnosis, Footwise experts carry out a number of checks, then video customers walking barefoot on a treadmill. Depending on the results, orthotic shoe inserts may be prescribed (custom-made or digitally fitted, which is the less expensive option).

● The painful foot condition plantar fasciitis can make people effectively disabled. One sufferer – a dog walker by trade – told us that, while cortisone injections didn't really help, orthotic inserts (although not cheap) brought about a major improvement in two weeks.

SHOW SOME SHOE SENSE

We really love pretty shoes, with pointy toes and high heels. But would we walk in them or wear them every day? Absolutely not. High heels should be treats like champagne and choccies. Nothing wrong with wearing them for high days and holidays but not on a daily basis. Bunions affect one person in three in the West, mainly because of our addiction to unsuitable shoes, and they are very difficult to deal with. So do your feet a favour and invest in footwear that cares for your feet. Our big faves, by several miles, are FitFlops, the sandals (and now boots, short and long) with the built-in gym, developed by beauty and fitness expert Marcia Kilgore, and extensively tested. They work out everything from your butt to your toes. We love them and so do all our friends. They're even glam!

FOOT REVIVERS

Feet deserve a medal: so please award them a reviving treat. For us, feet treats are a beauty essential and choosing natural is extremely important: Chinese medicine deems the soles of the feet highly absorbent. Our testers trialled oceans of lotions, soaks and scrubs, and found these to be the best

❀ ORIGINS REINVENTING THE HEEL
Score: 9/10
An amazingly high score for this product, which universally wowed our testers. It contains skin-sloughing salicylic acid, jojoba oil, shea butter and a put-the-spring-back blend of menthol, peppermint, nutmeg and pine essential oils.
Comments: 'Pure luxury: after a heavy day, this will lift up your feet – and you!' • 'it's divine – takes ten minutes to sink in but don't let that put you off' • 'big improvement: dry soles definitely softened, much easier to file off hard skin' • 'perfect – does what it claims, and more'.

❀ AVEDA FOOT RELIEF
Score: 8.8/10
With a similar texture to Aveda Hand Relief, this soothing, cooling cream targets even the roughest, toughest feet with active herbs combined with fruit acids and salicylic acid, which have a skin-sloughing action. Lavender and rosemary oils deodorise and refresh.
Comments: 'Really refreshing smell, feet instantly tingly and less achey and sore' • 'even my bunions are less painful and red' • 'the best ever – send up Fred Astaire please!' • 'reduced tenderness after high heels – took away that heavy feeling in legs'.

★ ❀ GILDEN TREE NOURISHING FOOT CREAM
Score: 8.17/10
US brand Gilden Tree specialise in foot care – so should we be surprised they have two winners in this category? Thick and very creamy, this bestseller is rich in aloe vera, shea butter, with healing comfrey and foot-reviving lemon peel and rosemary.
Comments: 'Large tub of cool, soft, light, fragrant cream instantly softened hard skin on feet; left legs refreshed and soft, calmed and reduced soreness' • 'better than any foot cream I've ever used' • 'magical – prolonged use has helped fade old scars and blotches' • 'loved it so much I used it all over my body' • 'fab for my dry, sensitive, blister-prone feet'.

★ ❀ GILDEN TREE EXFOLIATING FOOT SCRUB
Score: 8.11/10
This creamy, deep-cleansing scrub – the 'sister' product to Gilden Tree's Nourishing Foot Cream – performed really well in its own right. Along with their signature, certified-organic aloe vera, it has tiny particles of pumice to buff and smooth.
Comments: 'Fluffy texture and fresh fragrance; left my feet and legs clean, smooth and refreshed' • 'as a high-heels wearer, dry skin is problem – this was a gem!' • 'lovely, flowery, sensuous smell – feet soft and smooth, a lovely product' • 'left feet velvety – my five-year-old daughter loved it too'.

★ ❀❀ WELEDA FOOT BALM
Score: 8/10
This great value foot-saver (and deodoriser) is totally free of synthetic ingredients and features antiseptic calendula, disinfectant/antifungal lavender, rosemary and myrrh, with invigorating rosemary and sweet orange.
Comments: 'Loved this – absorbed really fast, no greasy residue' • 'gave me new feet – reviving and refreshing!' • 'my feet felt lighter' • 'liked that you could put on tights immediately'.

★ ❀❀ MOOM AROMATHERAPY FOOT SPA
Score: 7.94/10
Good for tired feet and weary legs, this rich cream is best rubbed into bare feet at night. It contains potent aromatic oils of tea tree (to help heal abrasions and fight athlete's foot), camphor (for joint stiffness), peppermint and disinfecting eucalyptus, plus vitamin A to help maintain the skin barrier, keeping infection at bay.
Comments: 'Thick soft cream with yummy coconut/minty smell – left skin refreshed, very soft and nourished' • 'reduced tenderness on poor feet!' • 'loved this at night – feet felt refreshed and silky-soft' • 'feet cooler, less sore and tender after hard day's shopping, almost instant improvement on hard skin areas'.

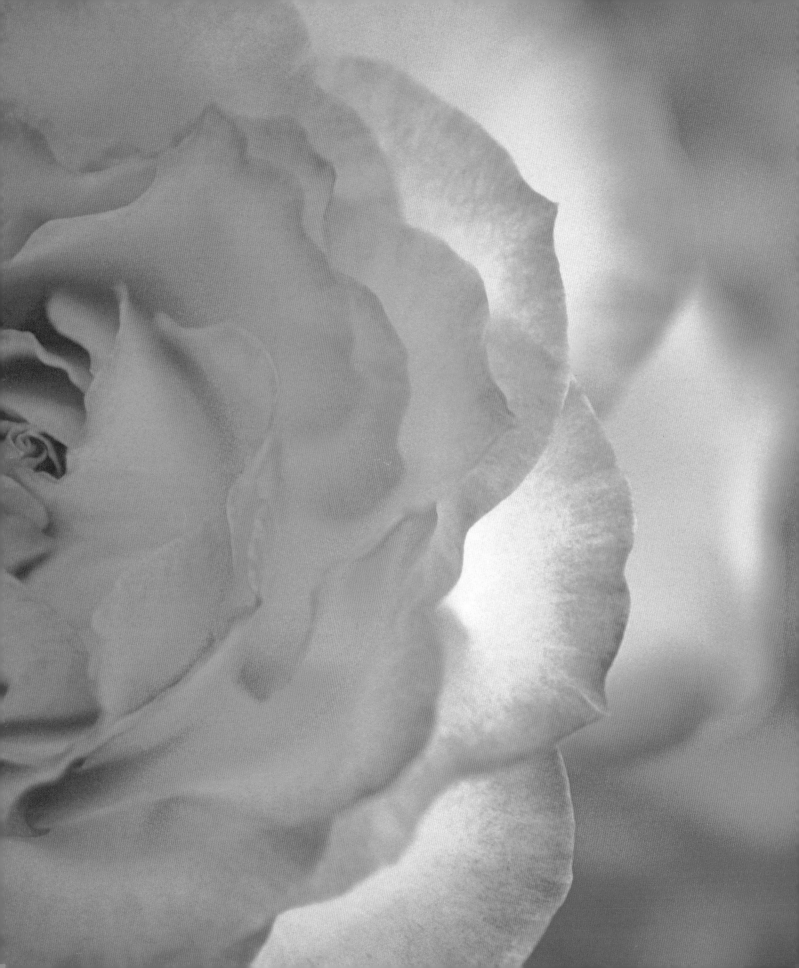

Fragrance

Fragrance can catapult us like a time machine through space, reviving precious memories of places and people. But today, we live in an over-fragranced world. (Really, who needs scented loo paper, tissues or wall paint?) We think it's time to make fragrance special again – rather than taking it for granted because it's everyday, everywhere. So here you will discover some of the greatest ways to fragrance your life more naturally – with world-class perfumes, exquisite essential oils and safer candles.

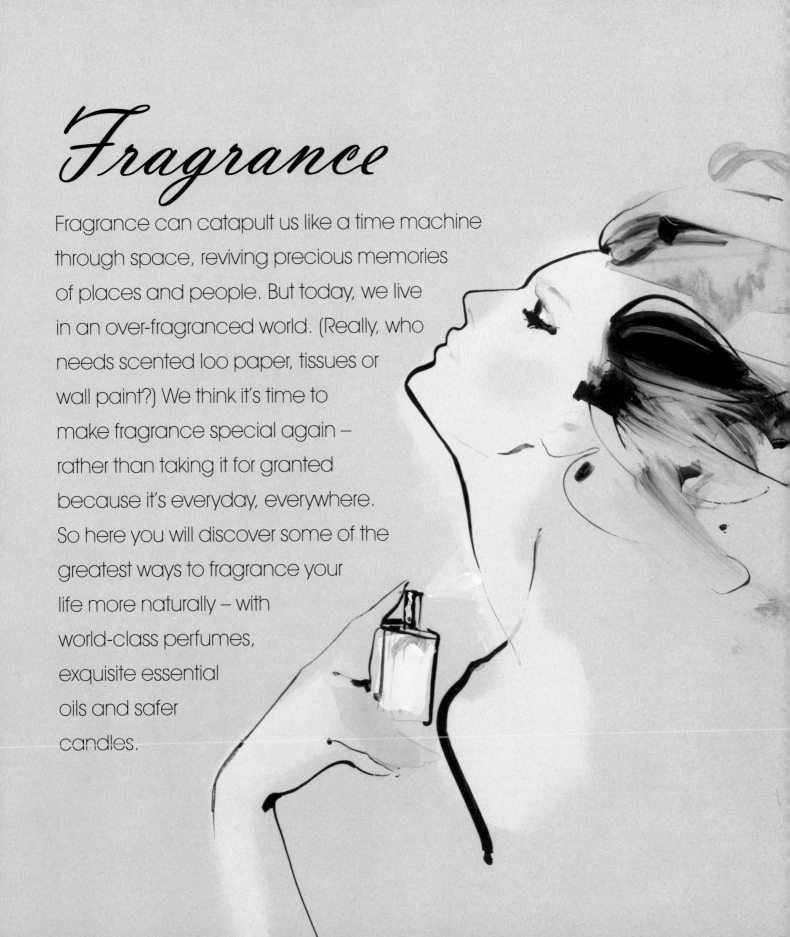

TALKING SCENTS

First, a few words about the meaning of 'green'. In fragrance-speak, 'green' perfumes are those with spring-like and grassy notes – although they may actually be a blend of hundreds of synthetic ingredients fused to mimic narcissus, lily of the valley or newly-mown hay. To us, though, 'green' fragrances are those that are genuinely close to nature: distilled from real plants or created from blends of essential oils

Frankly, there is more secrecy in the world of fragrance than in MI5 or the CIA, let alone a James Bond film plot. It is the one area of the beauty industry where we are still kept completely in the dark about what's in the bottle. To be fair, it's easy to see why the fragrance industry has lobbied so hard to be a 'special case' when it comes to labelling: if the Chanels and Guerlains of this world had to list the full ingredients of No 5 or Shalimar on their packaging, there'd be a mad scramble by copyists to re-create them, and sales of those legendary fragrances would plunge.

But there are, however, real question marks over the safety of some petrochemically derived ingredients in fragrances. (According to the US National Academy of Sciences, 95 per cent of chemicals used in fragrances are synthetic compounds derived from petrochemicals.) Synthetic musks, phthalates and glycol esters, for instance, are all endocrine disrupters: potentially, they play havoc with our hormones and, in some cases, long-term exposure is suspected of causing damage to the reproductive organs, liver and kidneys, and reducing male sperm count. And the impact of these hormone-disrupting ingredients travels far beyond our pulse points: synthetic musks, for instance, which are 'bio-accumulative' (ie, they build up in

the body) have even turned up in fish.

An increasing spritz-it-all-over lavishness with fragrance may also be linked, so experts believe, to the sky-rocketing number of asthma cases. One study by Louisiana State

'You spray a perfume on in the airport duty-free and feel as if you're poisoning your skin – like it has cheap ingredients. I'm fed up with it'

STELLA McCARTNEY,
who briefed perfumers that her
Stella fragrance should be more
natural than most

University found that the scented perfume strips in magazines triggered chest tightness and wheezing in asthmatics. (Personally, we've never liked our copies of *Vogue* to smell of Obsession or White Diamonds, and

always rip out the offending pages before we settle down to a good read.)

The fragrance industry is certainly not innocent of all this. Perhaps, for instance, you've noticed that your favourite fragrance has been tweaked, and just doesn't smell the way it used to. Chances are that this is actually the result of a directive that a specific ingredient can no longer legally be used (rather as, in gardening circles, we've seen a gradual withdrawal of particularly toxic pesticides such as lindane). Many thousands of the ingredients available to a perfumer for his or her alchemical art have never actually been tested for toxicity, and those that have may only have been scrutinised for allergic potential or phototoxicity (interaction with the sun to trigger skin reactions), rather than long-term effects on our nervous or reproductive systems. But in future, as more safety data is collected, we expect ongoing tweaking of some very famous fragrance formulas indeed. (To be fair, many natural ingredients are also being phased out or placed on the restricted list: limonene, for instance, from citrus oil, which gives scent that zesty whoosh of Mediterranean lemons, but which can trigger a reaction in the sun. Verbena and oak moss, both potential allergens, can only be used in the teensiest amounts too.)

Even if you're a tad rattled by this, we

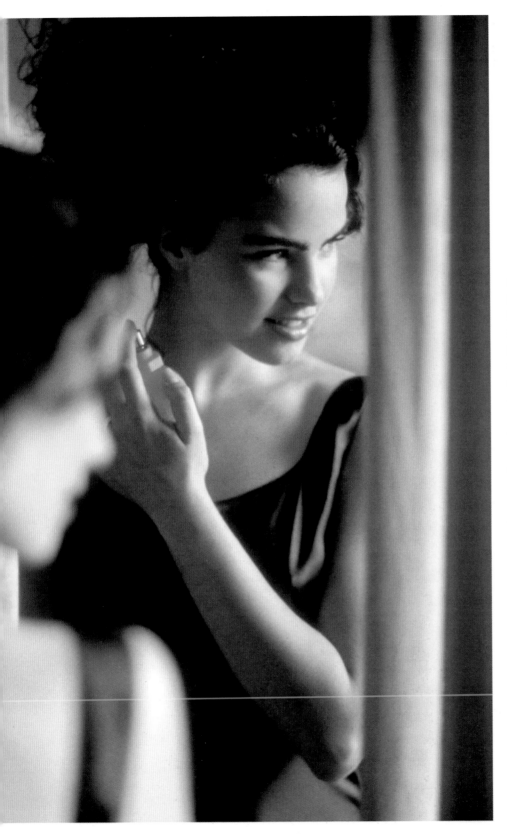

don't believe it's necessary to give up the indisputable pleasure of wearing fragrance. Personally, we love the stuff, and a dab of Shalimar, Mitsouko or Frederic Malle's Lipstick Rose makes us feel completely delicious. But rather than wallow in fragrance every single day, we now reserve it for special occasions – just like our mothers and grandmothers did. This isn't just prompted by health and environmental concerns. Ironically, what we've found is that this actually makes fragrance far more special than sloshing it on every morning out of sheer habit. You notice it more, enjoy it; it becomes linked with getting glammed up, with celebration and romance. Which is just what perfumers always intended, before fragrance became an everyday ritual like brushing your teeth or hair.

You may also like to know that – just as with all cosmetics – there is now a scramble to launch totally natural, 'green' fragrances. Some of them, frankly, are dreadful – and it's safe to say the Chanels of this world have nothing to fear from them, for now. But others do indeed make a delectable impact on the senses, without making such a big impact on the planet (or, perhaps, our health). So overleaf, we unstopper the truly natural fragrances which most definitely are to be sniffed at…

WONDERS OF THE NATURAL

When it comes to a sense of smell, nobody's is more fine-tuned than Roja Dove's. (Trust us: the sniffer dogs at Miami airport have nothing on Roja.) So we asked the *professeur de parfums* – who now has his own *haute parfumerie* boutique in Harrods, London – to spritz, splash and smell his way through more than 50 natural and organic fragrances, during a sniff-a-thon with Jo. Here are their favourites

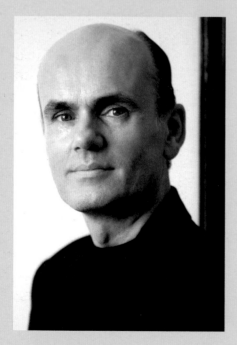

Overall, Roja was impressed – though perhaps that's not surprising, since he's always championed the use of natural ingredients in fragrances, believing them to give a richness in perfumery that most synthetics can't rival. 'The good ones we've tested here really are very good,' observed Roja. 'If you consider yourself to be quite a sophisticated fragrance connoisseur, you might turn your nose up at some of them – but I say: you do so at your peril, because you'll miss some really fabulous discoveries.'

Roja and Jo were pretty convinced that some of the so-called all-natural contenders did have synthetics in their blends – which isn't apparent from the ingredients list. 'You can pick them out instantly,' observed Roja, adding that one scent supposedly based on violets would be impossible to create naturally, as violets don't give up their odour. By comparison, synthetic contenders seemed cloying and almost to catch in the back of the throat of our two 'noses-for-an-afternoon'.

Innercalm Wind Down
BY INTELLIGENT NUTRIENTS

'A wonderfully cocooning fragrant oil: citrus and spicy, with lovely woody notes – slightly reminiscent of walking into a very luxurious, posh spa. I was surprised by some of the certified-organic fragrances launched by Intelligent Nutrients (the new range created by Aveda founder Horst Rechelbacher), but this is the one I think would work best on the skin – while totally restoring your spirits.'

Royal Jasmine BY AL QURASHI

'Traditionally in Arabia single oils are layered onto the skin: this is a truly stupendous jasmine pure oil – from the Rolls Royce of Arabian perfumers – which garlands you with its intoxicating, exotic fragrance, as if you're sitting in a jasmie-covered bower. Wear it alone, or 'custom-blend' by adding a drop of rose or oud-wood oil over it, for depth and extra warmth.'

Rock Star BY RICH HIPPIE

'The white floral heart is beautiful – it makes me think of a garland of soft, creamy blossoms worn around someone's neck – and the top notes remind me of gingerbread. I'd happily sit next to someone

fragrance WORLD

wearing this whereas I want to run a mile from most white florals. Totally narcotic.' Rich Hippie, a Californian natural fragrance company, claim to make their products 'with organic and wild-crafted ingredients, peace, love and harmony'.

Heaven Scent BY DEBORAH MITCHELL

'Lots of sandalwood – a unisex fragrance that smells like old-fashioned men's grooming products and old money – in the nicest possible way!' Created by a facialist and skincare expert, this also contains skin-softening oils, to spritz on the body.

Angel Water BY ENATA

'Like walking into a lovely spa; it instantly enhances your sense of wellbeing. I like this tons: there's a big bouquet of white flowers that is very multi-faceted, as in the most sophisticated fragrances – and you wouldn't tire of this because of its complexity. Very beguiling and uplifting.' Enata is founded by aromatherapist Glenda Taylor (see page 174 for her recipes for home-made perfumes), who is now working in the natural fragrance world.

Boisé BY PATYKA

'Tons of patchouli, but this is also lovely and airy – it reminds me of a summer's day when your hands are literally in and out of the plants. That beautiful leafiness reminds me of summer, sun and escapism. This is a very carefree scent.' The essential oils, plant absolutes and alcohol in Patyka fragrances are certified organic by Ecocert.

Monsieur Balode BY FLORASCENT

'One for the man in your life: this smells like man's skin, through a cashmere sweater. Warm and intimate, with a huge, chocolatey patchouli note. For a man who would charm you naturally, because he's not trying…' Florascent is a German range of vegan fragrances from perfumer Roland Tentunian. However, Jo and Roja were unconvinced that some of them could have been concocted 100 per cent naturally. Of 23 Florascent blends trialled, this was their top choice.

We love…

We readily admit, our dressing tables are still cluttered with perfume bottles: Chanel's divine, irisy 28 La Pausa (from their Exclusives collection), Mitsouko, Shalimar and Lipstick Rose. But increasingly, we are drawn to natural fragrances. Not everyone realises that 4711 by Meuhlens, the classic *eau de Cologne*, has always been created with totally natural ingredients, which may explain why we both love it. It belongs in every fragrance wardrobe: it's the ultimate pick-me-up – hugely uplifting without being over-stimulating, and you can layer almost any other fragrance over its citrus, aromatic freshness. (Also fabulous spritzed onto hankies and bedlinen: pull back the sheets, spray – then close again.) Jo wears a dab of exotic Aromatherapy Associates frankincense essential oil on her skin in winter (a trick she learned from *Vogue* beauty guru Kathy Phillips), or a touch of the patchouli or vetiver that she loved as a frustrated, too-young-to-be-a-hippy teenager. She is also a fan of Jo Wood's Amka, a zesty natural body spritz that is like being whisked back in time to a long-lost mandariny scent from Goya called Aqua Manda.

THE
do-it-yourself
PERFUMER

The most natural scent you can wear, of course, is the one you make yourself. So we asked Glenda Taylor – a leading aromatherapist and talented perfumer whose company Balm Balm designs one-off signature fragrances for a handful of lucky individuals each year – to create some essential-oil-based blends exclusively for *The Green Beauty Bible*

Explains Glenda: 'Essential oils are not recommended to apply directly on to the skin, so the following blends would work best in jojoba oil, or a very high-grade alcohol such as Absolut vodka. Perfumes can be anything from 15 per cent to 40 per cent dilution. Eau de parfum is 7 to 15 per cent and eau de toilette 3 to 10 per cent. The blends here give approximately 1ml of the fragrance ingredients, so add that to 10ml of jojoba oil or alcohol for a good-strength eau de parfum.' (10ml is approximately a dessertspoonful.) Glenda continues, 'This recipe is much stronger than an aromatherapy blend as it's not intended for massage – just for pulse-points. If you use jojoba oil, you will be creating what is known as a "perfumed oil", and this is absorbed very efficiently – so, again, use only on pulse-points.'

There are now several brands of organic essential oils and we do recommend you choose those to make your gorgeous perfumes. One supplier we like is Materia Aromatica, which is certified by The Soil Association.

A romantic blend
- 10 drops rose absolute essential oil
- 10 drops neroli
- 5 drops rose geranium

A sensual fusion
- 3 drops ylang-ylang essential oil
- 7 drops jasmine
- 7 drops sandalwood
- 3 drops clary sage

or

- 10 drops rose absolute essential oil
- 10 drops frankincense
- 5 drops black pepper

An uplifting blend
- 10 drops grapefruit essential oil
- 10 drops lemon
- 3 drops rosemary
- 4 drops verbena

Something breezy
- 3 drops peppermint essential oil
- 15 drops bergamot
- 7 drops lime

To soothe you
- 5 drops lavender essential oil
- 10 drops mandarin
- 5 drops petitgrain

or

- 10 drops frankincense essential oil
- 5 drops cedarwood
- 10 drops bergamot

A blend for the office
(to help you concentrate)
- 3 drops spearmint essential oil
- 12 drops grapefruit
- 10 drops bitter orange

Pregnancy perfume
- 10 drops mandarin essential oil
- 5 drops lime
- 10 drops lavender

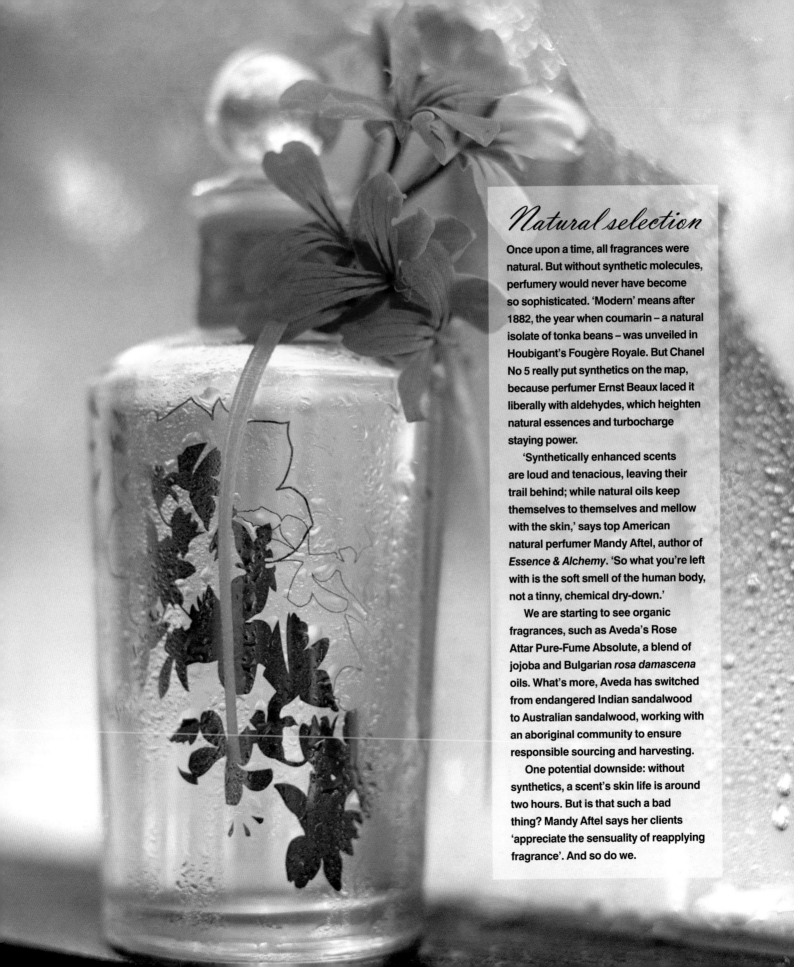

Natural selection

Once upon a time, all fragrances were natural. But without synthetic molecules, perfumery would never have become so sophisticated. 'Modern' means after 1882, the year when coumarin – a natural isolate of tonka beans – was unveiled in Houbigant's Fougère Royale. But Chanel No 5 really put synthetics on the map, because perfumer Ernst Beaux laced it liberally with aldehydes, which heighten natural essences and turbocharge staying power.

'Synthetically enhanced scents are loud and tenacious, leaving their trail behind; while natural oils keep themselves to themselves and mellow with the skin,' says top American natural perfumer Mandy Aftel, author of *Essence & Alchemy*. 'So what you're left with is the soft smell of the human body, not a tinny, chemical dry-down.'

We are starting to see organic fragrances, such as Aveda's Rose Attar Pure-Fume Absolute, a blend of jojoba and Bulgarian *rosa damascena* oils. What's more, Aveda has switched from endangered Indian sandalwood to Australian sandalwood, working with an aboriginal community to ensure responsible sourcing and harvesting.

One potential downside: without synthetics, a scent's skin life is around two hours. But is that such a bad thing? Mandy Aftel says her clients 'appreciate the sensuality of reapplying fragrance'. And so do we.

A BREATH OF
fresh air

Scented candles – preferably posh ones in heavyweight jars – have become the ultimate tasteful and acceptable gift to friends, hostesses and even to ourselves. We love them – but do we really need all the other 101 'fresh' (not) smells swirling round our homes in cleaning products of all kinds? And don't get us started on plug-in room fragrances or loo fresheners that are meant to smell like a florist's shop…

We live in an over-fragranced world. A world in which the interiors of our homes have become hugely polluted with chemicals – because the idea that everything should smell nice has permeated every layer of the market. Not so long ago, bathroom cleaner smelled of bathroom cleaner and nothing more. (And the distinctive tang was a signal of cleanliness.) Now we have bathroom sprays fragranced with wild orchid, window cleaning sprays designed to conjure up an ocean breeze, even loo paper that's scented with roses.

We say: enough, enough, enough! It not only amounts to a nasal assault, but they may be impacting negatively on our health. 'Not a lot is known about these perfumes and air-fresheners, which tend to be bought to improve air quality but just mask the problem while adding to the range of chemicals in the home – and there is

Why not?

Use a diffuser with a programmable timer – they plug into a wall socket – to help you wake up in the morning (lots of options if you Google). Instead of the sound of an alarm, you can be gently roused by a whiff of citrus oils. You could also place ceramic ring diffusers above the light bulbs in the lamps in your home and office; the gentle heat from the bulb slowly pulses the fragrance into the room (although be aware: this takes much longer with long-life light bulbs).

concern some might be carcinogens,' Dr Derrick Crump, an expert on the indoor environment at the Building Research Establishment, has observed.

We already live in a kind of 'chemical soup', a world in which we're assaulted with a barrage of volatile organic compounds – VOCs – which are 'off-gassed' by insulation, fibreboard, synthetic carpets, flooring and fabrics, paints, resins, varnishes and photocopiers. Even if you inhabit an old-fashioned country cottage surrounded by vintage fabrics, you may still be awash with VOCs from the lemony scent of your washing-up liquid or the pine-like whiff of spray-on furniture polish. Increasingly, hyperactivity, learning difficulties, asthma and eczema are all being linked with VOC pollution.

Now, we're absolutely not suggesting that you live in squalor. But we do recommend switching to a cleaning range such as Ecover, Bio-D, Method, Seventh Generation, Clear Spring, Earth Friendly, Natural House and Planet Pure (all pretty widely available retail and online), which are based on plant and mineral ingredients. And which, in our experience, get your washing-up/laundry/kitchen sink just as clean. Not only that, as we've mentioned before, Sarah's 30-year-long eczema cleared completely when she switched to Ecover and Bio-D.)

At the same time, if you're a scented candle fiend – as we are – you may like to experiment with some of the (mostly) new brands that are based on essential oils and natural waxes, rather than synthetic fragrances and petroleum-derived paraffin wax, and certainly to move away from any that have lead wicks. Our own particular favourite is the Natural Magic range (don't forget to recycle the glass jars afterwards) and also honey-scented, natural beeswax ranges such as Blossom Candles.

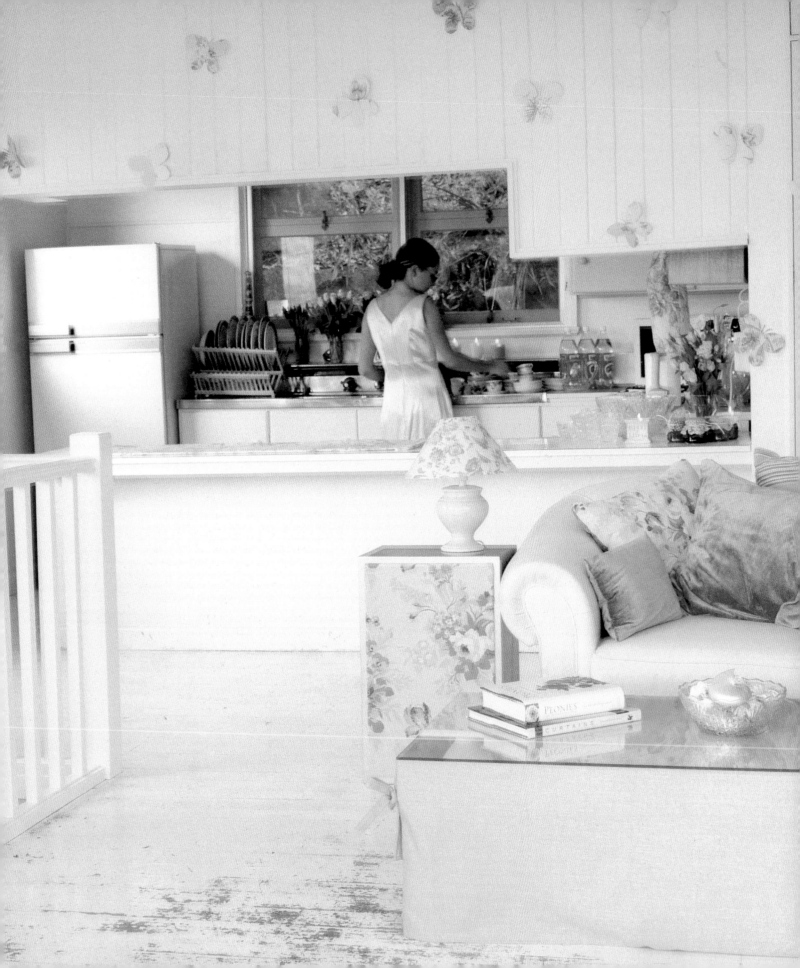

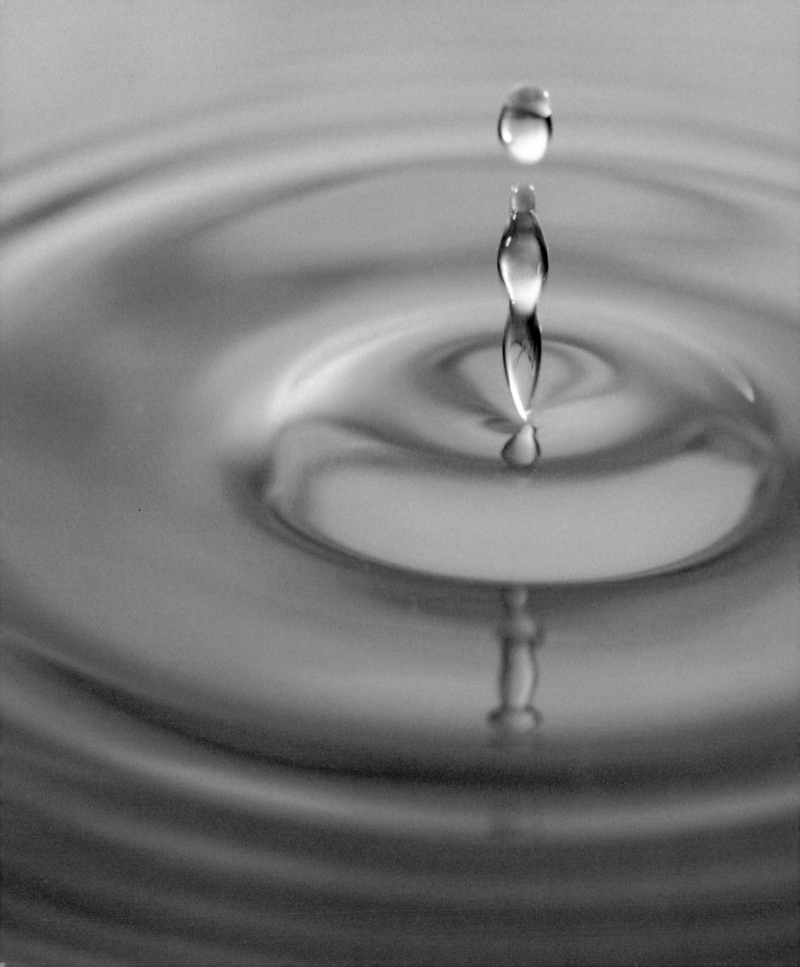

Natural living

Like the planet we're part of, we are all governed by natural cycles: light and dark, the lunar month, sunny days and dark ones, the seasons... While we love some of the advances of modern life – this book has been a five-centre production, thanks entirely to modern technology – we also love to live simply (though we never forgo glam sessions) and in tune with nature as much as possible. It keeps us happy, calm and, without wishing to sound precious, fulfilled.

LIZ EARLE

When we asked our *Green Beauty Bible* testers for nominations for their favourite 'green goddesses', skincare guru Liz Earle scored as highly as her products. So, one sunny lunchtime, we sat down with Liz, who's married to film-maker Patrick Drummond and the mother of four, to talk about what she does to green her lifestyle

It's all about making small changes when you can, and, for me, it's been a journey over 20 years or more that's still continuing. It would be almost impossible to be 100 per cent environmentally 'clean'. Our mantra both at work and at home is to 'aim for progress, not perfection'.

Little ways of cutting energy consumption include putting lids on saucepans, turning the refrigerator temperature up and washing machine temperature down, and switching off all stand-by lights at the mains (my children laugh because I am always crawling around the floors of hotel rooms looking for sockets).

I try to minimise environmental radiation wherever we are – so no TVs in the bedrooms. I took an EMF (electromagnetic field) detector around with me for a week. Every time we drove by a Tetra (mobile phone) mast there was a huge amount of disturbance. But, more worryingly, there was also a tremendous pulsing near a digital cordless phone. So we only have old-fashioned analogue phones. I'm also worried about the dangers of modern digital cordless baby monitors: you put them next to your baby's head 24/7 and, according to Powerwatch, an independent EMF information service, 'a DECT monitor placed in your baby's bedroom will expose them to more pulsing microwave radiation than living near to a mobile phone base station mast'. (For more information, visit www.powerwatch.org.uk)

We don't have a microwave in the house any more, partly because of the potential for radiation leakage, which may lead to a range of health problems, from cancer to headaches and increased stress, but also because they zap your lovely fresh food, seriously depleting the goodness.

'We grow most of what we eat on our organic farm, from traditional rare breed sheep, pigs and chickens, to fruit and veg in the kitchen garden'

Ideally, I'd buy organic locally produced food. But it's also very important to support small organic farmers overseas, particularly in developing countries where they rely on the extra premium for organic produce to stay alive. Curiously, the carbon footprint is often lower because the crops are grown in natural heat and light, picked by hand – and some even travel in the hold of tourist planes, which doesn't add extra carbon emissions. Whereas European produce is often grown under fossil-fuelled heat and light, and is machine-harvested before being trucked thousands of miles in refrigerated containers.

We have a total ban on most artificial additives and colourings, which definitely makes a difference to the children's behaviour, and also the sweetener aspartame: it's addictive, can cause neurological changes and affect your mood. My teenagers like Zapp chewing gum, which is sweetened with xylitol, a natural sweetener, and aspartame-free.

I love growing my own flowers and herbs for the house and for presents. In the winter we use foliage and berries, which saves a fortune too.

I try not to buy food packaged in plastic. You use it for a few minutes but it stays in the ground for hundreds of years. I have a total aversion to plastic food packaging and I think plastic carrier bags should be banned – now.

We use natural cleaning ranges such as Ecover, Bio-D and Earth Friendly, and Ecozone wash balls, which are as effective as conventional washing powders. For air fresheners, I use essential oils, such as lavender, neroli (orange blossom) and rose.

Magnets are an amazingly effective alternative to painkillers when treating muscle tension or bruising. I wear a magnetic necklace or bracelet, which I find particularly effective when travelling or sitting at the computer.

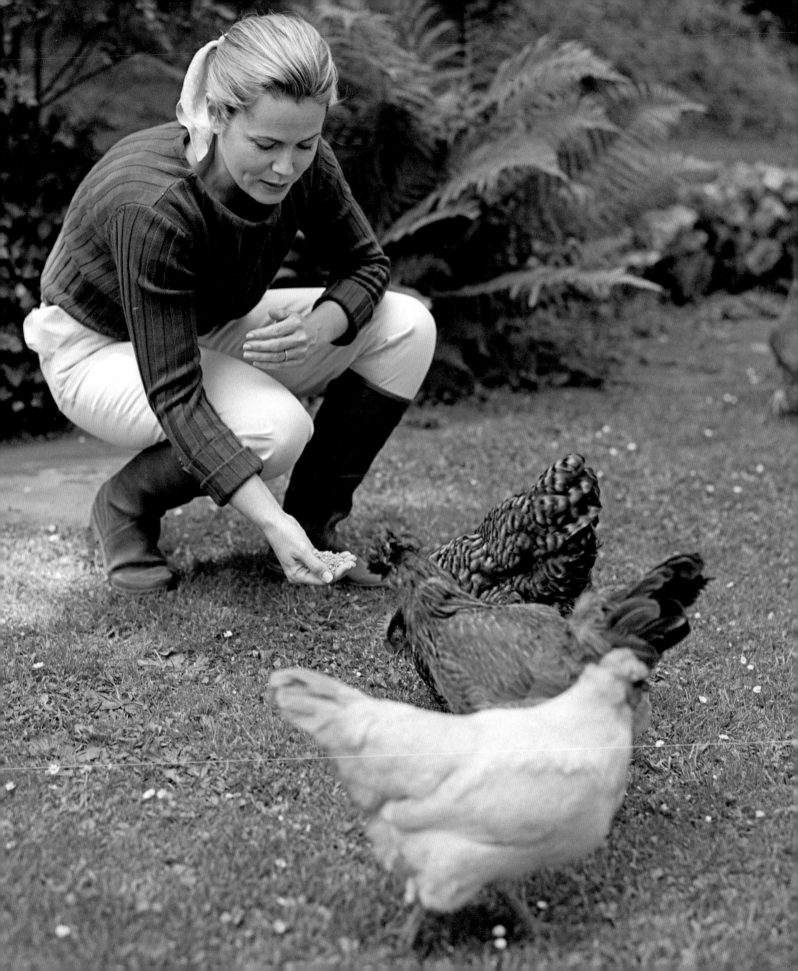

eating the
EVOLUTIONARY WAY

The sad truth is that the majority of diets don't work. You almost certainly won't enjoy your food, you won't feel well and if you do lose weight you'll probably pile it on again rapidly if (when) you come off the diet. But we want to tell you about a back-to-nature approach that's based on the evolutionary characteristics of your body, mind and spirit – and it works

Nearly ten years ago, Sarah came back blooming from a riding holiday in Colorado. She had mostly been eating meat and vegetables out there – but, indoctrinated with the notion that meat is bad, she put herself on a veggie diet. The digestive results were dire, from bloating to – well, we won't go into details, but just imagine everything you don't want.

One day shortly after, still feeling awful, she happened across a naturopath called Roderick Lane (who had looked after the late Diana, Princess of Wales). 'Hunter Gatherer,' murmured Roderick as he looked at Sarah and explained his theory about the five evolutionary biological types and the different diets that suit them. Sarah and Rod went on to write a book together called *The Adam & Eve Diet*. Jo was amazed when she read the description of Farmer Gardener and discovered that the lacto-vegetarian diet she naturally prefers was exactly the right one for her type.

The original paperback is currently out of print but one serially unsuccessful dieter, writing on www.amazon.co.uk, said: 'This is the first of 14 [diet] books that has worked

with ease and left me feeling well – and well-nourished. No headaches, no "detox symptoms", just weight loss and stability. My brother, a biochemist, sniffed at first, but later rather sheepishly admitted to the loss of about ten pounds without noticing it. This is a book for life.' We agree.

Essentially, your biotype is determined by the glandular biochemistry handed down to you through evolution. It's not a new concept: many traditional medical systems, which are thousands of years old, divide people into different types – Ayurveda for instance has three 'doshas'. Roderick found that patients in his naturopathic practice fell into five distinct patterns, which he then christened their 'biotypes'.

THE FIVE BIOTYPES

Your individual biotype is based on your dominant gland or glands. Glands are the biochemical factories in our bodies that produce hormones, the sophisticated chemicals that regulate the whole of our body chemistry and influence all of our

activities. Each gland is associated with a physiological function and this is what gives the five biotypes – Pathfinder, Hunter Gatherer, Pioneer, Farmer Gardener and Dancer – their individual physical, mental and emotional characteristics. This dietary approach is aimed at stabilising your body, the individual dominant gland in particular; but it's not simply about influencing your physique, it's a much more holistic approach that should help keep you looking and feeling at your best.

Remember that though they have distinct characteristics, the biotypes are all interdependent and may overlap to some degree, as well as having personal variations in physical and mental characteristics. Many people fit their biotype exactly, but others may have one feature that seems to belong to another type.

The most immediately recognisable characteristic is height, so we have listed the five biotypes in descending height order. Of course men fall into these categories too, with many of the same characteristics – we just haven't included them here on the score that they probably won't be reading a beauty bible.

Pathfinder (dominant gland: pituitary)

The trailblazer – self-contained and independent. As a biotype, the tall, rangy Pathfinder probably evolved after the Hunter Gatherer, to protect their communities when crises such as famine struck and the group needed to move on. The questing Hunter Gatherers would have adventured to a new terrain before the need became pressing. But when the time came to explore it properly, the practical Pathfinders would hack back the trail for the Pioneers and Farmer Gardeners. Today, Hunter Gatherers dream up a scheme, Pathfinders and Pioneers make it happen.

Pathfinder biotypes
Jerry Hall, Cameron Diaz
Uma Thurman, Venus
Williams

Body
- Over 5ft 10in (177cm) in height.
- Long body, legs and arms; flattish rather than curvy or contoured.
- Strong hands with pronounced joints.
- Large head, with longish face, bony nose, cheekbones and chin.
- Long, narrow feet with pronounced joints and long toes, almost like fingers.
- Medium to large breasts.
- May have a tendency to PMS and arthritis.
- When well, have great reserves of energy.

Mind and spirit
- Laid-back, more or less unflappable – the ultimate stoics.
- Often kind, but may be seen as uncaring because they tend not to be demonstrative.
- If interested in a subject, they will make themselves masters of detail.
- Great leaders, who seldom recognise limits.
- Tend to have a black and white view of life.

Pathfinder diet
This type functions best on the classic 'low allergen' diet: high in lean, low-fat protein, including poultry, fish and some red meat, green vegetables and salad, with complex carbohydrates in the form of ancient whole grains such as brown rice and low-gluten spelt and oats (modern wheat products, such as mass-produced bread, seldom suit them). They do not do well on processed foods such as refined carbs (white sugar and white flour); starchy root veg such as potatoes; dairy products such as milk, ice cream and cheese, although they can eat butter and yoghurt in moderation; and too much gluten (from wheat and other modern grains).

Eat lots of
- Protein: chicken, guinea fowl, turkey and other poultry and game; oily fish, such as salmon, tuna, mackerel, herrings, sardines; veggie protein – tofu and tempeh.
- Raw nuts and seeds: pine nuts, sunflower/ pumpkin seeds, linseeds, hazelnuts, almonds.
- Green vegetables that grow above the ground, 90 per cent cooked to 10 per cent raw.

Eat in moderation
- Lean red meat (but very little pork, ham or bacon).
- Brown rice, oats, millet, spelt, kamut and quinoa.
- Olive, corn and linseed oils.
- Butter.
- Live natural yoghurt.

Watch point...

Eat regularly, every three hours – Pathfinders tend to forget about food for days, and then eat lots, which puts a strain on their systems. If you are vegetarian or vegan, make sure you get enough protein.

Hunter Gatherer (dominant gland: thyroid)

The first three people who walked out of the cradle of Africa were probably Hunter Gatherers. Most in tune with nature's rhythms, Hunter Gatherers are nomads – movement is instinctive, they're designed to walk long distances, gathering food as they go. Even today, if you ask a Hunter Gatherer to sit still for long periods, they become fretful.

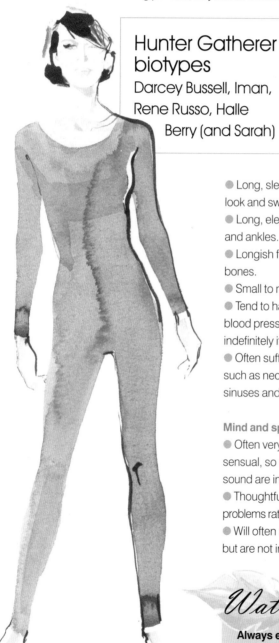

Hunter Gatherer biotypes
Darcey Bussell, Iman, Rene Russo, Halle Berry (and Sarah)

Body
● Height: 5ft 6in to 5ft 10in (167cm to 177cm).
● Overall long, lean tendency.
● Classically shaped hands, with delicate bone structure and fingers the same length as palms.
● Long, slender face with slightly classical look and swan-like neck.
● Long, elegant bones, with small wrists and ankles.
● Longish feet and toes, with delicate bones.
● Small to medium breasts.
● Tend to have a slow pulse rate and low blood pressure and can keep going almost indefinitely if well nourished.
● Often suffer chronic nagging problems such as neck or shoulder ache, blocked sinuses and skin rashes.

Mind and spirit
● Often very creative and romantic; highly sensual, so colours, shapes, textures and sound are important to them.
● Thoughtful, often need time to consider problems rather than give immediate answers.
● Will often negotiate and/or compromise, but are not ineffectual or weak.
● Very moral, usually acting on principle rather than pragmatism.
● Hunter Gatherers gather! Bowls of fruit and veg, pebbles, feathers, clothes, photos, friends, lame dogs: you name it, they collect it.
● Can be contradictory about displays of affection: sometimes demonstrative, other times reticent.
● Usually good listeners.

Hunter Gatherer diet
Of all the biotypes, these are the most sensitive to eating food that doesn't suit them. The aim of this high protein diet is to support the thyroid (which governs the body's metabolic rate) and enhance its ability to perform everyday tasks. If the thyroid is out of kilter, this naturally slim biotype gains weight rapidly. Hunter Gatherers should avoid refined carbohydrates, such as sugary products, white flour products and starchy root veg.

Eat lots of
● Proteins: eggs, poultry, fish, and veggie protein such as tofu.
● Vegetables that grow above the ground (ie, not root veg).
● Hard fruit such as apples and pears. (For both veg and fruit, eat 90 per cent cooked and 10 per cent raw.)

Eat in moderation
● Whole grains: brown rice, oats, spelt, rye and quinoa.
● Corn, flaxseed and olive oil.
● Butter.
● Other fresh fruits.
● Red meat (pork/bacon only if organic).

Watch point...
Always eat a good breakfast; cut down on quick-fix, 'naughty but nice' stimulants such as sugar, chocolate, coffee and alcohol. When you're tired, rest – going to the gym isn't the answer for exhausted Hunter Gatherers.

Pioneer (dominant gland: adrenal)

'Onward and upward' could be the Pioneer's mantra. Pioneers have an incredible will to get things done. The Pioneer is the person you want around when it's a question of survival, or achieving a deadline. If you want your spirits lifting, call a Pioneer: they'll help you sort your problems, organise a party and tell you jokes along the way.

Body

● Height: 5ft 4in to 5ft 9in (162cm to 175cm).
● Strong, usually curvy body with compact, muscular legs.
● Firm hands with squarish fingers.
● Strong joints and muscles.
● Square face, with a right-angled jawline.
● Medium to large breasts balanced by proportionately broadish hips.
● Capable of incredible bursts of concentration and energy.
● Tend to suffer from impact injuries such as damaged knees or backs; classic sufferers. of stress-related injuries that never repair fully, owing to their innate impatience.
● May be prone to heart problems and may have addictive personalities.

Mind and spirit

● Tend to be good organisers and motivators.
● Once a Pioneer says they're your friend (or lover), it's for life, but, unlike the romantic Hunter Gatherers, they may never tell you again.
● Pioneers tend to like simple food and neat-as-a-new-pin environments.
● Despite all this, they do have a romantic, creative soul – it just needs to be uncovered.

Pioneer diet

This biotype needs to establish a regular eating pattern that supports the adrenal gland. Pioneers do well on simple meals that follow the principles of food combining, the system based on separating proteins and carbs at main meals, and eating fruit on its own at least 30 minutes away from meals.

Food-combining meals consist of protein – meat, fish, cheese, eggs and dairy products – with non-root veg/salad, but not starches, such as grains, bread, pasta, pastry, pulses and rice. You can eat the starchy foods with 'neutral' veg and salads at a separate meal. Other neutral foods, which you can combine with protein or starch, include fats, oils, cream cheese, herbs and spices, and small quantities of nuts and seeds. You could also have a fruit/yoghurt/nuts and seeds meal.

For more information, read *The Complete Book of Food Combining* by Kathryn Marsden.

Choose a variety of these foods on a rotating basis
● Whole grains and grain products: brown rice, rye, barley, oats, buckwheat, millet, whole wheat, spelt, faro, kamut and quinoa.
● Pulses: beans, lentils, peas, chickpeas, tofu, tempeh, TVP (textured vegetable protein).
● Vegetables and salads in season: particularly green veg, raw salads, root veg, chicory and all bitter leaves, and tomatoes.
● Fruit in season (avoid bananas and grapes).

Eat in moderation
● Fish, particularly oily fish.
● Poultry, without skin.
● Eggs, no more than three a week.
● Olive, corn and linseed oils.
● Raw nuts and seeds; buy unshelled and unroasted.
● Potatoes.
● Organic cow's or goat's butter.
● Organic full fat cow's, goat's or sheep's milk and plain yoghurt.

Watch point...

Sit down peacefully for meals, rather than snatching a sandwich at your desk while making a phone call.

Pioneer biotypes: Catherine Zeta Jones, Susan Sarandon, Angelina Jolie, Isabella Rossellini

Farmer Gardener (dominant gland: gonads)

Although they're usually energetic, full-of-life characters, Farmer Gardeners represent the more stay-put nature of mankind. They're designed to nurture: to plant seeds, raise livestock and produce children. The caring professions are filled with this type, and they do TLC remarkably well. They can change their shape to that of a Dancer, see opposite, by exercising and dieting rigorously, but as soon as they stop, they return to their original shape.

Farmer Gardener biotypes
Drew Barrymore, Sophia Loren, Dolly Parton, Sarah Michelle Gellar (and Jo)

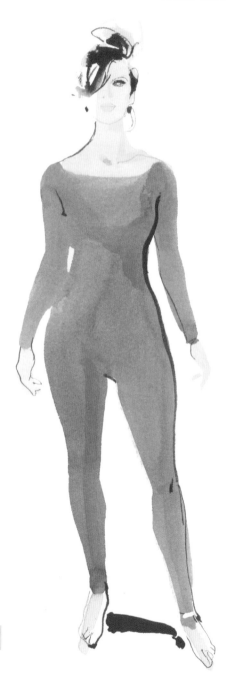

Body
- Height: 5ft 4in (162cm) and below.
- Hourglass figure with pronounced waist and hips, and often sloping shoulders.
- Dimply hands with tapered but slightly full fingers.
- Large head with rounded facial features.
- Short, thick bones and delicate but strong joints.
- Small feet with short toes.
- Full, soft-looking ribcage with medium to large breasts.
- Often eat poorly and put on weight; prone to bad backs and knees, also PMS.

Mind and spirit
- Their caring nature makes them the quintessential home-makers, with a social conscience that tends to be active in their own community.
- They have a high libido, so tend to crushes and passionate relationships.
- Ferociously protective of family.
- Loyal, reliable and hard-working – but can hold a grudge for eternity.
- Positive personality – seldom martyrs.
- Image-conscious, so expect designer labels – and collections of anything from china to paintings to Chanel earrings.

Farmer Gardener diet
This type tends to have high levels of oestrogen and testosterone, which may swing out of kilter. A lacto-vegetarian diet (dairy produce with lots of plant foods) helps hormonal balance. Farmer Gardeners also tend to be slow metabolisers, and this sort of easily absorbed food helps increase the rate at which food is turned into energy (metabolised) in the body. This is the only biotype that can thrive on a vegan diet.

Eat lots of
- Dairy products: cheese, hard and soft; preferably goat's or sheep's milk; goat's and sheep's milk yoghurt; full-fat organic milk; quark and crème fraîche (but not butter or cream).
- Green and root vegetables, salads, endive and Chinese leaves.
- Fruit: apples, pears, soft fruits, dates, figs, exotic fruits.
- Whole grains and grain products: brown rice, rye, barley, oats, buckwheat, millet, wheat, spelt, faro, quinoa and kamut.

Eat in moderation
- Oily fish: mackerel, herrings, kippers, pilchards, trout, salmon, sardines, fresh tuna, anchovies.
- Poultry: chicken, turkey, guinea fowl.
- Corn, linseed and olive oils.
- Eggs: no more than three a week.
- Nuts and seeds: hazelnuts, almonds, walnuts, pine nuts, sunflower seeds, linseeds, pumpkin seeds.

Avoid spicy foods such as curry; always have some protein at lunchtime.

Dancer (dominant glands: pituitary and gonads)

Dancers are the most recent type to emerge (albeit some 40,000 years ago). They are the product of Pathfinder and Farmer Gardener gravitating together – think of a towering footballer hand-in-hand with a diminutive Dolly Parton type. Dancers are the ultimate urbanites, who developed when mankind started living in villages, cities, kingdoms and, later, empires. Dancers are 'iron butterflies', who look fragile but are actually very strong.

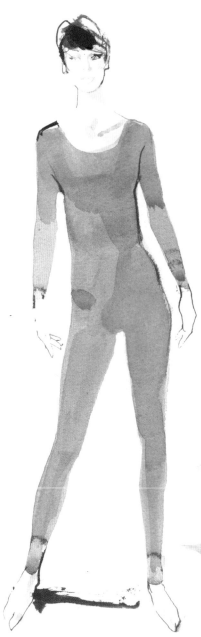

Dancer biotypes
Lucy Liu, Christina Ricci, Winona Ryder, Anne Robinson, Calista Flockhart

Body
● Height: 5ft 4in (162cm) and below.
● Straight, flat torso, with an almost adolescent physique that's actually very strong.
● Small hands with slender fingers.
● Small head with neat, sharp features.
● Small bones that are deceptively strong.
● Little, soft feet that taper towards the heel.
● Small, delicate-looking ribcage with medium to small breasts.
● Prone to damaged joints and aching muscles.

Mind and spirit
● Self-aware and image-conscious.
● Charming, quick-witted and usually very determined.
● Emotionally cool, holding everything inside until they explode.
● Good communication skills – unless people don't see their point of view.
● Combine the dynamic nature of the Pathfinder with the stability of the Farmer Gardener.
● Eminently adaptable and flexible.
● Work well in careers that demand strength, dedication and discipline.
● Weak spots – addictive behaviour (everything from shopping to alcohol and drugs) and tremendous volatility.

Dancer diet
These iron butterflies flourish on a demi-vegetarian diet containing elements of all the food groups and can break many food rules, such as not eating fruit at the end of a meal. The Dancer diet is similar to that for Farmer Gardeners, but they have a faster metabolism so need more 'slow burn' foods such as seeds and nuts, and lean protein such as chicken, turkey, fish or tofu at lunch to avoid suffering a mid-afternoon dip. Dancers don't do long-term planning, so opt for quick-cook food.

Choose a variety of these foods on a rotating basis
● Dairy products (but avoid cow's milk): goat's or sheep's cheese, yoghurt, quark and crème fraîche.
● Green and root vegetables, salads, endive and Chinese leaves.
● Fruit: apples, pears, soft fruits, dates, figs, exotic fruits.
● Whole grains and grain products: brown rice, rye, barley, oats, buckwheat, millet, wheat, spelt, faro, quinoa and kamut.

Eat in moderation
● Fish of all kinds.
● Poultry.
● Eggs, no more than three a week.
● Olive, corn and linseed oils.
● Nuts and seeds: pine nuts, sunflower/ pumpkin seeds, linseeds, hazelnuts, almonds, walnuts.

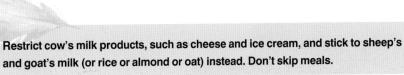

Restrict cow's milk products, such as cheese and ice cream, and stick to sheep's and goat's milk (or rice or almond or oat) instead. Don't skip meals.

just juice

Fresh fruit and vegetable juices are bursting with life power, a raw energy that is miraculous in its beneficial effect on the human body, according to natural health and beauty expert Leslie Kenton, a devoted juicer for more than 35 years

We agree with Leslie (one of our great heroines by the way): sometimes we get lazy – and we always regret it. Fresh fruit and veg juices are supercharged nourishment you can sip. If you wake up feeling blah, just down a juice (slowly, please, think of it as soup rather than water) and abracadabra: you have enough get-up-and-oomph for the whole day – and night. Drunk first thing in the morning, fresh juices kick-start your metabolism into working joyously. Do it daily, or as often as possible, and we've seen pallid, podgy, apathetic people transformed into vital, energetic human beings with bright healthy skin and sparkling eyes.

Juiced raw vegetables are high in natural vitamins, minerals and plant enzymes. 'There's no food or food product that can provide the same amount of vital nutrients at such a low cost – and no single vitamin or mineral supplement has such a synergistic balance of the essential components you need to keep you healthy,' points out naturopath Roderick Lane.

The Five-day Juice Detox (opposite), devised by Roderick, is designed to detox your body in less than a week. We also give you his recipe for the Ultimate Juice Formula, which will give you a lift at any time of day. If you're trying to give up nicotine, caffeine or alcohol, by the way, juicing can really help cut the craving. The regime doesn't include wheatgrass because many people really dislike it – if you like it, by all means include it.

You can incorporate the regime into your eating plan in different ways:
● Have a juice before breakfast every day, or at any time – if you come in from work famished, have a juice straight away to avoid raiding the fridge.
● Do a one-day fast, replacing meals with juices – best done at a weekend so you can rest – then continue with one juice daily, possibly replacing the evening meal if you are on a cleansing diet

Juices take about ten to 15 minutes to make and clear up. They're worth every second…

HOW TO MAKE FRESH JUICES
● Wash the raw vegetables or fruit under cold water.
● Scrub any root vegetable.
● Peel thick-skinned fruit, such as pineapple, melon, citrus fruit and kiwi; stone cherries, peaches, etc.
● Avoid fibrous fruit, such as bananas, rhubarb and apricots – they don't give very much juice and clog up the juicer.
● Chop up fruit and vegetables in small enough pieces to fit through the feeder tube (this is usually the most irritating bit).
● Roll up leaf veggies tightly; put parsley, celery and any other leafy-ended vegetables in stem-end first.

JUICERS
There are three types:
● Centrifugal: these use a circular filter basket with fine grating teeth to shred fruit and veg; when they're spun rapidly, centrifugal force separates the juice from the skin, pulp and pips. They're cheap to buy, but give you less juice than the other juicers.
● Masticating: these 'chew' the fruit and vegetables; they're more powerful, usually

'There's no food or food product that can provide the same amount of vital nutrients at such a low cost' **RODERICK LANE, naturopath**

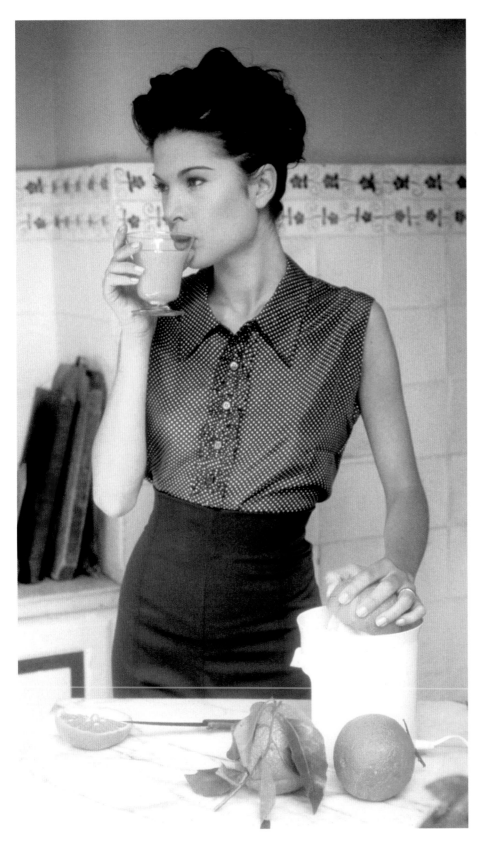

produce more juice and are much more expensive than centrifugal juicers.

● Triturating juicers: the latest generation of juicers are the most effective, quietest and most expensive; they crush the fruit and veg, including the cell walls.

FIVE-DAY JUICE DETOX

We haven't given precise quantities for each juice because individual juicers vary so much in the amount they give. You will be able to gauge the quantity your own juicer gives when you have tried out various combinations. As a rough guide, four large apples and the same weight of carrots give about 200ml (7fl oz) in a centrifugal juicer.

Day 1: melon (watermelon if possible, but any will do) and celery. Use a ratio of 3 parts melon to 1 part celery, by weight.

Day 2: celery and apple. Use 1:1, by weight.

Day 3: apple and carrot with ginger to taste. Use 1:1 by weight, with a 2.5cm (1in) chunk of peeled fresh ginger.

Day 4: carrot, celery and winter cabbage (or parsley, broccoli, spinach or chard): use 2 parts carrots and celery stalks to 1 part cabbage, by weight.

Day 5: carrot, celery, watercress, winter cabbage (or parsley, broccoli, spinach, chard), apple and ginger; use equal parts of each, with a 2.5cm (1in) chunk of peeled fresh ginger.

The Ultimate Juice Formula, for any time, anywhere

● **2 carrots**
● **2 handfuls of sprouted bean shoots**
● **4–6 stalks celery**
● **1 small beetroot**
● **small handful of parsley or watercress**
● **handful of spinach or any other dark green vegetable in season (spinach, chard, Savoy cabbage, beet tops, broccoli, etc)**
● **1 apple (eating or cooking) or pear**
● **ginger, 2.5cm (1in) peeled chunk**

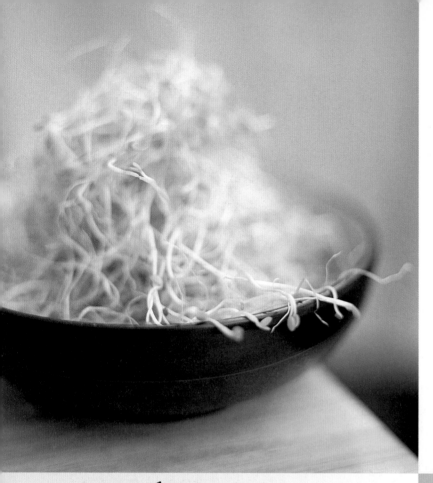
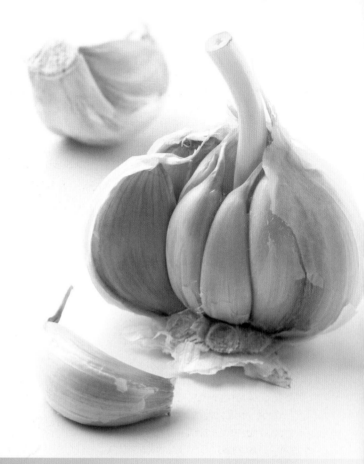

Alfalfa sprouts, garlic, honey and green tea are all superfoods

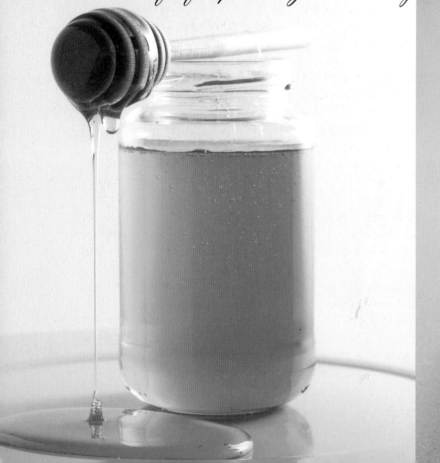
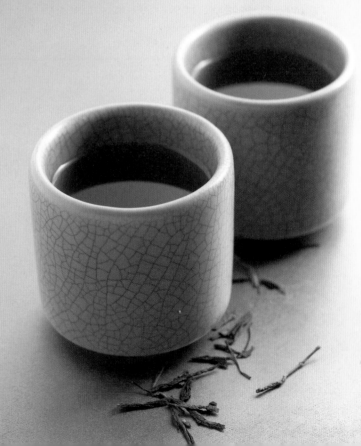

BRING ON THE SUPERFOODS!

Imagine if there was a medicine that could protect you against all the diseases of ageing, from cancer to loss of memory. Well, there is, but it's not a drug – it is the nutrients in fresh foods, traditionally grown without added chemicals. Here are the top anti-ageing superfoods to keep you healthy, slim and bursting with energy

Antioxidants These vitamins and minerals, mainly found in fruit and vegetables, prevent a damaging process called oxidative stress, caused by pollution, anxiety, ultraviolet light and smoking. This leads to the formation of excess free-radical molecules – the big villains behind disease and ageing. Antioxidants are now rated on the oxygen radical absorption capacity (ORAC) scale. The following are the top scorers (per 100g serving). Aim for 5,000 units a day, with lots of variety over the week.

Prunes: 5,770; raisins: 2,830; blueberries: 2,400; blackberries: 2,036; garlic: 1,940; kale: 1,770; strawberries: 1,540; spinach: 1,260; raspberries: 1,220; Brussels sprouts: 980; plums: 949; alfalfa sprouts: 930; broccoli: 890; beetroot: 840; avocado: 782.

Breakfast Always have a good breakfast, then eat every three hours to keep blood-sugar levels stable.

Organic eggs are the ultimate protein. They also contain nutrients that prevent fat deposits, help memory, concentration and emotional balance.

Green tea helps protect against heart disease, cancer, tooth decay, arthritis and bone loss. Also try white tea, which contains less caffeine and even more good chemicals.

Honey is a nutrient-rich alternative to sugar and sugary products (which contribute to all-round ageing); choose local, unprocessed honey or New Zealand manuka honey.

Organic milk contains calcium and magnesium for bones, plus conjugated linoleic acid (also found in organic beef), which helps with weight loss.

Millet is a nutritious, gluten-free seed that's rich in silica for hair, skin and nails.

Nuts Eat protein-rich, collagen-building almonds; brazil nuts for selenium to protect against cancer and improve thyroid function, and walnuts for a healthy heart.

Oats are a brilliant source of slow-release energy. They also lower cholesterol and blood pressure.

Olive oil helps reduce cholesterol and protect against heart disease; it also supports the liver.

Oily fish Mackerel, herrings, tuna, salmon, sardines and whole anchovies contain lots of omega-3 essential fatty acids (EFAs), which are vital for our brains and body health, from pregnancy to old age. A lack of omega-3 EFAs is strongly linked to low moods and depression, and many other mental and physical problems. Our bodies can't make these, so we have to get them from food sources. If you don't like fish, you can still get your omega-3s by eating a daily dose of flaxseed (linseed), flaxseed oil, rapeseed oil, walnuts, seaweed, spirulina or watercress, or from supplements.

Quinoa, 'the mother grain', is packed with fine-quality protein, plus calcium, iron, B vitamins and vitamin E.

Rhubarb, soya beans and yams contain plant oestrogens to help hormone function. (Don't exceed 50g soya daily.)

Seaweed is a rich source of calcium and other minerals that help bones, blood pressure, heart and menopausal symptoms.

Spices and herbs

Flavour foods or make infusions with rosemary and sage to help memory, and with revitalising thyme for lung function. Sprinkle on bright yellow turmeric to help prevent Alzheimer's and irritable bowel syndrome, reduce joint pain and boost immunity. Cook or make drinks with fresh ginger to reduce inflammation for conditions such as rheumatism and heart disease. Grind lots of black pepper on food to help your body absorb more nutrients.

Water Drink at least eight large glasses of still water a day between meals, for skin, brain, digestion – everything!

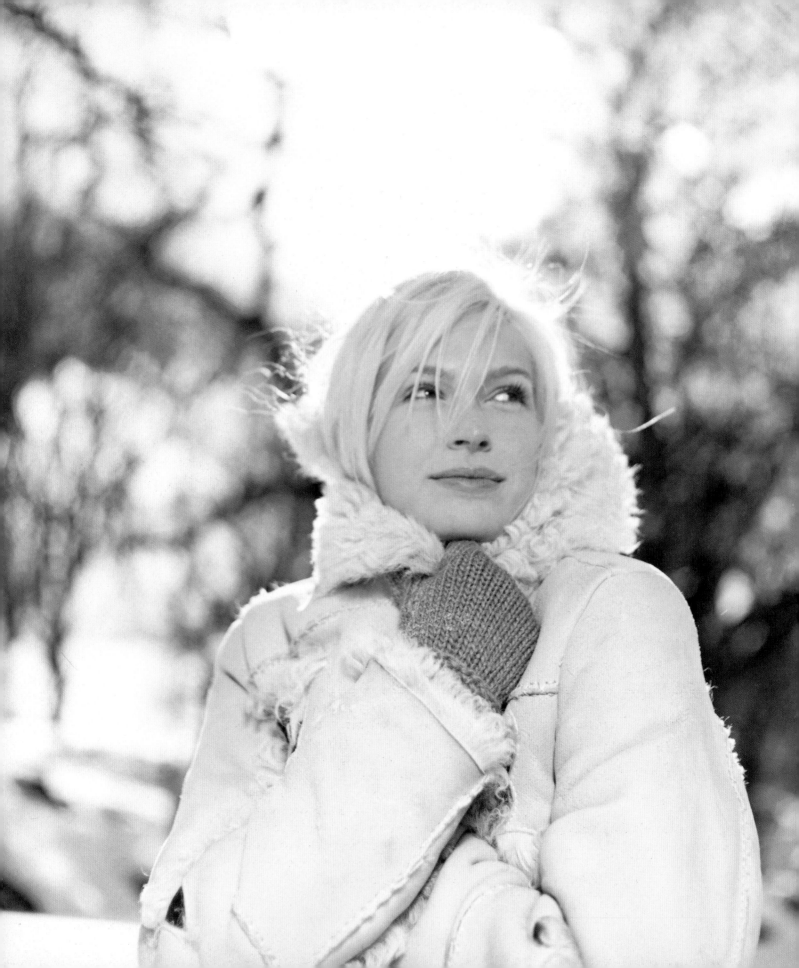

10 NATURAL WAYS TO BOOST YOUR *immune system*

Your immune system is your body's defence force, protecting you against all comers of a naughty nature and helping you fight disease – from colds and flu, to more serious conditions such as cancer. The bonus is that a healthy immune system helps you look and feel great. Here's advice from the experts we trust

All year round, you need to keep your immune system in the best possible condition so it can work at its very best to keep you well. As we explain on the previous pages, a really good diet will help enormously – so always start with that, plus carefully chosen supplements if you feel you need them. In the winter, or if you have been poorly, we suggest considering these simple tips to boost your immunity. NB: if you are pregnant, breastfeeding or have a medical condition, please check with your doctor before taking any herbs or supplements. Immune boosters are generally not recommended for anyone taking immuno-suppressive drugs.

1 Take astragalus

Top of most experts' lists is this Chinese native herb used by traditional Chinese medicine (TCM) for thousands of years – as part of the wonderfully named Jade Screen – to support and enhance the immune system. Astragalus is taken to prevent and treat common colds and upper respiratory infections, as well as for heart disease, chronic hepatitis and as an adjunctive therapy for cancer. According to the American National Center for Complementary and Alternative Medicine, which is researching the herb's effects on the immune system, it's considered safe for most adults (although it may interact with drugs that suppress the immune system so always check with your doctor).

When to take: as a three-week course in the winter or if you have been unwell; repeat if you feel rundown or tired.

Product: Astragalus Extract by Doctor's A-Z.

2 Get (magic) mushrooming

Dr Andrew Weil, the world's leading practitioner of integrated medicine, recommends taking a supplement providing five or more kinds of Asian mushrooms (such as maitake, shiitake, cordyceps, reishi, hericium and enoki), which have powerful immune-enhancing benefits. He also takes astragalus (see above) if it's a bad flu season or he is travelling.

When to take: daily.

Product: Dr Weil takes Host Defense by New Chapter, which contains 16 mushroom extracts.

3 Remember zinc

Your immune system won't function properly if there isn't enough zinc in your body. It's often deficient in the diet, especially in older people, and a two-year double-blind study suggested that zinc and selenium (another trace mineral), taken together, can reduce the number of infections. Recent research shows that including manganese can also help with preventing and treating viral infections.

When to take: daily.

Product: Mega Minerals Complex by Lamberts. This supplement contains 7.5mg zinc, 50mcg selenium and 2mg manganese, plus other minerals. Take one to two tablets (depending on how good your diet is).

4 ...and vitamin C

Research suggest that taking vitamin C regularly can help prevent colds. If you take it when you have a cold or flu, it may help reduce the symptoms and the time they last. (Vitamin C is also vital for the body to manufacture collagen, a key protein in our skin, connective tissue, cartilage and tendons.)

When to take: daily through the winter.

Product: try Camu-Camu Plus Vitamin C Complex by LifeTime Vitamins. Take 30ml daily for general health, 90ml daily to boost your immune system. This delicious drink, which also contains acai, raspberry, blueberry and mangosteen juices, is well-absorbed by the body and, unlike orange and other citrus juices, does not create an acid environment in the body in which virus and bacteria thrive. Or try a supplement such as Ester-C Complex by Life Time Vitamins, which provides buffered vitamin C over a 12-hour period and has very high absorption rates.

5 Have a spoonful of chywanaprash Ayurvedic tonic

This organic paste is a great immune-boosting, vitality-enhancing remedy containing fruit, spices, herbs and honey. Eat one to two teaspoons in the morning on toast, mixed with warm full-fat organic milk or straight from the spoon. Children love it and it's a good general tonic. (Legend has it that it was created by the Indian sage Chywana, who decided to start a family at 80 years old and so created this 'jam'.)

When: daily.

Product: Chywanaprash by Pukka Herbs.

Ancient Egyptian records suggest that the slaves who built the Pyramids were given onions and garlic for strength and to ward off infections

6 Eat spices

Herbalist Michael McIntyre recommends flavouring food with medicinal spices such as cinnamon, nutmeg and cardamom, as well as ginger, horseradish, garlic and onions. Ancient Egyptian records suggest that the slaves who built the Pyramids were given onions and garlic for strength and to ward off infections. Try blending equal quantities of fresh peeled garlic and ginger, keep in the fridge and use to flavour soups and stews. (Also see the Ayurvedic nightcap on page 205.)
When to take: all of it – often.
Product: Revitalising Cinnamon and Cardamom Herbal Tea by Pukka Herbs.

7 Drink fresh juices

As we say on page 188, fresh vegetable and fruit juices are supercharged nourishment. The concentration of antioxidants and other essential vitamins and minerals flooding through you stimulates your immune system as well as detoxing your body. If you want to give your immune system a boost, naturopath Roderick Lane recommends juicing equal amounts of washed carrots, celery, winter cabbage (or broccoli) and apples with ginger to taste (try a one-inch peeled chunk of ginger root for each batch).
When: every day.
Product: try the Intojuice, a low-speed masticating juicer which preserves nutrients and is easy to clean and reassemble (free UK delivery from www.intojuice.com). See page 188 for more information on the different types of juicers.

8 Think positively and laugh!

While excitement and challenges in your life are good for your health, too much pressure and too little support can lower your immunity to illness. Immune expert Dr Alex Concorde believes the key is preventing stress, rather than the popular concept of stress management: 'It's helpful to dissipate stress when you have it, but to safeguard your immune system, you need to stop yourself getting stressed in the first place.' Her tip for busy people – in addition to being organised – is not to focus on the relentless demands on your time but rather on what you can achieve by your actions, whether that's at home (creating a loving, stable environment, say), in your profession (being

successful) or in a voluntary organisation (helping other people and/or the environment). Also, try to do things in a way that's fun – both for you and others. Laughter has been shown to help the immune system, as has optimism – so share a joke and be positive!

9 Take action

Regular moderate exercise – 30 minutes to an hour a day of fast walking, for instance, preferably outdoors (see page 196) – can give substantial benefits to your immune system; it also helps you relax, which is vital. Yoga has also been shown to improve the immune system (turn to page 198 for some simple sequences that you can do at home).

10 Keep warm and eat comfort food

Up to 40 per cent of body heat can be lost if your head is bare so make woolly hats a style statement! Keeping warm and dry in the winter – with hats, scarves, layers of clothing, thick tights and boots – stops cold-related stress, according to the Center for Disease Control in America.

According to traditional Chinese medicine, we should eat warm food too, so tuck into those hot soups and stews. You might consider a couple of sessions of acupuncture to tune up your system for the winter.

Virus zappers

If you do get a sniffle, tickly throat or ear ache, take echinacea immediately – at the very first sign – until the symptoms are gone, suggests Michael McIntyre. Try Echinacea Tincture by Eclectic Herbals, take 15–30 drops in water four to five times daily. Also take an omega-3 supplement, which may help to conquer the virus. Try MorEPA by Healthy and Essential, take one capsule daily, or VegEPA by Igennus, take two capsules daily. Avoid citrus drinks such as orange juice which create an acidic environment in which infection thrives, and also dairy products (milk, cheese, etc), which may make mucus problems worse.

green exercise

Why pound a treadmill in a commercial gym redolent of hot bodies when you can satisfy body and mind getting fit in a natural environment?

We can't count the number of people we know who have shelled out hundreds, even thousands, of pounds for gym membership and end up going maybe three times a year. Of course, there are some who love it and really do get their money's worth, but not us for sure (or anyone we know). We've always preferred to take exercise outside (even yoga – to which we're both devoted – when it's fine).

Sarah discovered years ago that grooming her four horses and mucking out stables were better upper body and arm exercise than the 'pec' machine had even been. As well as swimming whenever possible, Jo and her husband Craig have walked every day without fail since they were married in 1991. And both of us love gardening: digging, weeding, potting and the rest give you top-to-toe activity and that wonderful release from stress we have come to expect from what is now called 'green exercise'.

'We're programmed as humans to be with the natural environment,' says Dr William Bird, a GP and strategic health adviser for Natural England. 'Increasing evidence suggests that both physical and mental health are improved through contact with nature. When we see trees, the sea, fields and woods we overwhelmingly feel at peace. Research shows that blood pressure and muscle tension drop significantly when we're in the presence of nature. It's to do with evolution: nature has a strong effect on a deep part of the brain. It gives us a sense of belonging and of wellbeing.'

For our very first book, *The Beauty Bible*, the leading social psychologist Professor Michael Argyle (who sadly died in 2002) recommended getting close to nature as one of the key ways to helping yourself feel happier. 'Seeing beautiful scenery, breathing clean air, watching animals and birds, and sitting in the sun are all effective blues beaters and help you sleep soundly,' he said. No wonder the new buzz word is 'ecotherapy', which could, according to many experts, help millions. (We'd certainly back it against addictive antidepressants in many cases.) In fact, according to psychiatrist Dr David Servan-Schreiber, author of *Healing Without Freud or Prozac*, regular exercise not only decreases depression but actively stimulates our pleasure mechanism: 'In addition to relishing sex and life's other big pleasures, people who exercise regularly get more pleasure out of the little things in life: friendship, meals, hobbies, even the smiles of passers-by. Essentially, it becomes easier for them to be satisfied.'

The British Trust for Conservation Volunteers (BCTV) has cunningly combined green exercise with voluntary work, another proven life-enhancer. Dr Bird set up the first BCTV Green Gyms in the mid 1990s; groups meet in their local area at least once a week for (free) sessions that last up to three hours. Activities range widely and can suit all ages and levels of fitness: think community gardening, tree planting and dry stone walling. There are lots of other community 'green gyms' run by volunteer organisations worldwide; these often take place on a seasonal basis such as clearing overgrown vegetation from small streams every autumn with local wildlife trusts.

Extraordinarily, exercising outside is more effective in terms of weight loss than doing the same thing indoors: a US study reports that exercising in the fresh air burns 12 per cent more calories than performing same activity indoors, and, according to the BCTV, you burn almost a third more calories in an hour doing some Green Gym activities than in a step aerobics class. Your figure benefits too, according to research, with waist-to-hip ratio and weight decreasing in the first three months.

Our message is this: walk, run, skip, ride, bike, swim – whatever you enjoy and can do easily and practically, within your budget. Try to get outside for at least 45 to 60 minutes a day, in chunks if that's more practical. (Remember, another benefit is getting a dose of vitamin D for healthy bones.) Add in treats, such as skiing or diving, as and when you are able. Make exercise social if you like: join a walking/hiking/rambling group, for instance, or go mountain climbing with a gang.

> *Research reports that exercising in the fresh air burns 12 per cent more calories than performing the same activity indoors*

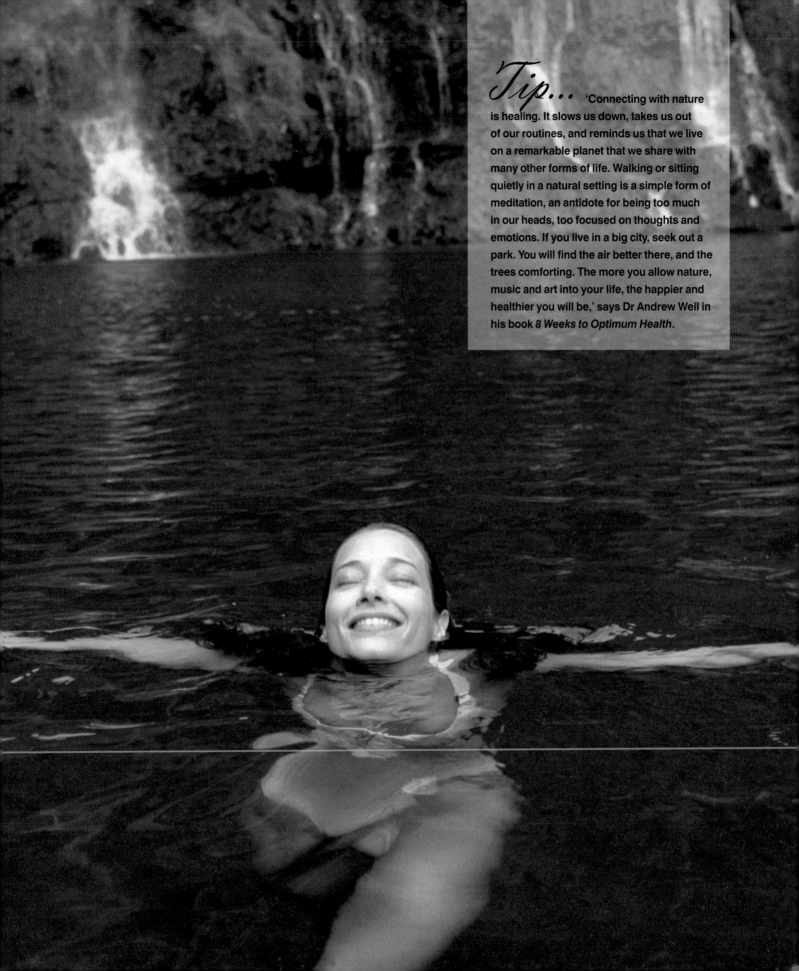

we love YOGA

We don't think there is any other discipline that offers such truly mind, body and spirit enhancing effects. We have both been practising it for years and can't imagine ever giving up – especially having seen octo- and nonagenarians in India with flowing movements and smooth faces curved into the most amazing shapes…

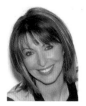

We asked our friend Kathy Phillips to suggest simple, short sequences for *The Green Beauty Bible*. Kathy, who is Condé Nast's international beauty director in Asia, has been practising yoga for 30 years and is a qualified teacher. (We very much like her bestselling book *The Spirit of Yoga*, now available in paperback.) Her interest in yoga inevitably led to the pursuit of a greener lifestyle, including an appreciation of alternative therapies and a passion for aromatherapy: indeed she gave up being health and beauty director at *Vogue* after seven years to found the aromatherapy company This Works.

Kathy says: 'Yoga can bring harmony and balance to your life. If you really can only devote ten minutes a day to practise it, this is certainly better than nothing. You can benefit from stretching your body in the right way, and taking time to breathe deeply – even for a short time – can have an accumulative effect.

'Too many people today use yoga as an aerobics class. It's better to focus on small but really practical physical postures and enjoy the clarity that deep, even breathing can give. Be precise with your movements. Listen to your body: think of it as a musical instrument and make sure that it is in tune with your life, your surroundings and your emotions.'

Simple poses to energise you in the morning

The morning is the time to do the standing poses, to help you to be 'alive' and energetic.

Mountain pose

Stand firmly, with your feet a hip-width apart and your toes turning slightly inwards. Press on the balls of your feet and then back into your heels: your weight should be evenly distributed. Then stand up, bottom tucked in, kneecaps lifted, shoulders back and ribs soft. Elongate the back of the neck but keep your arms relaxed. Breathe evenly in and out, keeping your facial muscles relaxed. When you are completely grounded, lift both arms up keeping everything else where it is.

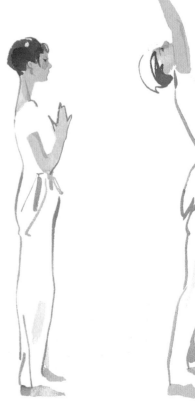

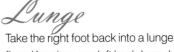

Lunge

Take the right foot back into a lunge, knee on the floor. Keeping your left heel down, bend your left leg and lengthen upwards with your trunk, head up, chin in, hands by your sides. Breathe and let your hips drop down. Repeat on the other side.

Standing forward bend

Stand straight as in Mountain pose. Exhale and bend forward keeping your knees straight. If your hands don't reach the floor, stretch forward and let them rest on a table. If your hamstrings are very tight, bend your knees a little but keep your back long. Breathe slowly as you hang and let gravity lengthen your spine. Come up on an exhalation, putting the weight into your heels.

Twist

or Sage's pose to a chair

Stand on your left leg with your right leg up on a chair, feet facing forward. Drop your tail bone and let your back grow upward. Exhale, feel the abdomen moving inwards, then turn towards your bent leg. Take your left arm and drop it over your right thigh. Twist as far round as you can, looking over your right shoulder. Take a few breaths in this position, then repeat on the other side.

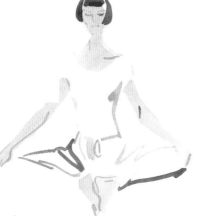

Child pose

Kneel, keeping your knees together and your sitting bones in contact with your heels. Exhale and fold your trunk forward to bring ribs to thighs and head to floor. Take your arms back to rest beside your body. If your buttocks don't touch your heels, put a cushion between the two.

Cobbler's pose

Sit up straight. Bend your knees and bring your feet as close in towards you as you can. Let your legs drop apart. If this is difficult, you can sit against a wall with a cushion under each thigh. Sit and breathe evenly allowing your thighs to drop down towards the floor. Keep shoulders down and hips relaxed.

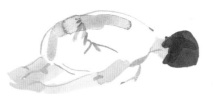

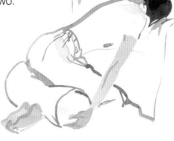

Simple poses to wind down in the evening

The evening is the time for inverted poses and stretches to help you relax

Wind-down warm-up

● Lie flat on the floor with your knees bent and hip-width apart, and feet parallel, flat on the floor.

● Take several deep breaths and enjoy feeling your shoulder blades and pelvis heavy on the floor. Gently breathe out and press into your feet, so that you can elongate your back flatter along the floor.

● Hold your right leg round the back of the thigh, exhale and gently draw it towards you. Keep your left foot firmly on the floor and then, if you are comfortable, stretch your left leg flat along the floor. Repeat with other leg.

● Finally bring both knees towards the chest together, holding around the backs of the thighs; keep your chin tucked in as you elongate the back of your neck and let your lower back muscles release with every slow breath.

Shoulder stand and plough

If you've been standing all day or hunched over a computer then the back of your neck, shoulders and upper back are likely to be tense. This is perfect to counteract all of that.

● Lie on your back, hands by your sides, palms facing down. Make sure you are straight. Roll the feet over to behind your head. Beginners should roll over on to a sofa, the end of a bed or a chair so that their feet can rest on that instead of the floor. Place your hands against your back to support it, keeping the elbows in. Your legs should be straight and your spine long.

● To go into shoulder stand, exhale and take your legs up so that your whole body from your shoulders to your feet is in a vertical line. Your weight should be on your elbows.

● Keep your face, neck and shoulders relaxed, and breathe.

● Gently roll down.

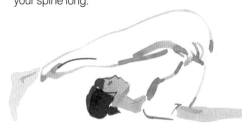
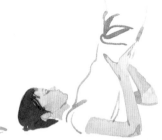

Spinal twist

Lie on your back with knees folded close to your chest. Loop your left arm under your knees, and let both legs roll gently over to the left while your head turns to look over your right arm, which should be outstretched at shoulder level. Breathe and relax. Repeat on the other side.

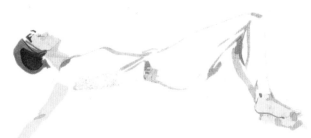

Corpse pose

Always end your stretching routine with some gentle breathing. This is not the time to sleep but to be centred and stable. Stretch out straight on the floor with arms relaxed at your sides, palms up. Rest your eyes, unclench the jaw, soften the throat and watch the breath move evenly along the spine, undoing tension and putting you in touch with the pull of gravity. Enjoy this stillness for ten minutes, if you can.

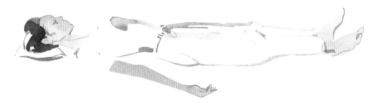

UPLIFTING BATH TREATS

We set our testers the challenge of trialling quite a few new entries in our quest to identify bath treats which really do restore get-up-and-go when it got-up-and-went – and are pleased to welcome two new entries right at the top of the energy-boosting chart (see below). We suggested they use them on sluggish mornings, when energy's crashed or the blues have set in – and these were their zingy faves…

❀ TAER ICELANDIC BATH OIL GLACIER

Score: 8.11/10

Whoooooah. When Taer (the little Icelandic brand) say 'Glacier', they ain't kidding. This is a powerful, sinus-clearing blend of sweet birch (great for aching muscles), spicy fennel, peppermint and fir needle. We love it – as did our testers! The peppermint delivers a sensory wake-up call as the oil diffuses to create an opulent, milky bath.

Comments: 'Divine smell, refreshing, calming, the ultimate bath oil; bathtime has become a highpoint; I feel re-energised' • 'as good as a power nap' • 'skin feels fresh, but glowing with warm zingy energy – amazing!' • 'even my beer-swigging, footie-loving brother was impressed by the smell' • 'Before: tired and grumpy. After: invigorated, happy, ready to take on the world!' • 'stunning packaging – and it worked: more energy and sharper reflexes!'.

❀ NEAL'S YARD REMEDIES SEAWEED & ARNICA FOAMING BATH

Score: 8.06/10

A 'classic' product which has lingered in the Neal's Yard range for ever (which is why, at 26 per cent, it's less organic than some of their more recent introductions). A lightly foaming bath, infused with mineral-rich seaweed, juniper and comfrey, it offers instant invigoration, from essential oils of lemon, lavender, pine, juniper – plus therapeutic arnica extract to ease aches and pains. Testers were divided about the smell.

Comments: 'Liked the fragrance; was much more relaxed after' • 'skin felt soft and pampered, and smelt pretty good too' • 'smelt natural, a bit woody – not unlike pine, did lift my mood and make me feel revived' • 'felt very relaxed and refreshed, and skin smooth, clean and hydrated'.

❀❀ DR HAUSCHKA ROSEMARY BATH

Score: 8/10

This totally natural bath oil, from a reasonably priced range based on biodynamically grown plants, features warming, head-clearing rosemary. In fact, it's so stimulating that Dr Hauschka warn you not to use it at night. Do also try a couple of drops in your morning face-washing water as a wake-up call for the senses.

Comments: 'I was tired, but felt invigorated, energised and my mood was enhanced' • 'skin beautifully soft and supple' • 'I bought three for presents' • 'my husband said, "What a beautiful smell" and now uses it himself' • 'very calming' • 'like a full body treatment'.

❀❀ THE ORGANIC PHARMACY NEROLI BATH OIL

Score: 7.72/10

Neroli is the sweet, breath-of-spring flower of the orange tree, which famously has the effect of uplifting the spirits. In this luxurious (and decidedly luxuriously priced) bath treat, it is blended with skin-nourishing oils of jojoba, rosehip, wheatgerm and sunflower. Strangely, a couple of testers said it relaxed them so much after bathing at night that they went to bed and fell asleep instantly.

Comments: 'Loved the unsweetened orange scent; felt recharged, alert and perkier' • 'left my skin delicately fragranced and moisturised; didn't need a body lotion' • 'I was amazed at the instant effect this had on my mood' • 'lifted my spirits and relaxed my body' • 'skin was much softer than usual' • 'very soothing and moisturising – and lasts for a long time' • 'I was feeling pumped up after a work-out; after the bath I felt deeply relaxed and chilled out emotionally'.

❀❀ THIS WORKS ENERGY BANK BATH AND SHOWER OIL

Score: 7.55/10

Our testers raved about this 'energy blockbuster', which our friend Kathy Phillips created in tandem with Aromatherapy Associates. It's a fusion of ylang-ylang, patchouli, geranium, sandalwood and rosemary essential oils.

Comments: 'Fantastic fragrance, and very natural – I felt uplifted, mentally clear, raring to go!' • 'this is the ultimate pamper product' • 'gorgeous aroma, not too overpowering, instantly invigorating and relaxing – all at once!' • 'expensive, but it lasts for ages'.

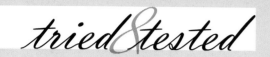

RELAXING BATH TREATS

Like us, our panellists share a passion for d-e-e-p relaxers – and awarded extremely high marks to several of the natural bath blends here, delighting in a new entry from Dr. Andrew Weil for Origins. Oh, we sincerely hope the day never comes when hot water is rationed. (We know that showers are more eco-friendly, but truly: nothing rivals the power of a glorious bath when you want to unwind…)

✿ REN MOROCCAN ROSE OTTO BATH OIL
Score: 9.27/10

Rose otto is one of the world's priciest and most precious essential oils, and Ren have decanted loads into this oil, accounting for the utterly gorgeous smell.

Comments: 'This product is heaven: if there are ten products to try before you die, this is one!' • 'when I feel low, I smell the bottle and that alone lifts me' • 'smells like my grandmother's rose garden: divine, romantic, old-fashioned' • 'my skin was soft and I felt very relaxed' • 'felt relaxed and rejuvenated' • 'definitely improved my sleep'.

✿✿ THIS WORKS DEEP CALM BATH AND SHOWER OIL
Score: 8.44/10

We're not surprised that this oil scored impressively well, as you'll find it on our own bathroom shelves. Made by Aromatherapy Associates for Kathy Phillips's range, it seems pricey until you discover a little really does go a l-o-n-g way – more than 20 baths per bottle, say testers – thanks to the super-high concentration of vetivert, camomile and high-altitude lavender essential oils, in a skin-nurturing pure coconut oil base. (Its Energy counterpart also triumphed in the Uplifting Bath Treats category, see page 201.)

Comments: 'Before: I felt tired, preoccupied; after: I was relaxed, untroubled!' • 'my skin felt wonderfully moisturised' • 'this is the ideal way to unwind after a stressful day, with candles, a good book and *The Archers*!' • 'a little of this bath oil went a long way' • 'the bath was easy to clean after' • 'it has such a fantastic smell, which wafted from the bathroom into the bedroom' • 'I loved the white glass bottle – it would make a fabulous present for a stressed-out friend'.

★✿✿✿ ORGANIC BLUE RELAXING BATH & MASSAGE OIL
Score: 8.25/10

Hats off to this Soil Association-certified organic product, which is very reasonably priced. With oils of lavender, geranium, Roman camomile and grapefruit in a moisturising base of sunflower, jojoba and coconut oils, it can double as a massage blend.

Comments: 'Loved it; skin felt so soft and didn't need a moisturiser for two days' • 'totally relaxed and calm after using it – and slept wonderfully' • 'left me relaxed and clear-headed, with soft skin'.

✿ INDIA HICKS ISLAND LIVING SPIDER LILY BATH SALT
Score: 8.25/10

The spider lily note in these fragrant bath salts was inspired by an exotic flower native to the Bahamian island where 'green goddess' India Hicks lives, and is blended with elements of citrus, orange blossom, tropical fruits, night-blooming jasmine and 'sea air' accords. (The fragrance itself isn't natural, but the Island Living range does exclude propylene glycol, mineral oil and parabens.) The salts, which come in a stylish, reusable wooden-lidded glass jar with a seashell scoop, contain a blend of coconut, avocado and soya oils, alongside seaweed, algae extract and Epsom and sea salts.

Comments: 'The exotic floral perfume was very pleasing; I was tired before, serene after' • 'this is really good for aching muscles and has a lovely softening effect on patches of dry and rough skin that I haven't found with any other bath treats' • 'I usually find salts drying, but these softened and moisturised my skin surprisingly well' • 'I loved the nice big glass jar with wooden top, and the real shell scoop' • 'these salts give bath oils and milks a run for their soothing and moisturising effects, with much less mess left in the bath'.

❀ ❀ ❀ AROMATHERAPY ASSOCIATES DEEP RELAX BATH AND SHOWER OIL

Score: 8.25/10

Some of you may have noticed that this product has risen up the score charts a notch or two – that's because Aromatherapy Associates accidentally resubmitted it for testing, and it gained an even higher score – so we've incorporated some of their comments, too. This is one of our all-time bath favourites, not least because a little bit (just a capful) goes such a long, long way – filling not just the bathroom but the whole house with powerfully de-stressing wafts of vetivert, camomile and sandalwood, diffused in its skin-softening coconut oil base. As an alternative to using this blissful blend in the bath, Aromatherapy Associates suggest sprinkling a few drops in a bowl of hot water next to the bed, or applying a drop to pulse points – a tip we'll be trying ourselves.

Comments: 'Lovely bottle; gorgeous fragrance, lovely silky smooth skin afer using it – I keep opening the bottle during the day just to have a little sniff. Felt so relaxed I drifted off quickly' • 'top marks; fragrance so beautiful I would wear it as a perfume, made me feel very calm and pampered; oil mixed into bath water completely; left skin perfectly moisturised' • 'have now had to hide the bottle from my husband and teenage son!' • 'definitely the best, I felt so relaxed I had a very good night's sleep'.

❀ DR. ANDREW WEIL FOR ORIGINS THE WAY OF THE BATH MATCHA TEA BODY SOAK

Score: 8.05/10

A great big green tub for the bath-side, filled with a green powder that swirls when scooped into water to release a fabulously stress-busting fragrance, derived from essential oils. It's rich in antioxidants and Japanese sea salts (those are said to be reviving, but our testers found this powder had the exact opposite effect). Dr. Andrew Weil suggests sinking into the green-tinged waters and reminding yourself 'of the tea philosophy of Ichigo Ichi-e: "We only have once chance to enjoy the present moment. Let's do our best."' A bath product with a dollop of philosophy, whose sentiments we can but echo.

Comments: 'Heaven in a pot, smells like the most perfect woodland, just what you want in a warm comforting bath; I felt relaxed and slightly pepped up in a calm way which is what I want to be everyday' • 'knackered and grumpy before, calm and serene after – literally!' • 'heavenly, beats everything else hands down' • 'simply the best bath soak I've used, like a warm watery hug, with delicious aromas drifting round the house; add a candle and a bath pillow and you have a spa moment at home!'

❀ ❀ ❀ LIZ EARLE NATURALLY ACTIVE SKINCARE COMFORT BATH OIL

Score: 7.8/10

One of a trio of Vital Oils for the Bath from this hugely popular brand (now truly international), Comfort Bath Oil combines warming, woody elements – myrtle, cypress, cedarwood, vetivert and vanilla – designed to relax and calm you as it soothes your senses.

Comments: 'Very natural calming fragrance, intense but not heavy; I was tired and irritated before, tired and calm after' • 'made me more relaxed and ready to sleep' • 'heavenly bathtime treat – felt less tired and relaxed after – comfortable' • 'surprised that such a small amount went so far – would definitely buy it again' • 'I really liked this – and so did my husband, so much so that he used it too' • 'felt very luxurious – I'm heavily pregnant and this really relaxed me; my skin was nicely moisturised and I slept like a baby after' • 'I was tired and ratty and this really relaxed me – very pleasantly mood-enhancing'.

We love...

For us, there is almost nothing as wonderful as sinking into a fragrant bath at the end of a long day (and, yes, we do try to recycle the water). Our favourite products don't change: This Works Deep Calm Bath & Shower Oil, and Aromatherapy Associates Deep Relax Bath and Shower Oil, both of which are guaranteed to send us slipping into the arms of Morpheus. But also try any body oil that you like: they work perfectly in the bath. Sarah's current blend is Trilogy Aromatic Body Treatment Oil which has rose, orange blossom and vanilla.

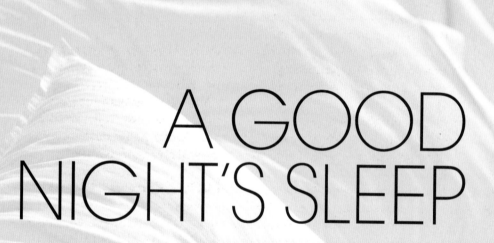

A GOOD NIGHT'S SLEEP

We love it, we want it – and we're just not getting enough… Sleep used to be called the sex of the 1990s, and in our experience the phenomenon has continued into the noughties – with no prospect of ending

An investigation by the National Sleep Foundation of more than 2,000 women between 18 and 64 found that they are much more likely to suffer from insomnia than men. Almost 70 per cent had several disturbed nights every week. As many of us have experienced, the study showed that chronic sleep deprivation led to fatigue and mood

'Life's too short not to sleep. Yul Brynner's wife gave me some earplugs 30 years ago.

swings, with more than half the participants feeling sad or depressed as a result. The most common sleep problem nowadays is not actually going to sleep so much as staying asleep; many people wake with a start between 4am and 5am, the time when underlying anxieties seem to surface like sea monsters and our brain just can't deal with them. We have talked to many experts over the years and here's what works for us.

Lifestyle factors that could disturb sleep

● Physical discomfort: check your mattress at least twice a year for signs of wear and tear and turn it every six months. Your pillow/s may be too large, too small or lumpy. Experiment with bedding changes. Try varying the bedroom temperatures – if you and your partner disagree, compromise.

● Intrusive noise or light: if blocking out sound is not possible, try a 'white noise' generator, an inexpensive device that mimics the sound of waves, waterfalls or rain (available from Victoria Health). You can also buy CDs that do the trick nicely – Sarah relied on Gregorian chant for years to block out an elephantine neighbour above. Soft foam earplugs can be useful, especially if your beloved snores. Block morning light with curtains or blinds, or eye masks (we like JetRest, which are moulded to rest above rather than on your eyes).

● Never work in your bedroom; and don't have any machines – except for a radio and/ or CD player – in the bedroom; it should be kept for sleeping (and the other kind of sex).

Prepare well for sleep

● Don't drink coffee, tea or cola after 6pm and avoid heavy fatty or sugary foods and excess alcohol, which your body has to process during the night. Cool your body by walking barefoot, opening a window, wearing light night clothes and having a warm, not hot, bath by candlelight.

● If you wake up frequently to go to the loo, reduce the amount of liquid you drink after 6pm.

● Try taking 500mg of magnesium as a supplement (Magnesium 500mg by Lifetime Vitamins) or a hot nightcap of full-fat organic milk (see right).

● Write down your priorities for the next day before you go to bed. Then keep a pen and pad on your bedside table and write down anything that pops into your mind.

● When you turn out the light, remember the nicest thing that happened to you that day – so you go to sleep thinking lovely thoughts; or write it down in a special book (before you turn out the light obviously) – at the end of a year you will have your own book of joy.

● Take regular daily exercise outdoors (see page 196): this will help your muscles to relax, and exposure to sunlight reinforces natural sleep/wake cycles.

● Try eating a portion of starchy food, such as a banana, a small pot of organic natural yoghurt or an oat- or rice-cake 30 minutes before bedtime – it may increase production of sedative brain chemicals. Keep a store beside your bed too, with your glass of water (with Sleep Well drops in it, see below).

● Take valerian, an effective sedative herb, half an hour before bedtime and/or if you wake in the night. (Try Valerian by Lamberts or Valerian and Ashwagandha Formula by Pukka Herbs – take one to two.)

● Try a flower remedy before bed and if you

SPICY NIGHTCAP

Ayurvedic practitioner Sebastian Pole recommends this delicious drink to calm the nervous system.

Over a gentle heat, stir together 1 cup organic full-fat cow's/almond/ rice milk, 2 teaspoons organic ground almonds, 2 cardamom pods, 5 strands saffron and a pinch of nutmeg. Strain, add 1 teaspoon honey, manuka if possible, and drink straight away.

wake in the night. 'Sleepy drops', as one stressed-out executive calls them, work on even hardened cases of insomnia.

● Do five or ten minutes of yoga (or a whole class if you can). It can have a remarkable effect. On page 200, you will find specific poses to help you slumber sweetly.

If you have a bad night

● The next day, avoid the temptation to eat sugary foods and drink coffee. Sip still cool water continuously, eat a protein-rich breakfast and snack on healthy foods. Take some gentle exercise and a nap in the afternoon if possible, then follow the suggestions above.

● If you toss and turn for more than 15 minutes, do something to divert your mind from obsessing about sleep: read a trashy novel (nothing stimulating), do the ironing or washing-up (nothing energetic).

Now I always travel with earplugs, a pillow and linen pillowcases' JANE BIRKIN

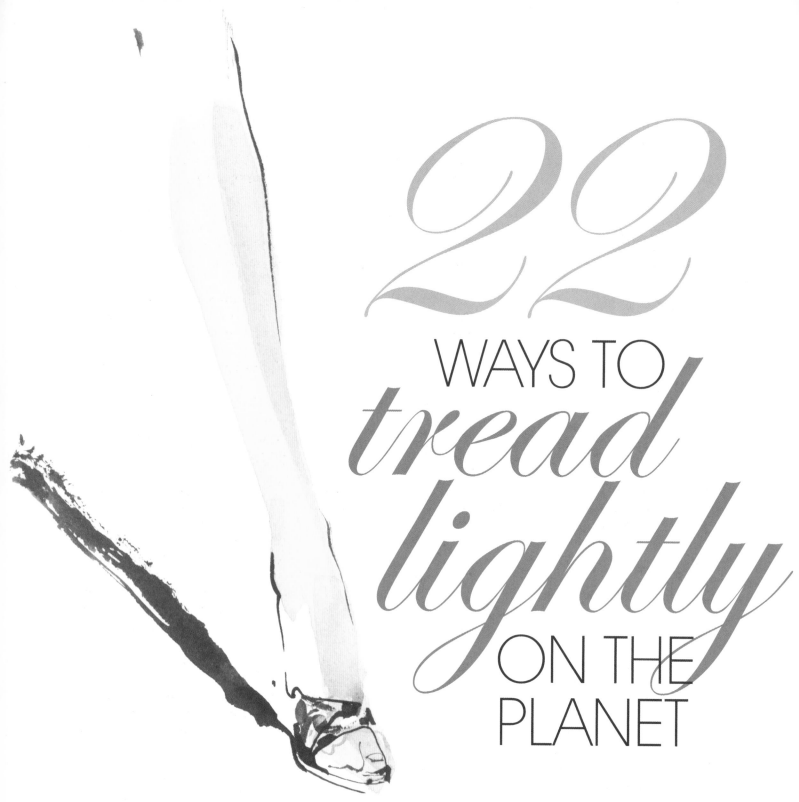

22 WAYS TO *tread lightly* ON THE PLANET

Softening your carbon footprint is far easier than you think. A few of these small changes can make a world of difference. And even your bank balance will be healthier as a result

1 Insulate your roof: it's the single most energy-effective thing you can do.

2 Switch to energy-saving compact fluorescent light bulbs. Each bulb produces the same amount of light as a conventional bulb but causes the emission of 70 per cent less carbon dioxide. Initially, they may cost more, but you save about £7 a year running costs on each one.

3 Draught-proof doors and windows and insulate your hot water tank.

4 Turn down your central heating, take up exercise and wear pretty thermal vests and gorgeous warm cardies.

5 To save water, never leave taps running, repair leaks and consider auto-spouts. These attach to your existing tap and can save 70 per cent of usual water consumption: infrared sensors activate the water flow only when you move your hands underneath. A budget option is DIY flow restrictors.

6 Take a train or boat wherever possible, rather than a plane or car.

7 Buy organic cotton goods. A quarter of the world's insecticides are used to grow conventional cotton and about 8,000 chemicals to process it.

8 Use natural candles instead of electric lights for evening meals: it saves energy and boosts romance! We love Natural Magic scented candles.

9 Say no to plastic carrier bags. We use about 17 billion annually – they're made from non-biodegradable polyethylene, which can last for up to 1,000 years. They're serial killers for marine life and land creatures. They can end up in the food chain and block drains. Take your own bag, and ask traders to use biodegradable bags, made from corn or potato starch. Also avoid buying goods in plastic wrapping.

10 Use real handkerchiefs rather than scrappy paper tissues.

11 Buy natural cleaning products, such as Ecover or Bio-D. Or, even cheaper and greener, use lemon juice (add to water for glasses), vinegar (spray on windows and wipe off with old newspaper), bicarbonate of soda (dissolve in warm water to clean fridges, etc). Recycle old toothbrushes for almost every fiddly job. For more ideas, get the *Simple Solutions* booklet, £1 from the National Federation of Women's Institutes (www.womens-institute.org.uk); also look at the *Household Cleaning* fact sheet from the Women's Environmental Network (www.wen.org.uk).

12 Mend something. It's a lost art because so much fashion is disposable – and badly made in the first place. Without wanting to sound like our own mothers, we like to buy clothes that will last, and mend them: get zips fixed, replace buttons, put hems up…

13 Never wash anything hotter than 30 degrees centigrade, and use a capful of white wine vinegar instead of fabric conditioner. It's just as effective (and doesn't smell like a salad dressing, honest!).

14 Always put lids on pans when cooking so food cooks quicker and you save energy.

15 Grow your own salad leaves, herbs and edible flowers (pots and window boxes are fine for these too). And make a compost bin.

16 If you don't have a dual flush on your loo, put a Hippo the Water Saver in the cistern (www.hippo-the-watersaver.co.uk).

17 Get an Ecube (www.ecubedistribution.com): it fits on to the temperature sensor in your fridge, and reduces the energy it uses switching itself on and off every time someone opens the door.

18 Recycle envelopes and boxes: you need a paper knife (to open them neatly), sticky tape, sticky address labels – and sealing wax for fun!

19 Buy an insulated mug and take it with you when you're out and about. Some coffee shops will make a cup of tea for you in your own cup, which will save on all that plastic and paper waste.

20 Stop junk mail. In the UK, you can contact Mailing Preference Service (www.mpsonline.org.uk).

21 Switch off standby lights (on TVs, etc). Turning off unneeded lights can save 10 per cent or more of your building's whole energy use. Unplug everything you can: appliances can still use electricity if they're plugged in.

22 Invest in a OneClick Intellipanel for your computer and peripherals (www.oneclickpower.com): when you close down your computer it automatically switches off the modem, printer, scanner, etc.

WHAT WE PREFER NOT TO FIND IN NATURAL PRODUCTS

These are the ingredients we don't really want to find in a natural product. In fact, our own choice is to avoid them altogether, if at all possible. That's because we eat organic food, live a natural lifestyle, use eco-paints – and so it goes on. It's a free country. You may choose to avoid these ingredients too, or you may be attracted to natural and green cosmetics not because of what they leave out, but because of what they include: that is, active natural ingredients that will help your face, body and hair look its healthy best, or which are produced locally to you, cutting 'beauty miles'.

There isn't room in this book to list all the 'questionable' ingredients in cosmetics, but we have listed here the ones that are most widely used, and widely acknowledged to have question marks over them. You'll find more information on our website if you log on to www.beautybible.com, as well as a longer list of other ingredients about which we have some concerns. No products with two daisies (or more) in this book contain any of these ingredients.

DEA (diethanolamine) and TEA (triethanolamine): you'll find them listed on labels as, for example, cocamide DEA or lauramide DEA, etc. These can cause allergic reactions, irritate the eyes and dry both hair and skin. They are 'amines' (ammonia compounds) which can react with nitrates to form carcinogens. Dr Samuel Epstein, chairman of the Cancer Prevention Coalition in the US, has petitioned for labelling which would read: 'Caution – this product may contain N-nitrosodi-ethanolamine, a known cancer-causing agent'.

Mineral oil: this is listed as paraffinum liquidum on European labels; petrolatum is basically the same thing. It's cheap, it's been plentiful – but now that the world's oil supply is peaking (or has peaked, depending on who you ask), all that is changing. Once oil's gone, that's it (for billions of years); other ingredients can do the same job, if not better, and be sustainably produced, crop after crop. We prefer them. It's that simple.

Additionally, some experts believe that because mineral oil acts as a very effective barrier on the skin, it can tamper with the body's own moisturising mechanism, ultimately leading to chapping and dryness – the very conditions it's used to alleviate.

Imidazolidinyl urea and diazolidinyl urea: the American Academy of Dermatology has found these widely used preservatives to be a key cause of contact dermatitis.

Methylisothiazolinone (MIT): this antibacterial agent is found in antimicrobial soaps, hand soaps and a surprising number of personal care products. Not only does it have the potential to cause irritation or allergic reactions, but it has also been linked with nerve damage. The quantities in cosmetics are teensy, but we avoid this ourselves, thanks.

Parabens: these ingredients have been around since the 1920s and have become the most highly-contentious in the beauty world, with companies scrambling to emblazon their packaging with 'paraben-free'. Parabens are widely-used preservatives, added to ward off bacterial growth, and are also found in food and drugs, in smaller amounts. They're actually a 'family' of preservatives which includes methyl-, propyl-, butyl- and ethyl-paraben, and the versions used in cosmetics are synthesised, rather than naturally occurring. But are they safe? The US Food and Drug Administration points to a review of studies that says they absolutely are, and that they have very low irritancy potential. Several of the studies that we have seen damning parabens are flimsy, at best (although some doctors are now recommending to patients they avoid parabens). We would certainly welcome more studies on the safety of parabens – and in particular, whether there could be any possible link to breast cancer, or to reduced sperm counts – but meanwhile, as the natural beauty world becomes more sophisticated, many brands are finding effective alternatives to these preservatives. If you feel at all concerned about any health question marks over this family of ingredients, it's easier than ever to avoid them.

Propylene glycol: although this may come from a natural source – vegetable glycerine, mixed with grain alcohol – it's more usually a synthetic petrochemical mix combined with a water-attracting humectant, and has been known to cause allergic reactions such as eczema.

PVP/VA copolymer: a petroleum-derived chemical common to hair sprays and styling products (the word 'polymer' gives a clue as to its plastic-like holding powers), it can be toxic when inhaled, and damage the lungs of sensitive individuals.

Sodium lauryl sulfate: this harsh detergent, mainly used as a foaming agent, is hugely controversial and you will find we have written lots on it throughout this book. We don't like it but we have to point out that there is some suggestion that the huge amount of publicity knocking SLS began as an unfounded 'whispering campaign'. The American Cancer Society actually took advertising to quash the widespread rumour that SLS causes cancer. However, it certainly is highly de-greasing, drying and irritating to skin, interfering with the skin's barrier system and making it easier for other ingredients to enter. It may also trigger some asthma attacks we are told by readers. Many natural shampoo companies now trumpet their use of 'laureth' ingredients, instead, but (like DEA and TEA) these can react to produce nitrosamines. The good news is that, increasingly, the savvier natural beauty companies are turning to gentle, non-irritating cleansing agents derived from corn and sugar.

Stearalkonium chloride: developed originally as a fabric softener, it's perhaps not surprising this is also now used in hair conditioners and creams. It can cause allergic reactions and natural cosmetics use proteins or herbal ingredients instead, which boost hair health.

Synthetic colours: these are labelled as FD&C or D&C on the label, followed by a colour and a number (for instance FD&C red no 6, or D&C green no 5). Derived from coal tar, they are potentially carcinogenic.

Triclosan: turn to page 117 for more information on this.

GLOSSARY
Here are some of the terms and symbols you'll find on packaging, demystified for you

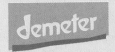

ORGANIC: this means ingredients have been sustainably produced, without agricultural chemicals and a long list of other chemical ingredients that are used in the cosmetics industry. Alas, the term 'organic' is widely abused in the beauty world because European guidelines are not yet governed by law. Personally, we're incensed to find non-certified brands with the word 'organic' used in their name and marketing; (sometimes products have absolutely no organic ingredients and the labelling is purely there for marketing). The only way to be sure a product contains genuinely organic ingredients is to look for one of the official logos on the packaging. Historically, there have been differences between standards because they were all developed independently, but the different bodies are now working towards complete harmonisation and from 2010, manufacturers and brands will have to work to a new European Standard called COSMOS (Cosmetics Organic and Natural Standard). This has taken many years, and compromises on all sides, but brands will continue to carry the Ecocert, Soil Association and BDIH symbols, so you can still look for these for reassurance that the organic claims made by brands really do stand up to scrutiny. Through the introduction of COSMOS, it's hoped that the standards will ultimately become law, so the term can't be abused without risk of prosecution – as in the food industry.

BIODYNAMIC: biodynamic farming is based on organic principles, but some people describe it as 'beyond organics', because not only does it exclude the use of synthetic fertilisers and chemicals in crop production, but also requires specific measures to strengthen life processes in soil and plants, such as planting by phases of the moon. (When you think that the moon has the power to move billions of gallons of water across the earth's surface, it makes sense that it has the power to affect plant growth too.) Demeter is the official body for biodynamic farming. Its logo certifies that a product contains biodynamically grown ingredients. Weleda and Dr Haushka are the best-known biodynamic ranges.

NATURAL: BDIH is a European organisation that certifies the naturalness – although not organic status – of beauty products. Materials should be plant-derived, minerals are allowed, and some nature-identical preservatives and natural preservatives are permitted. They do not allow synthetic dyes, colorants or fragrances, silicones, petroleum products, or any ingredient produced via 'ethoxylation', such as sodium laureth sulfate.

BEAUTY
without tears

The bad news? Animal testing of cosmetics may have been banned in the UK and some parts of the US, but companies can still go abroad to get their ingredients tested. The good news? More and more brands are making a cruelty-free pledge. Here's how to ensure that your make-up and skin creams are bunny-friendly

Many people think that animal testing is no longer used – but while animal testing of cosmetic ingredients in the UK ended in 1997, it continues elsewhere in the world. Now we are all for safety testing of the ingredients in cosmetics. Many of the ones in use today were introduced before 1981, when safety assessment became compulsory in Europe. But – big but – we are completely against animal testing in any form. Which is why the REACH initiative (the Registration, Evaluation, Authorisation and Restriction of Chemicals) may be bad news for bunnies (and rats and mice).

We applaud steps taken by the US states of New York and California to outlaw animal testing. In the UK, there's a complete ban on animal testing of both finished products and ingredients – which might seem like good news, but there's no ban on goods sold that have been tested overseas. And now there's REACH. Designed to assess the safety of up to 30,000 chemicals, REACH could banjax the valiant efforts many beauty companies have made to eliminate animal testing, because many cosmetics ingredients may have to be compulsorily re-tested if they are also used in other product categories, such as household care products.

The European Coalition To End Animal Experiments estimates that 8–12 million animals will die in the process, though thanks to lobbying from organisations such as BUAV (British Union for the Abolition of Vivisection in Animal Experiments) and FRAME (Fund for the Replacement of Animals in Medical Experiments), that number was cut from a proposed 45 million, and companies must share safety tests data and ensure that all non-animal tests have been explored.

Of course, you may think: but I want to know that the ingredients I slather on my skin, or use to froth away dirt and grime from my hair (or even to wash my floor) are safe. So do we. But the point is: animals don't necessarily have to suffer for safety to be determined – there are alternatives to many tests, but they often cost more to carry out. We are excited by L'Oréal's recent announcement of a viable, lab-grown alternative to human skin, and look forward to further breakthroughs of this kind. If you care about animal welfare, support the charities that continue to press for alternatives, such as FRAME in the UK, and Alternatives Research & Development Foundation in the US. We would also urge you to join organisations that campaign for animal welfare, such as People for the Ethical Treatment of Animals (PETA) and, in the UK, the RSPCA.

Many of you are keen to buy vegan cosmetics, as well as 'cruelty-free' cosmetics. Many ranges carry the appropriate 'leaping bunny' logos on their packaging to communicate their policies, but you may also want to visit brands' own websites, to determine where they stand on issues of animal welfare. But companies' statements can be as clear as fog, sometimes – so here's the lowdown on what those words mean. (If companies fall short of your expectations, e-mail or write to them to make your feelings felt.)

'We don't test our products or ingredients on animals.'
Cosmetics companies can distance themselves from animal testing by having outside labs conduct the testing for them. Companies that are truly serious about ending animal testing should put pressure on their suppliers, making sure they are not conducting testing on any of the ingredients they sell to them. (NB: even the most basic ingredients have undergone animal testing in the past, so no company can genuinely claim that none of their ingredients have been tested on animals.)

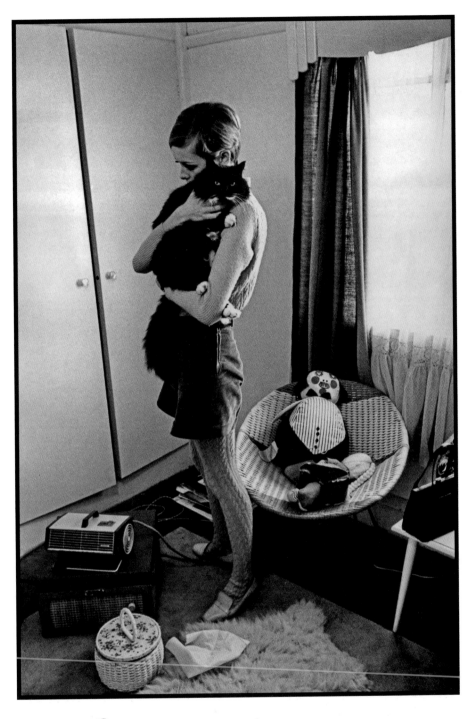

'It should be of great concern to us all that some companies continue to torture innocent creatures when there are other ways of testing' TWIGGY

'None of our ingredients have been tested on animals since the year xxxx.'
Companies can limit ingredients used to those developed before a certain 'cut-off' date, but re-testing of ingredients by suppliers is common – so companies need to have their own monitoring system to ensure suppliers are complying with their policy on animal testing. Look for 'fixed cut-off' dates (ie, a precise year) rather than a 'rolling rule', whereby companies say, for instance, 'we will not sell a product whereby the end product or ingredients have been tested on animals in the past five years'.

'We donate substantial funds to the development of alternative tests.'
Hurrah for companies that donate to humane research charities or establish their own non-animal testing facilities. But animal tests could be made redundant if companies were willing to rely on the thousands of ingredients already known to be safe.

A LUSH POLICY

We have to single out Lush for special praise on the animal-testing front. Not only do they actively campaign about animal testing, they also have the most robust of policies. They give suppliers incentives by saying that if they stop testing, Lush will start buying from them. And if a company starts to test, they will stop buying from them. They also point out alternatives to animal tests, some of which they've been involved in developing. As Lush say: 'We urge all cosmetics companies to adopt this policy to suppliers: "Stop testing today, say you will not test in the future and we will give you our business. Simple."' And simply brilliant.

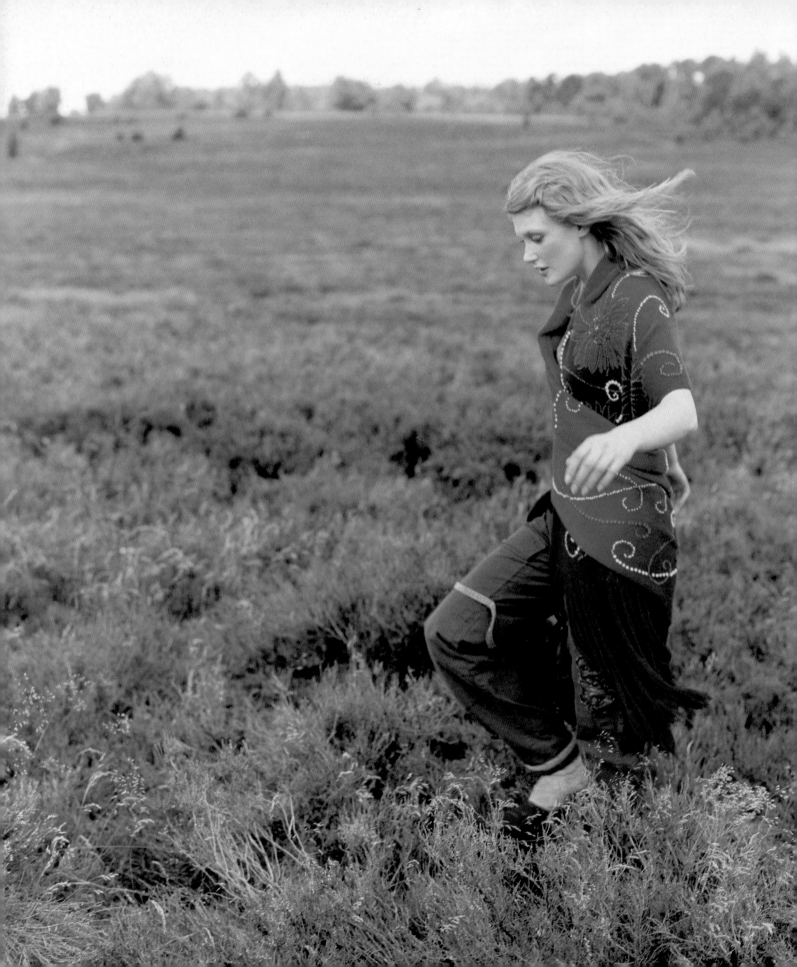

DIRECTORY

Many of the products from the beauty companies and natural health brands listed in this book are available in beauty departments, pharmacies or natural food stores – or you can try the following stockist/mail order numbers and website addresses; some stores listed also ship worldwide. All websites should direct you to a stockist/mail order source in your country. If you're still having trouble, try the search engine www.google.co.uk or www.google.com

All nutritional and herbal supplements, and many hair- and skincare products listed are available from Victoria Health, tel: 0800 389 8195, www.victoriahealth.com

www.beautybible.com (which we own 100 per cent, so it is totally independent) gives you access to exclusive discount and special offers from our approved suppliers. You can source all the products that won our 'Green Beauty Oscars' in the Tried & Tested sections of this book via the site. You will also find full ingredients listings of all these products, plus lots of other info. We regularly update the site with news, competitions, offers, a big Q&A section (and archive) and the products we love and use ourselves: it's literally your *Beauty Bible* online.

For more information on cruelty-free shopping, if you live in the UK, get hold of a copy of BUAV's *Little Book of Cruelty-Free* (www.buav.org) or Naturewatch's *The Compassionate Shopping Guide* (www.naturewatch.org). In the US, look at PETA's list of companies that don't test on animals, online at www.caringconsumer.com

If calling UK telephone numbers from abroad, dial 0044, then drop the first 0 of the following number.

A

Acupuncture:
  British Acupuncture Council, tel: 020 8735 0400, www.acupuncture.org.uk

AD Skin Synergy, tel: 01495 325284, www.adskinsynergy.com

Aesop, from Liberty, tel: 020 7734 1234, www.aesop.net.au

A'kin, tel: 0845 456 0639, www.mypure.co.uk

Dr Alex Concorde, tel: 0870 345 2255, www.the-concorde-initiative.com

Alida, tel: 01256 337660, www.alida.co.uk

Allergy:
  Allergy UK, tel: 01322 619898, www.allergyuk.org

Amanda Lacey, tel: 020 7351 4443, www.amandalacey.com

Andrew Chevallier, The Healthy Living Centre, tel: 020 7704 6900, www.thehealthylivingcentre.co.uk

Dr Andrew Tresidder, www.drandrew.co.uk

Dr Andrew Weil, www.drweil.com

Annemarie Börlind, from Simply Nature, tel: 01580 201687, www.borlind.com

Antipodes, tel: 020 8744 8050, www.antipodesnature.com

Aromatherapy:
  Aromatherapy Council, tel: 0870 774 3477, www.aromatherapycouncil.co.uk

Aromatherapy Associates, tel: 020 8569 7030, www.aromatherapyassociates.com

Avalon Organics, tel: 01782 567100, www.treeoflifeuk.com

Aveda, tel: 0870 034 2380, www.aveda.com

Avon, tel: 0845 601 4040, www.avonshop.co.uk

B

Bach Flower Remedies, A Nelson & Co Ltd, tel: 020 8780 4200, www.nelsonbach.com

Balance Me, www.balanceme.co.uk, e-mail: info@balanceme.co.uk

Balm Balm, tel: 020 8339 0696, www.balmbalm.com

Bare Escentuals, tel: 0870 850 6655, www.bareescentualsuk.com

Barefoot Botanicals, tel: 0870 220 2273, www.barefoot-botanicals.com

Bastien Gonzalez, tel: 07766 663271, www.bastiengonzalez.com

Bath Spa, tel: 01225 331234, www.thermaebathspa.com

Bio-D, tel: 01482 229950, www.biodegradable.biz

Blossom Candles, tel: 01444 487719, www.blossomcandles.com

Bobbi Brown, tel: 0870 034 2566, www.bobbibrown.co.uk

The Body Shop, tel: 01903 844554, www.bodyshopinternational.com

Braun Oral-B, tel: 0800 731 1792, www.oralb.com

British Trust for Conservation Volunteers, tel: 01302 388888, www.btcv.org.uk

C

Care by Stella McCartney, available from Selfridges, tel: 0870 837 7377

Chinese herbal medicine:
  Register of Chinese Herbal Medicine, tel: 01603 623994, www.rchm.co.uk

Chiropodists/podiatrists:
  The Society of Chiropodists and Podiatrists, tel: 0845 450 3720, www.feetforlife.org

Chung Shi, tel: 01675 430115, www.ljmsports.co.uk

Circaroma, tel: 020 7359 1135, www.circaroma.com

Clarins, tel: 0800 036 3558, www.clarins.co.uk

Clarymist, tel: 0845 060 6070, www.clarymist.co.uk

Colette Prideaux-Brune, tel: 01963 23204

Couleur Caramel, tel: 020 7512 0872, www.couleur-caramel.com

Cowshed, tel: 020 7851 1169, www.cowshedonline.com

Crystal, tel: 01784 460622, www.thecrystal.com

Cuttlefish, tel: 01273 622662

D

Daniel Galvin Junior, tel: 01795 581151, www.danielgalvinjnr.com

Deborah Mitchell, tel: 0870 166 5544, www.heavenskincare.com

Decléor, tel: 020 7313 8780, www.decleor.co.uk

Dental Miracle, from Victoria Health, tel: 0800 389 8195, www.victoriahealth.com

Derma E, from Victoria Health, tel: 0800 389 8195, www.victoriahealth.com

Dermatologists:
  British Association of Dermatologists, tel: 020 7383 0266, www.bad.org.uk

Desert Essence, from Victoria Health, tel: 0800 389 8195, www.victoriahealth.com

Dr Hauschka, tel: 01386 791022, www.drhauschka.co.uk

Dr Organic, tel: 0870 606 6605, www.hollandandbarrett.com

E

Earthbound Organics, tel: 01597 851157, www.earthbound.co.uk

Earth Friendly, www.naturalcollection.com

Ecco Bella, www.eccobella.com

Ecolani, from Victoria Health, tel: 0800 389 8195, www.victoriahealth.com

Ecover, tel: 0845 130 2230, www.ecover.com

Ecozone, tel: 0845 230 4200, www.ecozone.co.uk

Elemis, tel: 01278 727830, www.elemis.com

Elizabeth Arden, tel: 020 7574 2714, www.elizabetharden.com

Eminence Organic Skin Care, tel: 01527 834904, www.eminenceorganics.com

Emma Hardie, tel: 0800 389 8195, www.emmahardie.com

Enata, tel: 020 8339 0696, www.enata.co.uk

Ergoform, from Victoria Health, tel: 0800 389 8195, www.victoriahealth.com

Espa, tel: 01252 352231, www.espaonline.com

Essential Care, tel: 01638 716593, www.essential-care.co.uk

Eve Lom, tel: 020 8740 2076, www.evelom.co.uk

F

Farouk CHI, www.farouk.com

Florascent, from The Natural Store, tel: 01273 746781, www.thenaturalstore.co.uk

Footwise, tel: 020 7937 9993, www.footwiseuk.com

Fushi, tel: 0845 330 1880, www.fushi.co.uk

G

Gengigel, tel: 01480 862080, www.gengigel.co.uk

Gilden Tree, from Victoria Health, tel: 0800 389 8195, www.victoriahealth.com

Gillian Hamer, the Wren Clinic, tel: 020 7283 8908

Green Hands, tel: 01568 612426, www.greenhands.co.uk

Green People, tel: 01403 740350, www.greenpeople.co.uk

H

Dr Hap Gill, tel: 0845 225 0040, www.drhapgill.com

Hard Candy, www.hardcandy.com

Harrods Urban Retreat, tel: 020 7893 8333, www.urbanretreat.co.uk

Healing:
Confederation of Healing Organisations (Government-recognised body),

www.confederation-of-healing-organisations.org

Herbalists:
National Institute of Medical Herbalists, tel: 01392 426022, www.nimh.org.uk

Homeopaths:
The Society of Homeopaths, tel: 0845 6611, www.homeopathy-soh.org

Honeybee Gardens, www.honeybeegardens.com

Hypnotherapy:
National Register of Hypnotherapists & Psychotherapists, tel: 01282 716839, www.nrhp.co.uk

I

Imedeen, tel: 0845 555 4499, www.imedeen.co.uk

India Hicks Island Living, Crabtree & Evelyn, tel: 020 7361 0499, www.crabtree-evelyn.co.uk

Inika, tel: 0845 045 0664, www.inikacosmetics.com

Inlight, from Victoria Health, tel: 0800 389 8195, www.victoriahealth.com

J

Jane Iredale, tel: 020 8450 7111, www.janeiredale.com

Jason, tel: 0845 072 5825, wwwkinetic4health.co.uk

JetRest, tel: 0870 739 1591, www.thejetrest.com

John Frieda, tel: 020 7491 0840, www.johnfrieda.com

John Masters Organics, for products, tel: 020 7318 3538, www.johnmasters.co.uk; US salon: 001 212 343 9590

John Yiannis Tsagaris, tel: 0871 903 0000, www.energybodies.co.uk

Dr Joseph Mercola, www.mercola.com

Jo Wood Organics, tel: 0845 607 6614, www.jowoodorganics.com

Jurlique, tel: 0870 770 0980, www.jurlique.co.uk

K

Kimberly Sayer, from Love Lula, tel: 0870 242 6995, www.lovelula.com

Kimia, tel: 01706 836565, www.kimia.co.uk

Kiss My Face, www.kissmyface.com

Korres, tel: 020 7581 6455, www.korres.com

L

Label M, tel: 0870 770 8080, www.labelm.co.uk

Lavera/Laveré, tel: 01557 870203, www.lavera.co.uk, www.lovelula.com

Lily Lolo, tel: 0161 408 4732, www.lilylolo.co.uk

Living Nature, tel: 01794 323222, www.livingnature.com

Liz Earle Naturally Active Skincare, tel: 01983 813913, www.lizearle.com

Logona, tel: 0870 199 9220, www.logona.co.uk

L'Oréal, Available Nationwide

Louise Galvin, tel: 020 7289 5131, www.louisegalvin.com

Lush, tel: 01202 668545, www.lush.co.uk

M

Dr Marilyn Glenville, tel: 0870 532 9244, www.marilynglenville.com

Materia Aromatica, tel: 020 8392 9868, www.materiaaromatica.com

MBT, tel: 020 7684 4633, www.swissmasai.co.uk

Method, available from John Lewis, Tesco and Waitrose, www.methodhome.com

Michael McIntyre, tel: 01993 830419

Moom, tel: 080 8393 3581, www.moom-uk.com

MOP, tel: 01282 613413, www.mopproducts.com

Dr Mosaraf Ali, The Integrated Medical Centre, tel: 020 7224 5111, www.drali.com

Mother Earth, tel: 01539 435166, www.motherearth.co.uk

N

Nars, at Selfridges, tel: 0800 1234000, www.narscosmetics.co.uk

Natural Magic, tel: 0870 460 4677, www.naturalmagicuk.com

The Natural Toothbrush, www.naturaltoothbrush.com

Naturetis, tel: 0845 052 2484, www.naturetis.com

Neal's Yard Remedies, tel: 0845 262 3145, www.nealsyardremedies.com

Dr Nicholas Lowe, The Cranley Clinic, tel: 020 7499 3223

No-Miss, www.nomiss.com

Nude, tel: 0800 634 4366, www.nudeskincare.com

Nutritional therapists:
British Association for Nutritional Therapy, tel: 0870 606 1284, www.bant.org.uk

Nvey Eco, tel: 01617 185 905, www.nveyeco.co.uk

O

Olivia Garden, www.oliviagarden.com

Organic Blue, from Healthquest, tel: 0845 310 4411, organicblue.com

Organic food:
The Soil Association, tel: 0117 314 5000, www.soilassociation.org

The Organic Pharmacy, tel: 020 7351 2232, www.theorganicpharmacy.com

Origins, tel: 0800 731 4039, www.origins.co.uk

P

Palladio, tel: 0800 980 6665, www.beautynaturals.com

Patyka, www.patyka.com

Perfect Sweet, from Victoria Health, tel: 0800 389 8195, www.victoriahealth.com

Philosophy, tel: 0870 990 8452, www.philosophy.com

Phytologie, tel: 020 7620 1771, www.phyto.com

PitRok, tel: 0845 013 3145, www.pitrok.co.uk

Pozzani, tel: 0845 165 1250, www.pozzani.com

Preserve, from Victoria Health, tel: 0800 389 8195, www.victoriahealth.com

Primavera, tel: 01373 467103, www.primavera.co.uk

Priti, www.pritiorganicspa.com

Pukka, tel: 0845 375 1744, www.pukkaherbs.com

Pure Lochside, tel: 01436 810801, www.purelochside.com

R

Reflexology:
The British Reflexology Association, tel: 01886 821207, www.britreflex.co.uk

Reiki:
The Reiki Association, tel: 07704 270727, www.reikiassociation.co.uk

Ren, tel: 0845 225 5600, www.renskincare.com

Revlon, tel: 020 7391 7484, www.revlon.com

Rich Hippie, www.rich-hippie.com

Roderick Lane, tel: 0845 094 3224, www.rodericklane.co.uk

S

Sally Hansen, tel: 01233 656 366, www.sallyhansen.co.uk

Santé, tel: 0870 199 7838, www.santecosmetics.co.uk

Sea-Band, tel: 01455 639750, www.sea-band.co.uk

Sebastian Pole, Pukka, tel: 0845 375 1744, www.pukkaherbs.com

Seventh Generation, www.seventhgeneration.com

Sevi Vegan Cosmetics,
www.sevicosmetics.com

ShiKai, www.shikai.com

Shower Coach, from Nigel's EcoStore, tel:
0800 288 8970, www.nigelsecostore.co.uk

Soapods, tel: 020 8208 8826,
www.soapods.com

Soladey, from Evolved Products,
tel: 0845 055 1616, www.soladey.com

The Spa, tel: 01276 486100,
www.exclusivehotels.co.uk,
www.thespa.uk.com

Spa Illuminata, tel: 020 7499 7777,
www.spailluminata.com

Suncoat, from Green Hands,
tel: 01568 612426, www.greenhands.co.uk

Susan Posnick, tel: 020 8997 8541,
www.susanposnick.com

T

Taer Icelandic, from Harvey Nichols
Beyond Beauty, tel: 020 7235 5000,
www.taer.com

This Works, tel: 0845 230 0499,
www.thisworks.com

Titanic Spa, tel: 0845 410 3333,
www.titanicspa.com

Trevarno, tel: 01326 555977,
www.trevarnoskincare.co.uk

Trilogy, tel: 01737 822361,
www.trilogyproducts.com

Tulsee, tel: 0870 360 0399,
www.tulsee.com

U

Urban Decay, from Boots,
tel: 0845 070 8090, www.urbandecay.com

Urtekram, widely available from health food
stores, and Love Lula, tel: 0870 242 6995,
www.lovelula.com

V

Vaishaly Patel, tel: 020 7224, 6088,
www.vaishaly.com

VioClean, tel: 0845 800 1111,
www.vioclean.co.uk

W

WalaVita, tel: 01386 791022,
www.drhauschka.co.uk

Weleda, tel: 0115 944 8222,
www.weleda.co.uk

Wellington Centre, tel: 01424 442520,
www.wellingtonnaturalhealth.com

Y

Yes to Carrots, Debenhams Stores
nationwide, www.yestocarrots.com

Yin Yang, tel: 01993 822 800,
www.yinyangskincare.co.uk

Yoga teachers:
    British Wheel of Yoga,
    tel: 01529 306851, www.bwy.org.uk

Z

Zapp, www.zappgum.com

Zoya, tel: 0800 111 6647,
www.zoyapolish.co.uk

ZyloSweet, from Victoria Health,
tel: 0800 389 8195, www.victoriahealth.com

BEAUTY BOOKSHELF

The Cellulite Solution by
Dr Howard Murad (Piatkus)

*The Complete Book of Food
Combining* by Kathryn Marsden
(Piatkus)

Cosmetics Unmasked by Stephen
and Gina Antczak (out of print, but
copies are sometimes available on
www.amazon.co.uk)

8 Weeks to Optimum Health by
Dr Andew Weil (Ballantine)

Essence & Alchemy by Mandy Aftel
(Bloomsbury)

The Fragrant Pharmacy by
Valerie Ann Worwood (Bantam)

Healing Without Freud or Prozac
by Dr David Servan-Schreiber
(Rodale International)

*I Feel Bad about My Neck and Other
Thoughts on Being a Woman* by
Nora Ephron (Doubleday)

Living Beauty by Bobbi Brown
(Headline Springboard)

*Molecules of Emotion: Why You Feel
the Way You Feel* by Dr Candace B
Pert (Pocket Books)

Smart Medicine for Your Skin by
Dr Jeanette Jacknin (Avery)

The Spirit of Yoga by Kathy Phillips
(Cassell Illustrated)

Solve Your Food Intolerance by
Dr John Hunter (Vermilion)

The Ultimate Natural Beauty Book by
Josephine Fairley (Kyle Cathie)

INDEX

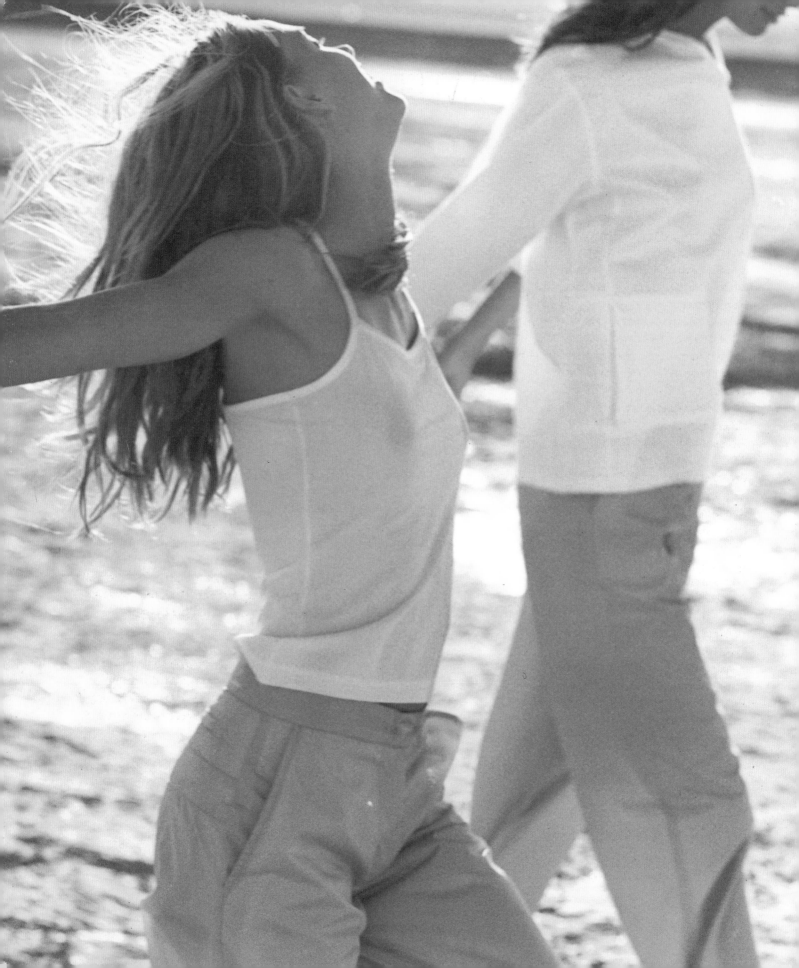

ACKNOWLEDGEMENTS

Thank you to all our experts and everyone who has contributed to this book, sometimes simply by smoothing the path:

Dr Mosaraf Ali, Integrated Medical Centre, London
Naomi Andersson, Green Hands salon
Edward Baldwin
Susan Baldwin, head of colour, John Frieda, London
Bobbi Brown
Andrew Chevallier, herbalist, UK
Juliet Cornwell, Lancôme, London
Kim D'Amato, organic nail expert, New York City
Shabir Daya, pharmacist, Victoria Health
Jessica de Bene, Origins UK
Roja Dove, *professeur de parfums*, London
Liz Earle
Professor Samuel Epstein, University of Illinois at Chicago School of Public Health
Dr Christopher Flower, Cosmetic, Toiletry & Perfumery Association
Noella Gabriel, Elemis
Daniel Galvin Junior, hairstylist
Dr Hap Gill, dentist, London
Dr Marilyn Glenville, nutritionist, London
Sheherazade Goldsmith
Bastien Gonzalez, medical pedicurist
Gillian Hamer, nutritionist, London
Dr Charlotte Hawkins, footcare expert, London
India Hicks
Susan Hope, researcher, *You* magazine, London
Amanda Lacey, facialist, London
Roderick Lane, naturopath, London
Lula Lewis, lovelula.com
Margo Lieber, Spa Illuminata, London
Kathryn Marsden, nutritionist, Spain
John Masters, the organic hairdresser, New York City
Tracey McLeod, facialist
Laura Mercier, make-up artist, New York City
Vaishaly Patel, facialist, London
Kathy Phillips, founder of This Works and yoga teacher, London
Sebastian Pole, Ayurvedic practitioner, Bath
Colette Prideaux-Brune, colour light therapist, Dorset

Sarah Raven, gardener, author and TV presenter, UK
Craig Sams, deputy chair of The Soil Association, UK
Dr David Servan-Schreiber, psychiatrist and author, France
Gill Sinclair, Victoria Health
Hana Sutherland, make-up artist, UK
Glenda Taylor, aromatherapist, UK
Helen Taylor, The Soil Association, UK
Dr Andrew Tresidder, UK
John Yiannis Tsagaris, doctor of traditional Chinese medicine, London
Abi Weeds, Essential Care, UK
Dr Andrew Weil, author and director of the Program for Integrative Medicine, University of Arizona
Andreas Wild (our hairdresser at John Frieda, who kept us smiling through the pain!)

Eternal thanks once more to **David Downton**, illustrator extraordinaire (and now a global superstar).

Several big bouquets to our wonderful team: designer **Jenny Semple**, copy editor **Catherine Sheargold** and picture editor **Kellee Hubbert**; to our fab Tried & Tested coordinator **Jessie Lawrence**, and the 'beauty elves' who put in hundreds of hours in our 'beauty dungeon': **Roxy Walton**, **Rose Eastell**, **Elizabeth Guy**, **Sacha Burrows**, **Lily de Kirgeriest** and our fabulous and tireless www.beautybible.com assistant, **Amy Eason**.

And, of course, huge thanks to our 1,200 testers, who slathered, spritzed, smoothed and scrubbed their way through so many products, giving us the all-important verdicts. And a round of applause, too, for **Dave Edmunds** and **Nikki** at the (now sadly closed) Hastings Old Town Post Office, for getting a mountain of parcels out to them.

Sue Peart, editor of *You* magazine, and **Catherine Fenton**, deputy editor, have again supported us wholeheartedly – thank you so much.

And, always, more thanks than we can say to our agent **Kay McCauley** and publisher **Kyle Cathie** (and **Julia Barder** and **Paul Game** at Kyle's office).

We dedicate this book to our lovely friend and inspiration Anita Roddick –
and to Gordon, Justine and Sam, in her memory

This revised paperback published in Great Britain in 2009 by Kyle Cathie Limited,
122 Arlington Road, London NW1 7HP
www.kylecathie.com

First published in hardback in 2008

10 9 8 7 6 5 4 3 2 1

ISBN 978 1 85626 851 6

Text copyright © Josephine Fairley and Sarah Stacey 2008

Illustrations copyright © David Downton 2008
Layout and design copyright © Kyle Cathie Limited 2008

Josephine Fairley and Sarah Stacey are hereby identified as the authors of
this work in accordance with Section 77 of the Copyright, Designs and Patents
Act 1998

A Cataloguing in Publication record for this title is available from the British Library

Book design by Jenny Semple
Edited by Catherine Sheargold
Picture research by Kellee Hubbert
Production by Sha Huxtable

Colour reproduction by Scanhouse
Printed and bound in Great Britain by Butler Tanner and Dennis Ltd, Frome

PHOTOGRAPHIC ACKNOWLEDGEMENTS

**The publishers wish to thank the
following organisations for their
kind permission to reproduce
photographs in this book:**

Jupiter Images
Camera Press/figarophoto.com
Getty Images
Corbis
Contour
Folio-id.com
Photolibrary
Alamy
Magnum
Scope Beauty
Charlotte Murphy